Imaging of the Lower Extremity

Editor

KATHRYN J. STEVENS

RADIOLOGIC CLINICS OF NORTH AMERICA

www.radiologic.theclinics.com

Consulting Editor
FRANK H. MILLER

May 2013 • Volume 51 • Number 3

ELSEVIER

1600 John F. Kennedy Boulevard • Suite 1800 • Philadelphia, Pennsylvania, 19103-2899

http://www.theclinics.com

RADIOLOGIC CLINICS OF NORTH AMERICA Volume 51, Number 3
May 2013 ISSN 0033-8389, ISBN 13: 978-1-4557-7327-5

Editor: Adrianne Brigido
Developmental Editor: Donald Mumford

Radiologic Clinics of North America (ISSN 0033-8389) is published bimonthly by Elsevier Inc., 360 Park Avenue South, New York, NY 10010-1710. Months of issue are January, March, May, July, September, and November. Periodicals postage paid at New York, NY and additional mailing offices. Subscription prices are USD 438 per year for US individuals, USD 685 per year for US institutions, USD 210 per year for US students and residents, USD 511 per year for Canadian individuals, USD 858 per year for Canadian institutions, USD 630 per year for international individuals, USD 858 per year for international institutions, and USD 302 per year for Canadian and foreign students/residents. To receive student and resident rate, orders must be accompanied by name of affiliated institution, date of term and the signature of program/residency coordinatior on institution letterhead. Orders will be billed at individual rate until proof of status is received. Foreign air speed delivery is included in all *Clinics* subscription prices. All prices are subject to change without notice. **POSTMASTER:** Send address changes to *Radiologic Clinics of North America*, Elsevier Health Sciences Division, Subscription Customer Service, 3251 Riverport Lane, Maryland Heights, MO63043. **Customer Service: Telephone: 1-800-654-2452** (U.S. and Canada); **1-314-447-8871** (outside U.S. and Canada). **Fax: 1-314-447-8029. E-mail: journalscustomerservice-usa@ elsevier.com** (for print support); **journalsonlinesupport-usa@elsevier.com** (for online support).

Reprints. For copies of 100 or more of articles in this publication, please contact the Commercial Reprints Department, Elsevier Inc., 360 Park Avenue South, New York, New York 10010-1710. Tel.: (+1) 212-633-3812; Fax: (+1) 212-462-1935; E-mail: reprints@elsevier.com.

Radiologic Clinics of North America also published in Greek Paschalidis Medical Publications, Athens, Greece.

Radiologic Clinics of North America is covered in *MEDLINE/PubMed (Index Medicus), EMBASE/Excerpta Medica, Current Contents/Life Sciences, Current Contents/Clinical Medicine, RSNA Index to Imaging Literature, BIOSIS, Science Citation Index,* and *ISI/BIOMED.*

Printed in the United States of America.

Contributors

CONSULTING EDITOR

FRANK H. MILLER, MD
Professor of Radiology; Chief, Body Imaging
Section and Fellowship Program and GI
Radiology; Medical Director MRI, Department
of Radiology, Feinberg School of Medicine,
Northwestern University, Chicago, Illinois

EDITOR

KATHRYN J. STEVENS, MD
Associate Professor of Radiology and
Orthopaedic Surgery (by courtesy),
Department of Radiology, Stanford University
Medical Center, Stanford, California

AUTHORS

SUZANNE E. ANDERSON, FRANZCR, PhD
School of Medicine, University of Notre Dame,
Darlinghurst, Australia; Department of
Radiology, Monash University, Clayton,
Melbourne, Australia

**BRENDAN R. BARBER, MBChB, MRCS,
FRCR**
Musculoskeletal Radiology Clinical Fellow,
Department of Radiology, Nuffield Orthopaedic
Centre, Oxford University Hospitals
NHS Trust, Headington, Oxford,
United Kingdom

LUIS S. BELTRAN, MD
Assistant Professor, Department of Radiology,
NYU Hospital for Joint Diseases, NYU Langone
Medical Center, New York, New York

JENNY T. BENCARDINO, MD
Associate Professor, Department of Radiology,
NYU Hospital for Joint Diseases, NYU Langone
Medical Center, New York, New York

HILLARY J. BRAUN, BA
Departments of Radiology and Orthopaedic
Surgery, Stanford University, California

DAVID BRAZIER, FRANZCR
Department of Radiology, Royal North Shore
Hospital, St Leonards, New South Wales,
Australia

MIRIAM A. BREDELLA, MD
Associate Professor of Radiology,
Division of Musculoskeletal Imaging and
Intervention, Department of Radiology,
Massachusetts General Hospital,
Harvard Medical School, Boston,
Massachusetts

ERIC CHANG, MD
VA Healthcare San Diego, San Diego,
California

CHRISTINE B. CHUNG, MD
Department of Radiology, University of
California-San Diego, San Diego, California

**SIMON DIMMICK, BPTHY, MBBS (Hons),
FRANZCR**
Department of Radiology, Royal North Shore
Hospital, St Leonards, New South Wales,
Australia; School of Medicine, University of
Notre Dame, Darlinghurst, Australia

JASON L. DRAGOO, MD
Department of Orthopaedic Surgery, Stanford University, California

HOWARD R. GALLOWAY, BM, BS, FRANZCR
Griffith ACT, Australia

DANIEL GEIGER, MD
Department of Radiological, Oncological and Pathological Sciences, Sapienza University of Rome, Rome, Italy

GARRY E. GOLD, MD, MSEE
Departments of Radiology, Orthopaedic Surgery and Bioengineering, Stanford University, California

BRIAN A. HARGREAVES, PhD
Departments of Radiology and Bioengineering, Stanford University, California

MARC E. LEVENSTON, PhD
Department of Mechanical Engineering and (by courtesy) Bioengineering, Stanford University, California

JAMES LINKLATER, MBBS, FRANZCR
Castlereagh Sports Imaging, St Leonards, New South Wales, Australia

EUGENE G. MCNALLY, MB Bch, BAO, FRCPI, FRCR
Musculoskeletal Radiology Consultant and Honorary Senior Lecturer University of Oxford, Department of Radiology, Nuffield Orthopaedic Centre, Oxford University Hospitals NHS Trust, Headington, Oxford, United Kingdom

ANNA NAZARENKO, MD
Radiologist–in-training (R3), Department of Radiology, Maimonides Medical Center, Brooklyn, New York

SIMON OSTLERE, FRCR
Department of Radiology, Nuffield Orthopaedic Centre, Oxford University Hospitals, Oxford, United Kingdom

JUDONG PAN, MD, PhD
Fellow, Division of Musculoskeletal Imaging and Intervention, Department of Radiology, Massachusetts General Hospital, Harvard Medical School, Boston, Massachusetts

MINI PATHRIA, MD
Department of Radiology, University of California-San Diego, San Diego, California

LYNNE S. STEINBACH, MD
Professor of Clinical Radiology and Orthopaedic Surgery, University of California San Francisco, San Francisco, California

KATHRYN J. STEVENS, MD
Associate Professor of Radiology and Orthopaedic Surgery (by courtesy), Department of Radiology, Stanford University Medical Center, Stanford, California

Contents

Femoroacetabular impingement (FAI) of the hip is a well-recognized entity that can cause hip pain and limit range of motion. Although there are 2 types of FAI (cam and pincer), these 2 entities most commonly coexist. Plain radiographs and magnetic resonance imaging are commonly used to assess FAI, and play an integral role in diagnosis in conjunction with patient symptoms and clinical examination. Treatment of FAI is also evolving, with arthroscopic management becoming increasingly more popular. This review provides an overview of the proposed etiology, mechanisms, clinical history, imaging, and treatment of FAI.

Soft tissue abnormalities about the hip represent a common clinical problem. Although the signs and symptoms of some of these abnormalities are clinically evident, other entities are frequently overlooked. This article provides an overview and discusses the role of major imaging modalities, especially MR imaging, the primary modality for evaluation of many soft-tissue abnormalities. An introduction to fundamental imaging anatomy and functional roles of soft tissue structures about the hip is provided, recognizing their importance in making the correct diagnosis. Intra-articular and extra-articular soft tissue abnormalities reviewed systematically according to their mechanism of injury and anatomic or functional compartments.

Meniscal injuries are common. Magnetic resonance imaging is considered the imaging modality of choice in diagnosing meniscal pathologic conditions in the nonoperative knee. Meniscal-preserving surgery is becoming more frequent, with a resultant increase in postoperative meniscal imaging, which is particularly challenging for the reporting radiologist. This article provides a review of the anatomy, pathologic conditions, and diagnostic pitfalls of meniscal injury, with a synopsis of the issues faced with postoperative meniscal imaging.

Disorders related to the knee extensor mechanism are common and rarely require imaging. Non specific anterior knee pain, fracture, dislocation, overuse tendinopathy and chronic patellofemoral instability are the commonest conditions encountered. Imaging is used in acute trauma, and for the assessment of cases of anterior knee pain resistant to conservative measures. The role of the radiograph is now largely restricted to cases of suspected fracture. Ultrasound is the optimum technique for suspected tendon and bursal pathology and MRI is widely used for the assessment of dysplasia and instability of the patellofemoral joint, including acute dislocation.

Posterolateral (PLC) and posteromedial (PMC) corners of the knee represent complex anatomic regions because of intricate soft tissue and osseous relationships in small areas. Concise knowledge of these relationships is necessary before approaching their evaluation at imaging. Magnetic resonance imaging offers an accurate imaging diagnostic tool to establish normal anatomy and diagnose and characterize soft tissue and osseous injury. It is important to carefully evaluate the PLC and PMC structures on magnetic resonance imaging before planned surgical intervention to avoid potential complications resulting from occult injury.

Cystic lesions are common around the knee and are often encountered as an incidental finding on routine magnetic resonance imaging examinations. The clinical presentation of cysts and other fluid collections is variable, depending on their size, location, and relationship to adjacent anatomic structures. This article reviews the anatomy, etiology, clinical presentation, and imaging features of commonly occurring cystic lesions around the knee and discusses some of the potential pitfalls that may be encountered in clinical practice.

Sports ankle injuries are very common worldwide. In the United States, it is estimated that 2 million acute ankle sprains occur each year, averaging to $318 to $914 per sprain. Magnetic resonance imaging is excellent for depicting normal ankle anatomy and can elegantly demonstrate ligamentous injuries of the ankle and associated conditions after ankle sprain. This article encompasses epidemiology, biomechanics, normal anatomy, and pathologic conditions of the ankle and foot ligaments. The specific ligaments discussed include the syndesmotic ligaments, lateral ligament complex of the ankle, deltoid ligament, spring ligament, ligaments of the sinus tarsi, and the Lisfranc ligament.

Impingement is a clinical syndrome of end-range joint pain or motion restriction caused by the direct mechanical abutment of bone or soft tissues. Impingement syndromes at the ankle may occur after acute macrotrauma or repetitive microtrauma. Modern imaging modalities can show underlying diseases and anatomic variations and assist with patient management. Implicit in the definition of impingement as a clinical syndrome is that the diagnosis remains clinical, because imaging changes alone do not reliably predict symptoms or clinical relevance. This article reviews the anatomy, pathogenesis, clinical features, differential diagnosis, imaging, and management of various impingement syndromes around the ankle.

Overuse injuries are a common and important cause of morbidity in elite and recreational athletes. They are increasingly recognized in the sedentary population. This article reviews the major classes of overuse injuries of the lower extremity. The underlying pathologic condition is correlated with the imaging appearances, and the often variable relationship between the imaging appearances and patients' symptoms are reviewed. Attempts at imaged-based grading systems and the ability of imaging to predict patients' prognosis are considered. Image-guided injection therapy for tendinopathy is an important and rapidly changing area; the indications, risks, and potential benefits of these interventions are reviewed.

This article reviews current magnetic resonance imaging (MR imaging) techniques for imaging the lower extremity, focusing on imaging of the knee, ankle, and hip joints. Recent advancements in MR imaging include imaging at 7 T, using multiple receiver channels, T2* imaging, and metal suppression techniques, allowing more detailed visualization of complex anatomy, evaluation of morphologic changes within articular cartilage, and imaging around orthopedic hardware.

PROGRAM OBJECTIVE

The objective of the *Radiologic Clinics of North America* is to keep practicing radiologists and radiology residents up to date with current clinical practice in radiology by providing timely articles reviewing the state of the art in patient care.

TARGET AUDIENCE

Practicing radiologists, radiology residents, and other health care professionals who provide patient care utilizing radiologic findings.

LEARNING OBJECTIVES

Upon completion of this activity, participants will be able to:

1. Describe imaging evaluation of traumatic ligamentous injuries of the ankle and foot.
2. Discuss overuse injuries of the lower extremity.
3. Review the application of advanced MRI techniques in evaluation of the lower extremity.

ACCREDITATION

The Elsevier Office of Continuing Medical Education (EOCME) is accredited by the Accreditation Council for Continuing Medical Education (ACCME) to provide continuing medical education for physicians.

The EOCME designates this journal-based CME activity for a maximum of 10 *AMA PRA Category 1 Credit*(s)™. Physicians should claim only the credit commensurate with the extent of their participation in the activity.

All other health care professionals completing continuing education credit for this activity will be issued a certificate of participation.

DISCLOSURE OF CONFLICTS OF INTEREST

The EOCME assesses conflict of interest with its instructors, faculty, planners, and other individuals who are in a position to control the content of CME activities. All relevant conflicts of interest that are identified are thoroughly vetted by EOCME for fair balance, scientific objectivity, and patient care recommendations. EOCME is committed to providing its learners with CME activities that promote improvements or quality in healthcare and not a specific proprietary business or a commercial interest.

The planning committee, staff, authors and editors listed below have identified no financial relationships or relationships to products or devices they or their spouse/life partner have with commercial interest related to the content of this CME activity:
Suzanne E. Anderson, FRANZCR, PhD; Brendan R. Barber, MBChB, MRCS, FRCR; Luis S. Beltran, MD; Jenny T. Bencardino, MD; Hillary J. Braun, BA; David Brazier, FRANZCR; Miriam A. Bredella, MD; Adrianne Brigido; Eric Chang, MD; Christine B. Chung, MD; Nicole Congleton; Simon Dimmick, Bpthy, MBBS (Hons), FRANZCR; Jason L. Dragoo, MD; Howard R. Galloway, BM, BS, FRANZCR; Daniel Geiger, MD; Sandy Lavery; Marc E. Levenston, PhD; James Linklater, MBBS, FRANZCR; Jill McNair; Frank H. Miller, MD; Anna Nazarenko, MD; Simon Ostlere, FRCR; Judong Pan, MD, PhD; Mini Pathria, MD; Lynne S. Steinbach, MD; Kathryn J. Stevens, MD; Karthikeyan Subramaniam.

The planning committee, staff, authors and editors listed below have identified financial relationships or relationships to products or devices they or their spouse/life partner have with commercial interest related to the content of this CME activity:
Garry E. Gold, MD, MSEE has a research grant from GE Healthcare and is a consultant/advisor for Zimmer and Isto.
Brian A. Hargreaves, PhD has a research grant from GE Healthcare and his spouse has an employment affiliation with Abbott Vascular.
Eugene G. McNally, MB, Bch, BAO, FRCPI, FRCR has a research grant from Arthritis Research UK and Health Technologies Assessment Uk and has royalties/patents with Elsevier Publishing.

UNAPPROVED/OFF-LABEL USE DISCLOSURE

The EOCME requires CME faculty to disclose to the participants:

1. When products or procedures being discussed are off-label, unlabelled, experimental, and/or investigational (not US Food and Drug Administration (FDA) approved; and
2. Any limitations on the information presented, such as data that are preliminary or that represent on-going research, interim analyses, and/or unsupported opinions. Faculty may discuss information about pharmaceutical agents that is outside of FDA-approved labelling. This information is intended solely for CME and is not intended to promote off-label use of these medications. If you have any questions, contact the medical affairs department of the manufacturer for the most recent prescribing information.

TO ENROLL

To enroll in the *Radiologic Clinics of North America* Continuing Medical Education program, call customer service at 1-800-654-2452 or sign up online at http://www.theclinics.com/home/cme. The CME program is available to subscribers for an additional annual fee of USD 288.

METHOD OF PARTICIPATION

In order to claim credit, participants must complete the following:

1. Complete enrolment as indicated above.
2. Read the activity.
3. Complete the CME Test and Evaluation. Participants must achieve a score of 70% on the test. All CME Tests and Evaluations must be completed online.

CME INQUIRIES/SPECIAL NEEDS

For all CME inquiries or special needs, please contact elsevierCME@elsevier.com.

RADIOLOGIC CLINICS OF NORTH AMERICA

Preface

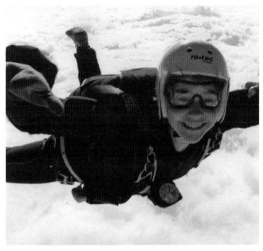

Kathryn J. Stevens, MD
Editor

We are increasingly becoming a health-conscious nation, with large numbers of people of all ages now participating in a variety of sporting activities. Sports-related injuries of the lower extremity are extremely common, accounting for a large percentage of patients currently referred from sports medicine clinics for diagnostic imaging. Although MRI is primarily the imaging modality of choice for the investigation of sports injuries, plain radiographs still play an important role in the diagnostic workup and can identify small avulsion fractures and soft tissue calcification that may not be readily apparent on MRI. Radiographs may also demonstrate anatomic variants that can predispose to soft tissue or osseous pathology. However, with its multiplanar imaging capabilities and excellent soft tissue contrast resolution, MRI is ideal for evaluating musculoskeletal disorders of the lower extremity. With the introduction of high-field MRI, improved surface coils, and new pulse sequences, MRI can now provide exquisite anatomic detail, allowing us to identify pathologic changes in increasingly small anatomic structures that would not have been possible a decade earlier. This requires musculoskeletal radiologists to continually improve their knowledge of anatomy and pathology in order to keep pace with technical advances.

When I was invited to be a guest editor for an edition of *Radiologic Clinics of North America* on imaging of the lower extremity, I wanted to provide a balanced selection of topics covering the hip, knee, ankle, and foot. In recent years, femoroacetabular impingement has been recognized as a leading cause of premature osteoarthritis in the hip. It is therefore vitally important to recognize some of the predisposing anatomic variants, as well as the resultant labral and osteochondral pathology. In the opening article, Dr Simon Dimmick has written a comprehensive article on the role of imaging in the diagnosis and treatment of femoroacetabular impingement. Drs Judong Pan and Miriam Bredella write an excellent accompanying article on soft tissue pathology around the hip, including some more recently recognized entities such as ischiofemoral impingement.

Knee pain is extremely common, with the majority of patients eventually referred for an MRI scan. Meniscal tears are one of the most commonly seen injuries in the knee, and Drs Brendan Barber and Eugene McNally describe the differing types of meniscal tears, with some of the potential pitfalls in diagnosis and strategies for imaging the postoperative meniscus. Dr Simon Ostlere subsequently reviews disorders of the extensor mechanism in the knee, including both acute traumatic lesions and chronic conditions such as patellar maltracking. Dr Geiger and colleagues write an outstanding article on posterolateral and posteromedial corner injuries of the knee, which commonly occur in conjunction with cruciate and collateral ligament tears. Drs Lynne Steinbach and Kathryn Stevens write a comprehensive review of cysts and bursal fluid collections occurring around the knee.

Radiol Clin N Am 51 (2013) xi–xii
http://dx.doi.org/10.1016/j.rcl.2013.03.001
0033-8389/13/$ – see front matter © 2013 Published by Elsevier Inc.

Ankle sprains are commonly encountered in clinical practice, and Dr Anna Nazarenko and colleagues provide an elegant review on the different patterns of ligamentous injury occurring in the ankle and foot. Long-term sequelae of ligamentous injuries in the ankle include ankle impingement syndromes, and Drs Simon Dimmick and James Linklater subsequently write an excellent review article on impingement syndromes occurring around the ankle.

In an effort to tie the various anatomic regions together, Dr Howard Galloway reviews the diagnosis and treatment of overuse injuries occurring in the lower extremity. The issue concludes with an article by Hillary Braun and colleagues describing the use of advanced MRI techniques in evaluating disorders of the lower extremity, including imaging of patients with orthopedic hardware.

I hope that this series of review articles will provide up-to-date information on some of the more commonly encountered injuries of the lower extremity, as well as raise awareness about less well recognized pathologic entities, and some of the advanced imaging options available. I am profoundly grateful to my colleagues, who generously contributed their time, efforts, and expertise into producing high-quality review articles, as I realize that the time available for such academic pursuits is increasingly scarce nowadays.

Kathryn J. Stevens, MD
Department of Radiology
Stanford University Medical Center
300 Pasteur Drive
Grant Building Room S-062A
Stanford, CA 94305-5105, USA

E-mail address:
kate.stevens@stanford.edu

Femoroacetabular Impingement

Simon Dimmick, BPTHY, MBBS (Hons), FRANZCR[a,b,*],
Kathryn J. Stevens, MD[c], David Brazier, FRANZCR[a],
Suzanne E. Anderson, FRANZCR, PhD[b,d]

KEYWORDS

- Hip • Femoroacetabular impingement • Cam • Pincer

KEY POINTS

- There are 2 types of femoroacetabular impingement: cam and pincer. These 2 entities coexist in 86% of cases.
- Magnetic resonance (MR) imaging and plain film imaging are the modalities of choice for the investigation of femoroacetabular impingement. MR arthrography is optimal for the assessment of articular cartilage and acetabular labral pathology.
- Findings associated with cam-type include bony excrescences/bumps at the lateral head-neck junction on an anteroposterior pelvic radiograph and the anterosuperior femoral head-neck junction on the lateral radiograph. On MR images, increased alpha angle, anterosuperior acetabular labral tears, and cartilage delamination may be visualized.
- Findings associated with pincer-type include coxa profunda, acetabular protrusio, retrotorsion of the femoral head, and acetabular retroversion on plain radiographs. On MR images, anterosuperior and posteroinferior articular cartilage injury, and anterosuperior labral tears may be visualized.
- Findings common to both types include reactive ossification of the labrum, fibrocystic change at the femoral head-neck junction, fragmentation of the acetabular rim, and an os acetabuli.

INTRODUCTION

Impingement of the native hip was first described in 1936 by Smith-Petersen.[1] An exponential increase in research into the causes, diagnosis, and management of hip impingement has occurred in the past 10 to 15 years. As a consequence, femoroacetabular impingement (FAI) is now a recognized cause of hip pain and restriction of hip motion in young adults, and a major cause of early primary osteoarthritis of the hip.[2–5] FAI is caused by morphologic abnormalities of the femoral head-neck junction and/or acetabulum, resulting in abnormal contact between the proximal femur and the acetabular rim. Hypermobility of the hip and reduced femoral antetorsion can also predispose individuals to this condition.[6] These changes result in recurrent microtrauma to the hip, leading to degeneration and tearing/avulsion of the acetabular labrum and articular cartilage damage. As a consequence, FAI is a recognized cause of early osteoarthritis of the hip, especially in the young and active individuals (aged 20–45 years).[7]

Pincer and cam impingement are the 2 main types of impingement that have been described. Pincer impingement is the acetabular cause of

Disclosure: The authors have nothing to disclose. There is no conflict of interest.
[a] Department of Radiology, Royal North Shore Hospital, St Leonards, New South Wales 2065, Australia; [b] School of Medicine, University of Notre Dame, Darlinghurst 2010, Australia; [c] Department of Radiology, Stanford University Medical Center, 300 Pasteur Drive, Grant Building Room S-062A, Stanford, CA 94305, USA; [d] Department of Radiology, Monash University, Clayton, Melbourne 3168, Australia
* Corresponding author. Department of Radiology, Royal North Shore Hospital, Pacific Highway, St Leonards, New South Wales 2065, Australia.
E-mail address: sdimmick@gmp.usyd.edu.au

Radiol Clin N Am 51 (2013) 337–352
http://dx.doi.org/10.1016/j.rcl.2012.12.002

FAI, and occurs as a result of focal or general over-coverage of the femoral head. Cam impingement is the femoral cause of FAI, occurring secondary to an aspherical femoral head-neck junction. These 2 types of FAI commonly coexist, and a combination of pincer and cam impingement is identified in 86% of cases.[8]

FAI causes limitation of range of motion in the hip, typically flexion and internal rotation. Initially, hip pain is experienced during specific activities. With progression of degenerative change and osteoarthritis, pain may become severe and continuous, and can affect activities of daily living.[7]

Early diagnosis of FAI is essential to facilitate treatment before significant labral and chondral damage has occurred. Medical imaging is at the forefront in the diagnosis of FAI. Magnetic resonance (MR) imaging and plain film imaging are currently the most used imaging modalities for the assessment of morphologic abnormalities associated with FAI, and for identification of underlying degenerative change.

This article reviews the pathophysiology of FAI, the imaging findings, and current treatment strategies.

ETIOLOGY OF FAI

Certain morphologic abnormalities of the acetabulum or femoral head-neck junction may predispose individuals to FAI. In most cases, cam-type impingement is caused by a primary osseous variant of the femoral head-neck junction. This is considered to be caused by delayed separation of the common femoral head and greater trochanteric physis, or eccentric closure of the femoral head epiphysis, leading to abnormal lateral extension of the physeal scar.[9] Subclinical slipped capital femoral epiphysis in adolescence, Legg-Calve-Perthes disease, and posttraumatic deformity of the femoral neck are also considered potential predisposing factors.[10–13]

Reduced femoral antetorsion can also impair internal rotation of the hip, leading to decreased joint clearance during flexion and internal rotation.[6,14,15] This may be congenital or secondary to a healed femoral neck fracture. Coxa vara may also be associated with cam-type impingement[16] caused by an abnormally located femoral neck that is situated more superiorly than normal.

Pincer impingement most commonly occurs as a result of abnormalities of the acetabulum. Acetabular retroversion (posteriorly orientated acetabulum) may predispose individuals to focal over-coverage, and is defined as the anterior acetabular margin lying lateral to the posterior margin. General over-coverage occurs as a result of coxa profunda or protrusio acetabuli. Both entities relate to increased depth of the acetabulum and are defined radiographically (see section on plain radiographs).[7] Acetabular protrusio can occur in patients with osteoporosis, osteomalacia/rickets, rheumatoid arthritis, Paget disease, or hypophosphatemia, or may be idiopathic (Otto disease).[17]

Pincer impingement can also be seen in individuals with excessive hip motion, typically in hypermobile young women (eg, ballet dancers), in the absence of morphologic abnormalities of the acetabulum.[18] Certain occupations such as carpet laying may also predispose to impingement caused by repetitive flexion, adduction, and internal rotation.[17]

Genetic factors in the etiology of FAI have been proposed, after a study on the siblings of patients with both cam-type and pincer-type FAI showed that the sibling had an increased risk of having the same cam or pincer deformities as the patient.[19] A link has also been demonstrated between aggressive adolescent sports training and the development of the bony changes of FAI.[20,21]

Abnormal morphologic changes in isolation may not necessarily produce symptoms of FAI. It is recognized that individuals with symptomatic FAI undertake specific activities or occupations that place the hip under stress, and may have an underlying vulnerability of the labrum and articular cartilage in addition to morphologic abnormalities.[19]

MECHANISMS OF FAI

Cam impingement occurs more commonly in young athletic men (average age 32 years).[7] This type of FAI is caused by an osseous excrescence/bump on the femoral head-neck junction, associated with a reduction in the offset at the femoral head-neck junction.[17] The offset is defined as the difference between the maximal anterior radius of the femoral head and the anterior radius of the adjacent femoral neck. Mechanical impingement of the nonspherical portion of the femoral head against the acetabulum and labrum during hip motion causes abnormal forces on the acetabular cartilage and subchondral bone in the anterosuperior acetabular rim area.[2,5,6,8,22] Recurrent microtrauma from athletic activity may result in abrasion of the acetabular cartilage or avulsion of cartilage from the subchondral bone.[7] As a consequence, this may lead to large areas of articular cartilage delamination or fissuring (greater than 1 cm). The surface area of chondral damage associated with cam-type FAI is usually greater than in pincer impingement.[7] Focal cartilage delamination (the so-called carpet phenomenon) is also more commonly seen with cam impingement.

Pincer impingement is more common in middle-aged women (average age 40 years).[7] Morphologic abnormalities of the acetabulum or hypermobility may result in abnormal contact between the acetabular rim and the femoral head, resulting in pincer-type impingement. Recurrent microtrauma may lead to ganglion formation or ossification of the acetabular rim, which then further deepens the acetabulum, thereby worsening the degree of over-coverage.

Impingement occurs at the anterosuperior rim of the acetabulum. The most common site of abnormality is therefore the anterosuperior rim, which includes labral tears/avulsion and articular cartilage lesions.[2] With further flexion, the femoral head subluxes posteriorly causing increased pressure between the posteromedial aspect of the femoral head and the posteroinferior acetabulum. A resulting contre-coup lesion may occur; 62% involve the femoral head and 31% the posteroinferior acetabulum.[2] Damage to the articular cartilage of the acetabulum is usually restricted to a thin (<5 mm) circumferential band near the labrum.[8]

In both cam-type and pincer-type FAI, although there is significant and potentially irreversible pre-arthritic damage of the articular cartilage in the early stage of the disease, typically no visible joint space narrowing is seen radiographically.

CLINICAL FINDINGS

Most patients with FAI are young and physically active. Although morphologic abnormalities associated with FAI are often bilateral, most patients present with unilateral symptoms.[7] Anterior hip or groin pain and limitation of hip flexion and internal rotation are commonly reported.[2,23] Less commonly, pain may be described in the region of the greater trochanter, radiating to the lateral thigh, or may be referred to the knee.[2] Painful clicking and locking of the hip may be experienced by patients with FAI and acetabular labral avulsion. Aggravating factors may include climbing stairs, prolonged periods of sitting, or when significant stress is placed on the hip.[24] Sports that require hip flexion in association with variable torque or axial loading may either cause or aggravate symptoms in individuals predisposed to FAI.[25,26] Individuals with abnormal femoral and acetabular morphology may or may not be symptomatic. However, the combination of morphologic abnormalities and precipitating activities (particularly sport) can result in repetitive microtrauma to the hip, which in turn leads to labral and chondral damage and subsequent symptoms.

Clinical examination alone may have low diagnostic accuracy.[27] In cam-type FAI, pain is usually elicited on hip flexion and internal rotation, with or without adduction. In pincer-type FAI, pain may be produced on external rotation of the hip in maximal extension (posterior impingement test).[2,28]

IMAGING TECHNIQUE
Plain Radiographs

- Anteroposterior (AP) pelvis
- Cross-table lateral view of the proximal femur
- Dunn/Rippstein view (optional)

MR Imaging

- Variable protocols available; discussion with referring clinicians is paramount.
- The gold standard for the assessment of articular cartilage and the acetabular labrum is MR arthrography.
- Pulse sequences include bilateral coronal short tau inversion recovery (STIR); unilateral standard axial T2; an axial oblique sequence acquired parallel to the longitudinal axis of the femoral neck; oblique coronal and oblique sagittal images (the latter with fat saturation), and a radial proton density-weighted acquisition.
- At 3T, acquire three-dimensional volumetric sequences to assess bony, articular cartilage and labral anatomy.

RADIOGRAPHIC FINDINGS
Plain Radiographs

Plain film imaging is used to assess the hips for features or abnormalities associated with FAI and to exclude osteoarthritis, avascular necrosis, or other joint conditions.[7] The morphologic abnormalities of FAI are often bilateral; however, many patients are only symptomatic on one side. Thorough assessment of both hips is therefore recommended.

The radiographic assessment of FAI includes a true AP pelvic view and a cross-table lateral view of the proximal femur. A Dunn/Rippstein view may also be performed in 45° of hip flexion.[29] This elongates the femoral neck and provides visualization of the anterior femoral head-neck junction.

In cam-type impingement, osseous excrescences or bone bumps are identified at either the lateral or anterosuperior femoral head-neck junction, and can be visualized on the AP radiograph of the pelvis and the cross-table lateral view of the proximal femur, respectively (**Fig. 1**). A pistol grip deformity is caused by an abnormal extension of the more horizontally orientated femoral epiphysis, and is characterized on radiographs by flattening of the usually concave surface of the lateral aspect of the femoral neck (**Fig. 2**).[9,30,31]

Coxa profunda is diagnosed when the floor of the acetabular fossa is touching or overlapping the ilioischial line medially (**Fig. 3**).[7] In acetabular protrusion, the femoral head overlaps the ilioischial line medially (**Fig. 4**).[7] Radiographic findings of acetabular retroversion on an AP projection include the crossover/figure-of-eight sign and the posterior wall sign. The crossover/figure-of-eight sign occurs when the anterior aspect of the acetabular rim is directed more horizontally and medially, crossing over the more straight and vertical posterior aspect of the acetabular rim (**Fig. 5**).[32,33] The posterior wall sign occurs when the posterior wall of the acetabulum is medial to a point drawn through the center of the femoral head (**Fig. 6**).[33] A false-positive or false-negative diagnosis of acetabular retroversion may be made when the pelvic radiograph is either rotated or has pelvic tilt.[7]

The most sensitive measurement technique for the assessment of pelvic tilt on an AP radiograph is the distance between the sacrococcygeal articulation and the superior aspect of the pubic symphysis.[34] A cadaveric radiographic study demonstrated that the neutral pelvic tilt in 32 mm in men and 47 mm in women.[35] In a well-centered radiograph, the tip of the coccyx should be between 0 and 2 cm above the top of the pubic symphysis.[36]

Over-coverage of the acetabulum can also be quantified using the lateral center edge angle (LCE) or the femoral head extrusion index. The

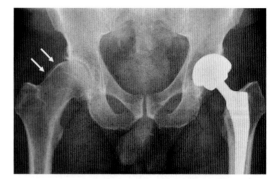

Fig. 2. AP radiograph of the pelvis in a 52-year-old man with right hip pain demonstrating moderate joint space narrowing superiorly in the right hip, compatible with osteoarthritis. There is flattening of the femoral head-neck junction laterally (*arrows*) indicating preexisting cam-type FAI. A total hip replacement has already been performed on the left.

LCE angle is defined as the angle formed by a vertical line and a line connecting the center of the femoral head with the lateral edge of the acetabulum. The normal range is between 25° and 39°.[7] An LCE angle less than 25° is defined as acetabular dysplasia and an angle greater than 39° is defined as acetabular over-coverage (**Fig. 7**).[14,37] Projection of the ischial spines into the pelvic cavity has also been described in pincer-type impingement in individuals with acetabular retroversion (see **Fig. 6**).[36]

The alpha angle and anterior offset are 2 measurements used for the quantification of the degree of asphericity of the femoral head. The alpha angle is defined as the angle between the axis of the femoral neck and a line connecting the center of the femoral head with the point of beginning asphericity of the head-neck contour. An angle greater than 50° is considered abnormal.[7] Anterior offset is defined as the difference in radius between the anterior femoral head

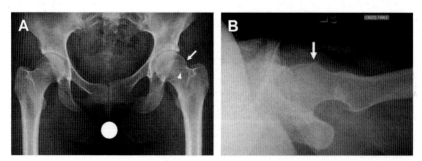

Fig. 1. (*A*) AP radiograph of the pelvis in a 22-year-old woman with left hip pain demonstrates bony convexity of the femoral head-neck junction laterally in the left hip (*arrow*). Fibrocystic change is seen in the left femoral neck (*arrowhead*). (*B*) Cross-table lateral radiograph of the left hip demonstrates a prominent bony excrescence on the femoral head-neck junction anteriorly. The *arrows* in *A* and *B* indicate the bony excrescence.

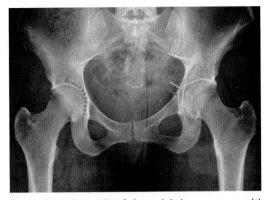

Fig. 3. AP radiograph of the pelvis in a woman with bilateral coxa profunda. The medial wall of the acetabulum (A) indicated in red (*dotted line* on the *right* and *arrow* on the *left*) either touches or projects medial to the ilioischial line (IL) indicated in blue (*line* on the *right* and *arrow* on the *left*).

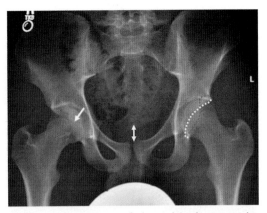

Fig. 5. AP radiograph of the pelvis demonstrating bilateral acetabular retroversion. On the right, there is a crossover sign of the acetabular margins, where the posterior wall (*red arrow*) crosses over the anterior wall (*white arrow*). On the left, the posterior acetabular rim is indicated by a dotted red line and the anterior rim by a dotted white line, to illustrate the resultant figure-of-eight configuration. The tip of the coccyx is less than 2 cm from the top of the pubic symphysis indicating neutral pelvic tilt (*double arrow heads*).

and the anterior femoral neck on a cross-table lateral view of the proximal femur. An anterior offset measuring less than 10 mm is a strong indicator for cam impingement.

The normal angle between the femoral neck and shaft is 120°. In coxa vara, the angle between the femoral neck and shaft measures less than 120°, and as stated previously, is a recognized cause of cam-type impingement.

Radiographic findings that are identified in both cam and pincer FAI include reactive ossification of the labrum, fibrocystic change/synovial herniation pits at the femoral head-neck junction, fragmentation of the acetabular rim, and an os acetabuli.[38–40] Recurrent irritation of the acetabular labrum may cause reactive ossification, particularly of the labrum.[23] In advanced cases, additional reactive bone apposition at the osseous rim leads to further deepening of the acetabulum increasing the

impingement problem. On radiographs, this may be visualized as a double contour of the acetabular rim.[7]

Fibrocystic change may be located in the femoral neck and is visualized in up to 33% of patients with FAI. These pits are seen as radiolucencies with a thin sclerotic margin (see **Fig. 1**). The site of fibrocystic change, which is found in the proximal superior/anterior quadrant of the

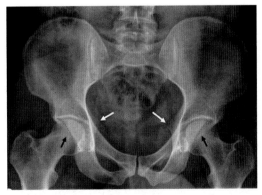

Fig. 6. AP pelvic radiograph in a man with bilateral acetabular retroversion, as indicated by a posterior wall sign, where the center of the femoral heads (*black arrows*) lies lateral to the posterior acetabular margins in both hips (*dotted red line*). The ischial spines are prominent (*white arrows*), and project into the central pelvis, a sign associated with acetabular retroversion.

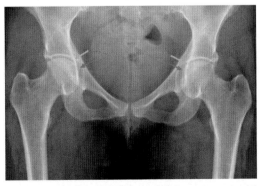

Fig. 4. AP radiograph of the pelvis in a woman with bilateral acetabular protrusio. The medial aspect of the femoral head (*red arrows*) projects medial to the ilioischial line (*blue arrows*).

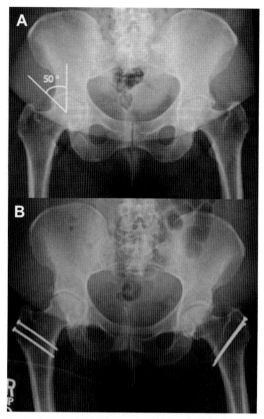

Fig. 7. (A) AP radiograph of the pelvis in a 33-year-old woman with bilateral acetabular over-coverage. The LCE angle is increased and measures 50° on the right. This angle is formed by a vertical line drawn through the center of the femoral head and a line drawn from the center of femoral head to the edge of acetabular roof. (B) AP radiograph of the pelvis of the same patient after bilateral acetabuloplasty. Screw-fixated trochanteric osteotomies are seen bilaterally, indicating an open procedure.

femoral neck, corresponds directly with the typical location of impingement in FAI.[7]

Abnormal stress or frank impingement in the setting of FAI may lead to an acetabular rim fracture, with a resultant prominent acetabular bony fragment, an os acetabuli (Fig. 8).[33] Os acetabuli may also represent unfused secondary ossification centers at the acetabular rim. Although these 2 conditions are morphologically similar, the cartilaginous growth plate is more parallel to the joint surface when the os is an unfused secondary ossification center and is perpendicular to the joint surface when secondary to FAI (see Fig. 8).[41]

MR Imaging

Plain radiographs and MR imaging are complimentary imaging modalities used in the diagnosis of FAI. MR imaging is essential in the assessment of the labrum and articular cartilage. Pulse sequences should preferably include 1 sequence that images both hips, such as coronal STIR, to assess for pathologic conditions within the remainder of the pelvis, and in particular the contralateral hip. Dedicated imaging of the symptomatic hip is then performed. MR arthrography is currently the imaging modality of choice for identifying subtle, early, articular cartilage lesions and labral tears.[42]

Radially acquired MR images, perpendicular to the femoral axis, enable comprehensive review of labral and articular cartilage pathology, and assessment of bone contours and configurations of the acetabulum and femoral head. This sequence also allows for measurement of the alpha angle in different locations.[43,44] At 3 T, three-dimensional sequences, allowing three-plane reformation are increasingly being used.[42]

Femoral torsion can be estimated from axial computed tomography (CT) or axial MR imaging images performed through the proximal and distal femur.[6,45] The angle of femoral antetorsion is the angle formed between a line drawn through the center of the femoral head and neck, and a line drawn along the posterior femoral condyles (Fig. 9). Patients with pincer-type FAI have significantly increased femoral antetorsion compared with patients with cam-type FAI.[6]

Assessment of articular cartilage is evolving using biochemical/physiologic sequences. Delayed gadolinium-enhanced MR imaging of cartilage, T1 rho and T2 mapping are potential tools for more detailed assessment of morphologic changes within the articular cartilage.[46–48]

Cam Impingement

The osseous excrescence/bump at the femoral head-neck junction may also be visualized on MR imaging in the coronal or axial oblique planes. This is identified as a bony excrescence either lateral, superolateral, or inferolateral to the physeal scar at the femoral head-neck junction. The alpha angle may be used to quantify a morphologic abnormality of the femoral head-neck junction.[49] Using an oblique axial image through the center of the femoral neck, a circle is drawn around the femoral neck (including the articular cartilage) and a line is drawn along the long axis of the femoral neck. The alpha angle is the angle between this line and a line drawn from the center of the circle to the point at which the femoral head protrudes anteriorly beyond the circle (Fig. 10). An alpha angle of greater than 50° is considered abnormal and suggestive of FAI.[49]

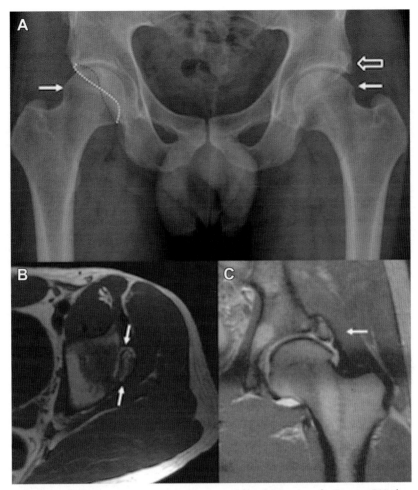

Fig. 8. (*A*) AP radiograph of the pelvis in a man with features of both pincer and cam-type FAI; there is a crossover sign of the acetabular margins (posterior wall, *red line*; anterior wall, *white line*). Bilateral bony excrescences are present (*white arrows*) and there is an irregular bony fragment along the left acetabular margin (*open arrow*) causing over-coverage of the femoral head. (*B*) Axial T1 and (*C*) coronal proton density-weighted images demonstrate a large bony fragment (*arrows*) parallel to the acetabular margin, compatible with an os acetabuli/stress fracture.

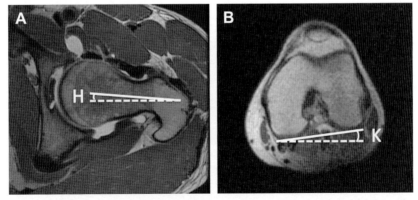

Fig. 9. Measurement of femoral antetorsion on MR Imaging. (*A*) Axial T1-weighted image through the left femoral neck. A line is drawn passing through the center of the femoral head and neck, and angle H is the angle between this and a line drawn parallel to the MR table (*dotted line*). (*B*) Axial T1-weighted image through the left knee shows a line drawn along the posterior margin of the femoral condyles, and angle K is the angle between this and a line drawn parallel to the MR table (*dotted line*). Calculation of the degree of antetorsion: (1) if the knee is internally rotated, as in this example, the angle of antetorsion = angle H + angle K; (2) if the knee is externally rotated, the angle of antetorsion = angle H − angle K.

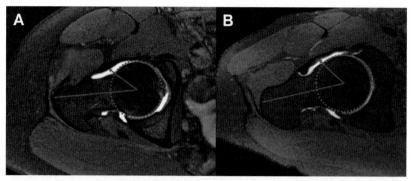

Fig. 10. (*A*) Axial oblique fat-saturated T1-weighted (T1 FS) image from an MR arthrogram in a patient with a normal alpha angle of less than 50°. (*B*) Axial oblique T1 FS image from an MR arthrogram in a patient with cam-type FAI. There is bony prominence of the femoral head-neck junction anteriorly, and the alpha angle measures approximately 65°.

Articular cartilage damage/lesions in cam impingement involve the anterosuperior quadrant of the femoral head and acetabulum, and may measure up to 10 mm in width. Cartilage delamination is common, ranging from 2 to 30 mm.[40] MR arthrography may be superior to standard MR imaging for the assessment of chondral delamination (**Fig. 11**).

Anterosuperior labral tears/avulsions are the most common in cam-type impingement.[50,51] Labral avulsions most commonly occur at the chondrolabral interface and are identified when fluid or contrast extends under the labrum (**Fig. 12**).[23] Paralabral cyst formation may herald an underlying labral tear.

Other findings associated with both pincer-type and cam-type FAI may also be visualized on MR imaging. Fibrocystic change may be identified on proton density-weighted or T2-weighted sequences with fat saturation in the anterosuperior

femoral head-neck junction at the site of impingement (**Fig. 13**). Os acetabuli are best visualized on coronal or sagittal T1-weighted sequences (see **Fig. 8**; **Fig. 14**). Subchondral edema involving the acetabular rim and femoral head likely corresponds to the site of impingement (**Figs. 15** and **16**). Ossification of the labrum or labral-acetabular junction may also be visualized, but this is more commonly seen in pincer-type impingement.

In advanced cases, osteoarthritic change may be present within the hip, with cartilage thinning, subchondral cyst formation, marginal osteophytosis, and subchondral sclerosis (see **Fig. 14**).

PINCER-TYPE FAI

Acetabular over-coverage may be seen on coronal MR images (**Fig. 17**). Acetabular retroversion is identified on axial MR images. The anterior rim of

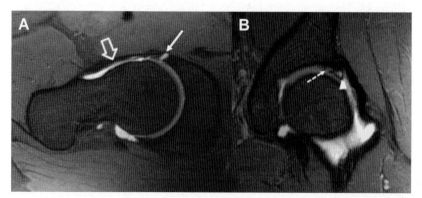

Fig. 11. A 21-year-old male runner with increasing left hip pain. (*A*) Axial oblique fat-saturated T1-weighted image from an MR arthrogram demonstrates a cam deformity of the femoral head-neck junction anteriorly (*open arrow*), with chondrolabral separation of the anterior labrum (*arrow*). (*B*) Coronal T2 fat-saturated image demonstrates intralabral cyst formation in the superior labrum (*arrowhead*), with a subtle area of delamination in the adjacent cartilage (*dotted arrow*).

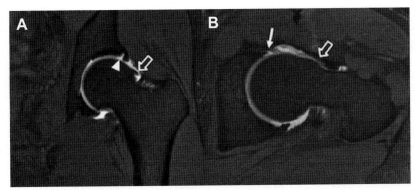

Fig. 12. (*A*) Coronal and (*B*) axial oblique fat-saturated T1-weighted images in a 29-year-old patient with left hip pain demonstrate a cam deformity of the femoral head-neck junction both laterally and anteriorly (*open arrows*). There is chondrolabral separation superiorly (*arrowhead*) and a labral tear anteriorly (*arrow*). The measured alpha angle was 66°.

the acetabulum is located lateral to the posterior rim on the most cranial image that includes the femoral head.[33]

Acetabular depth is assessed using oblique axial images. At the level of the center of the femoral neck, a line is drawn from the anterior to the posterior acetabular rims. The distance between this line and the center of the femoral head delineates the acetabular depth. If the center of the femoral head lies lateral to the line connecting the acetabular rims, such as in patients with pincer impingement, this indicates an increased acetabular depth.[44]

As previously stated, the most common site of labral pathology in pincer-type impingement involves the anterosuperior labrum. The posterior labrum, however, may also be involved. The labrum may be torn or avulsed, or may be partially or completely ossified. Articular cartilage damage

is most commonly present anterosuperiorly and posteroinferiorly (contre-coup lesion) (**Fig. 18**). Damage to the articular cartilage of the acetabulum is usually restricted to a thin circumferential band (<5 mm) near the labrum. Os acetabuli, fragmentation of the acetabular rim, or ossification of the labrum may also be identified (see **Fig. 8**; **Fig. 19**), and correlation with plain radiographs can be of assistance. Occasionally, a linear indentation may be evident at the head-neck junction.

Diagnostic Criteria

- Appropriate clinical history
- Identification of radiological features associated with:
  - Classic pincer form of impingement: overcoverage of the acetabulum, bony appositional change of the acetabular margin,

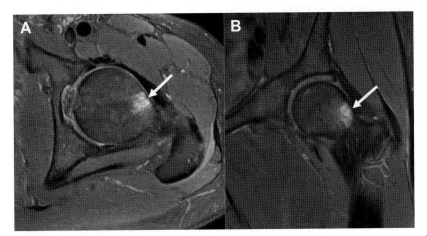

Fig. 13. Axial (*A*) and sagittal (*B*) proton density-weighted images with fat saturation in a 41 year-old man with right hip pain demonstrate fibrocystic change within the anterior-superior aspect of the femoral head-neck junction (*arrows*).

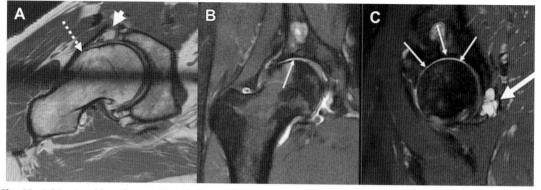

Fig. 14. A 24-year-old professional footballer with increasing hip pain. (*A*) Radial proton density-weighted image demonstrates an os acetabuli (*arrowhead*) and an aspherical femoral head (*dashed arrow*). Coronal (*B*) and sagittal (*C*) proton density-weighted images with fat saturation demonstrate significant degenerative changes with a joint effusion, posterior ganglion cyst (*thick arrow*) and extensive articular cartilage loss (*thin arrows*). These findings represent cam-type impingement with advanced osteoarthritis.

deep acetabular fossa, acetabular protrusio, coxa profunda
- ○ Classic cam form of impingement: pistol grip deformity, sloping femoral head-neck junction, sloping femoral head growth plate, lack of offset of the head-neck junction, fibrocystic change, os acetabuli (stress fracture/reaction)

Differential Diagnosis/Mimics of FAI

Clinically, mimics of FAI include ankylosing spondylitis or other inflammatory arthropathies of the

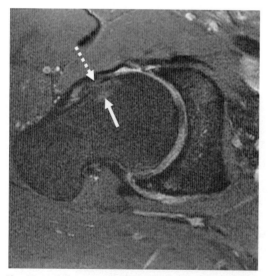

Fig. 15. Axial proton density-weighted image in a 43-year-old man demonstrates an osseous excrescence at the anterosuperior femoral head-neck junction (*dashed arrow*). Focal bone edema in this region (*arrow*) may be secondary to impingement between the acetabulum and the osseous excrescence.

hip (**Fig. 20**), diffuse idiopathic skeletal hyperostosis (DISH), and developmental dysplasia of the hip (DDH). Radiographically, these entities can be differentiated relatively easily.[7] Review of the sacroiliac joints and the thoracolumbar spine may identify changes associated with ankylosing spondylitis and DISH, respectively. Occasionally, pathologic conditions such as hydroxyapatite deposition disease of the hip or pelvis may mimic or coexist with FAI (**Fig. 21**). As stated previously, progression of FAI to secondary osteoarthritis and its severity are also important for diagnosis, management, and prognosis.

Pearls and Pitfalls

Coexisting/dual pathologies may be found in conjunction with FAI, and must be considered when interpreting imaging of the hip. These pathologies include hydroxyapatite deposition disease in young individuals, bone contusion (after trauma), gluteal enthesopathy, partial avulsion of the hamstring tendons, ischiofemoral impingement, intervertebral disc prolapse/herniation with referred pain, and advanced secondary osteoarthritis. FAI may be bilateral, although only 1 hip is symptomatic at the time of presentation/investigation, and FAI may be more prevalent in certain populations and families.

The main pitfalls of FAI imaging are not recognizing DDH or advanced secondary osteoarthritis. FAI surgery undertaken in the presence of underlying DDH may exacerbate an unstable joint, and is difficult to correct surgically. In cases of advanced secondary osteoarthritis caused by FAI, surgery may not slow down the rate of osteoarthritis, and the risk of a need for joint replacement increases.

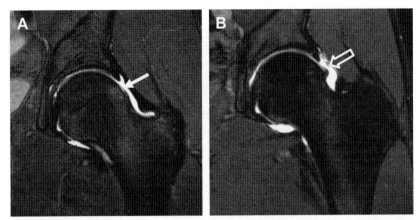

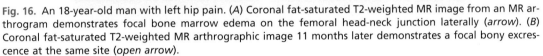

Fig. 16. An 18-year-old man with left hip pain. (*A*) Coronal fat-saturated T2-weighted MR image from an MR arthrogram demonstrates focal bone marrow edema on the femoral head-neck junction laterally (*arrow*). (*B*) Coronal fat-saturated T2-weighted MR arthrographic image 11 months later demonstrates a focal bony excrescence at the same site (*open arrow*).

A neutral AP radiograph of the pelvis is essential for the diagnosis of FAI. Neutral pelvic rotation is defined as the tip of the coccyx pointing toward the midpoint of the superior aspect of the symphysis pubis.[7] The appearance of acetabular morphology may vary considerably depending on pelvic tilt and rotation.[52] An AP radiograph centered over the hip overestimates acetabular version and is therefore not reliable for the assessment of acetabular retroversion.[7] In certain hips, it is difficult to distinguish between the 2 lines of the acetabular rim. As a helpful guideline, the posterior rim line can always be readily identified when starting from the inferior edge of the acetabulum.

WHAT THE REFERRING PHYSICIAN NEEDS TO KNOW

- Does the imaging fit the clinical diagnosis; is this consistent with FAI?
- Have other potential causes/potential coexisting pathologies been excluded? Ensure all anatomic regions have been reviewed (includes the hamstrings, iliopsoas tendon, gluteal tendons, and other tendons and soft tissues such as the external rotators of the hip). Exclude inflammatory arthropathy in the sacroiliac joints and calcification in the pubic symphysis.
- Is secondary osteoarthritis present? If present, describe the extent and site of

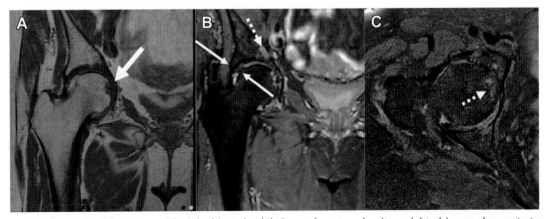

Fig. 17. A 40-year-old woman with right hip pain. (*A*) Coronal proton density-weighted image demonstrates acetabular protrusio (*thick arrow*). Coronal (*B*) and axial (*C*) proton density-weighted images with fat saturation show associated degenerative change with subchondral edema (*dashed arrows*) and marginal osteophyte formation (*thin arrows*).

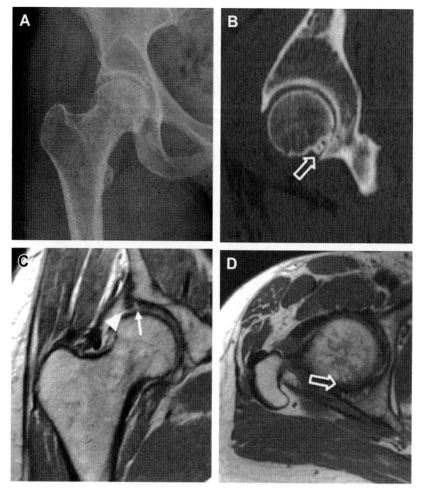

Fig. 18. A 49-year-old female cyclist with pincer impingement. (*A*) AP radiograph of the right hip demonstrates coxa profunda, with narrowing of joint space medially, and marginal osteophytosis. (*B*) Sagittal CT reformation demonstrates joint space loss posteroinferiorly (*open arrow*), with subchondral cystic change and osteophytosis. (*C*) Coronal proton density and (*D*) axial T1-weighted MR images demonstrate truncation and irregularity of the anterosuperior labrum (*arrowhead*), with fissuring of adjacent cartilage (*arrow*). Prominent cartilage thinning and bony reactive change is seen in the posteroinferior joint (*open arrow*).

changes (eg, osteophytes and geodes; describe site and size).

- What main features of FAI are evident: cam (ie, where is the lack of head-neck junction offset) versus pincer features?
- What is the state of the articular cartilage and labrum? Is there any cartilage delamination, focal defects (describe the site and extent; a clock face may be used for description)?
- Is there hip joint effusion or bone marrow changes?
- Incidental findings of FAI-like features on a plain radiograph; report these findings, suggest they may be associated with FAI, and recommend clinical review for orthopedic assessment of the hip.

MANAGEMENT OF FAI

Conservative management includes activity modification, core muscle strengthening, antiinflammatory medication, and intraarticular local anesthetic and corticosteroid injections.[19] Unfortunately, conservative management has been reported to be of limited benefit.

The goal of surgical management is to relieve impingement by removing the morphologic abnormalities involving the acetabulum and/or the femoral head-neck junction. An improvement in the patient's pain, an increase in range of motion, and a reduction or cessation in degenerative change can be expected. This is achieved by reshaping the acetabular rim (see **Fig. 7**) or recontouring the femoral head-neck junction

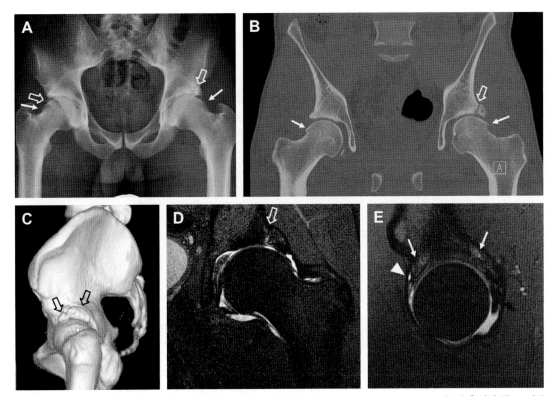

Fig. 19. A 23-year-old man with long-standing bilateral hip pain, recently worsening on the left. (*A*) The pelvic radiograph demonstrates over-coverage of the femoral heads bilaterally, with adjacent os acetabuli (*open arrows*), as well as bony prominence of the femoral head-neck junctions laterally in both hips (*arrows in A and B*). The appearance suggests mixed cam and pincer-type FAI. (*B*) Coronal CT reformat and (*C*) three-dimensional CT reconstruction demonstrates an irregular ossicle adjacent to the acetabular margin in the left hip (*open arrow*), compatible with a stress fracture. (*D*) Coronal T2-weighted image with fat saturation again demonstrates a fracture through the acetabular margin (*open arrow*). (*E*) Sagittal fat-saturated T2-weighted image demonstrates cartilage thinning in the superior joint both anterior and posteriorly, with subchondral cystic change (*arrows*). There is a tear of the anterosuperior labrum, with an early paralabral cyst (*arrowhead*).

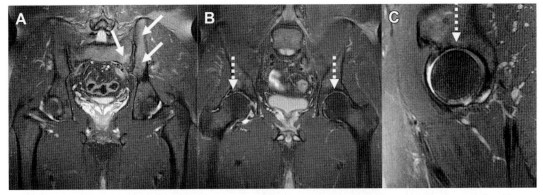

Fig. 20. A 45-year-old man with bilateral hip pain. (*A, B*) Coronal fat-saturated proton density-weighted images of the pelvis demonstrate an inflammatory arthropathy involving the left sacroiliac joint (*thick arrows in A*) and bilateral hip joints with secondary degenerative change (pseudo-FAI). (*C*) Sagittal proton density-weighted image with fat saturation of the right hip further demonstrates the articular cartilage loss. Dashed arrows in (*B, C*) indicate foci of articular cartilage loss.

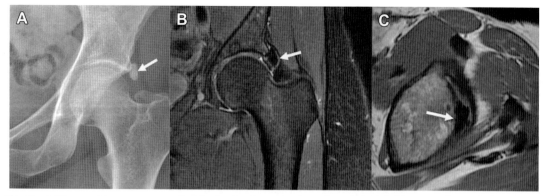

Fig. 21. A 38-year-old woman presented for further investigation of a painful left hip. AP radiograph (*A*) demonstrated a focus of calcification adjacent to the lateral aspect of the left acetabulum (*arrow*). (*B*) Coronal proton density-weighted image with fat saturation and (*C*) axial proton density-weighted image also identifies the focus of calcification (*arrow*). These findings represent hydroxyapatite deposition disease.

(femoroplasty) (**Fig. 22**). This procedure can be performed with open surgery, which necessitates a dislocation technique, allowing for optimal visualization. However, arthroscopic surgery is increasingly being used, enabling a speedier recovery. In specific cases, reorienting the acetabulum via a reverse periacetabular osteotomy is performed.

The labrum may either be repaired or debrided if there is extensive damage. The former is preferred, given the physiologic protective cuff impact on joint preservation. Refixation of the labrum after osseous correction may be associated with a better clinical outcome.[53] Articular cartilage lesions of the femoral head and acetabulum may be debrided and microfracture performed, or stabilized with thermoplasty or fibrin glue.[19]

Surgical approaches currently include a classic open dislocation technique, an anterior arthroscopic approach, or a combination of the 2 techniques. Although an open approach remains the gold standard, hip arthroscopy potentially has fewer complications and a shorter recovery time.[54] The current recommendations for achieving an optimum long-term outcome are based on early intervention, before irreversible joint damage has been sustained.

Complications of surgery for correction of FAI include minor ectopic calcification, nonunion of the greater trochanteric osteotomy, fracture, nerve damage, adhesions, avascular necrosis, and persisting pain.[55] Persisting symptoms and adverse outcomes may also be associated with surgical under correction or over correction.[7]

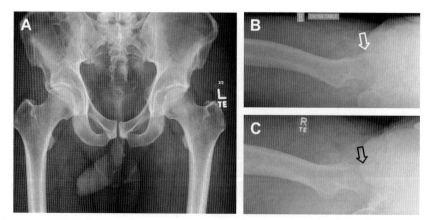

Fig. 22. Male patient with right hip pain and decreased femoral head-neck offset laterally in both hips on the AP radiograph (*A*). (*B*) Convexity of the femoral head-neck junction anteriorly is seen on a cross-table lateral view of the right hip (*white open arrow*). (*C*) After femoroplasty, the bony excrescence is no longer visualized (*open black arrow*).

SUMMARY

FAI is a recognized cause of hip pain, restriction of movement, and primary osteoarthritis in young individuals. Cam-type and pincer-type impingement may occur exclusively, but occur as a mixed pathology in 86% of cases. Plain radiographs and MR imaging form an essential component of assessment and diagnosis of FAI in conjunction with patient symptoms and clinical examination. Identification of FAI may allow early intervention to reduce or stop the progression of osteoarthritic change.

REFERENCES

1. Smith-Petersen MN. Treatment of malum coxae senilus, old slipped upper femoral epiphysis, intrapelvic protrusion of the acetabulum, and coxa plana by means of acetabuloplasty. J Bone Joint Surg Am 1936;18:869–80.
2. Ganz R, Parvizi J, Beck M, et al. Femoroacetabular impingement: a cause for osteoarthritis of the hip. Clin Orthop Relat Res 2003;417:112–20.
3. Murphy SB, Tannast M, Kim YJ, et al. Debridement of the adult hip for femoroacetabular impingement: indications and preliminary clinical results. Clin Orthop Relat Res 2004;429:178–81.
4. Tanzer M, Noiseux N. Osseous abnormalities and early osteoarthritis. Clin Orthop Relat Res 2004;429:170–7.
5. Jäger M, Wild A, Westhoff B, et al. Femoroacetabular impingement caused by a femoral osseous head-neck bump deformity: clinical, radiological, and experimental results. J Orthop Sci 2004;9:256–63.
6. Sutter R, Dietrich TJ, Zingg PO, et al. Femoral antetorsion: comparing asymptomatic volunteers and patients with femoroacetabular impingement. Radiology 2012;263(2):475–83.
7. Tannast M, Siebenrock KA, Anderson SE. Femoroacetabular impingement: radiographic diagnosis—what the radiologist should know. Am J Roentgenol 2007;188(6):1540–52.
8. Beck M, Kalhor M, Leunig M, et al. Hip morphology influences the pattern of damage to the acetabular cartilage: femoroacetabular impingement as a cause of early osteoarthritis of the hip. J Bone Joint Surg Br 2005;87:1012–8.
9. Siebenrock KA, Wahab KH, Werlen S, et al. Abnormal extension of the femoral head epiphysis as a cause of cam impingement. Clin Orthop 2004;418:54–60.
10. Goodman DA, Feighan JE, Smith AD, et al. Subclinical slipped capital femoral epiphysis. Relationship to osteoarthrosis of the hip. J Bone Joint Surg Am 1997;79(10):1489–97.
11. Eijer H, Myers SR, Ganz R. Anterior femoroacetabular impingement after femoral neck fractures. J Orthop Trauma 2001;15(7):475–81.
12. Leunig M, Casillas MM, Hamlet M, et al. Slipped capital femoral epiphysis: early mechanical damage to the acetabular cartilage by a prominent femoral metaphysis. Acta Orthop Scand 2000;71:370–5.
13. Snow S, Keret D, Scarangella S, et al. Anterior impingement of the femoral head: a late phenomenon of Legg-Calvé-Perthes' disease. J Pediatr Orthop 1993;13:286–9.
14. Tonnis D, Heinecke A. Acetabular and femoral anteversion: relationship with osteoarthritis of the hip. J Bone Joint Surg Am 1999;81(12):1747–70.
15. Tonnis D, Heinecke A. Diminished femoral antetorsion syndrome: a cause of pain and osteoarthritis. J Pediatr Orthop 1991;11(4):419–31.
16. Millis MB, Kim YJ, Kocher MS. Hip joint-preserving surgery for the mature hip: the Children's Hospital experience. Orthopaedic Journal at Harvard Medical School 2004;6:84–7.
17. Beall DP, Sweet CF, Martin HD, et al. Imaging findings of femoroacetabular impingement syndrome. Skeletal Radiol 2005;34:691–701.
18. James SL, Ali K, Malara F, et al. MRI findings of femoroacetabular impingement. Am J Roentgenol 2006;187:1412–9.
19. Pollard TC, Villar RN, Norton MR, et al. Genetic influences in the aetiology of femoroacetabular impingement: a sibling study. J Bone Joint Surg Br 2010;92:209–16.
20. Siebenrock KA, Ferner F, Noble PC, et al. The cam-type deformity of the proximal femur arises in childhood in response to vigorous sporting activity. Clin Orthop Relat Res 2011;469:3229–40.
21. Murray RO, Duncan C. Athletic activity in adolescence as an aetiological factor in degenerative hip disease. J Bone Joint Surg Br 1971;53:406–19.
22. Anderson SE, Siebenrock KA, Tannast M. Femoroacetabular impingement: evidence of an established hip abnormality. Radiology 2010;257(1):8–13.
23. Ito K, Leunig M, Ganz R. Histopathologic features of the acetabular labrum in femoroacetabular impingement. Clin Orthop Relat Res 2004;429:262–71.
24. Banerjee P, McLean CR. Femoroacetabular impingement: a review of diagnosis and management. Curr Rev Musculoskelet Med 2011;4(1):23–32.
25. Nepple JJ, Brophy RH, Matava MJ, et al. Radiographic findings of femoroacetabular impingement in National Football League combine athletes undergoing radiographs for previous hip or groin pain. Arthroscopy 2012;28(10):1396–403.
26. Philippon M, Schenker M, Briggs K, et al. Femoroacetabular impingement in 45 professional athletes: associated pathologies and return to sport following arthroscopic decompression. Knee Surg Sports Traumatol Arthrosc 2007;15(7):908–14.

27. Tijssen M, van Cingel R, Willemsen L, et al. Diagnostics of femoroacetabular impingement and labral pathology of the hip: a systematic review of the accuracy and validity of physical tests. Arthroscopy 2011;28(6):860–71.

28. Ganz R, Gill TJ, Gautier E, et al. Surgical dislocation of the adult hip. A technique with full access to femoral head and acetabulum without the risk of avascular necrosis. J Bone Joint Surg Br 2001;83: 1119–24.

29. Meyer DC, Beck M, Ellis T, et al. Comparison of six radiographic projections to assess femoral head/ neck asphericity. Clin Orthop Relat Res 2006;445: 181–5.

30. Harris WH. Etiology of osteoarthritis of the hip. Clin Orthop Relat Res 1986;213:20–33.

31. Resnick D. The "tilt deformity" of the femoral head in osteoarthritis of the hip: a poor indicator of previous epiphysiolysis. Clin Radiol 1976;27:355–63.

32. Siebenrock KA, Schoeniger R, Ganz R. Anterior femoro-acetabular impingement due to acetabular retroversion. Treatment with periacetabular osteotomy. J Bone Joint Surg Am 2003;85(2):278–86.

33. Reynolds D, Lucas J, Klaue K. Retroversion of the acetabulum. A cause of hip pain. J Bone Joint Surg Br 1999;81(2):281–8.

34. Tannast M, Murphy SB, Langlotx F, et al. Estimation of pelvic tilt on anterosuperior X-rays – a comparison of six parameters. Skeletal Radiol 2006;35(3):149–55.

35. Siebenrock KA, Kalbermatten DF, Ganz R. Effect of pelvic tilt on acetabular retroversion: a study of pelves from cadavers. Clin Orthop Relat Res 2003; 407:241–8.

36. Kalberer F, Sierra RJ, Madan SS, et al. Ischial spine projection into the pelvis: a new sign for acetabular retroversion. Clin Orthop Relat Res 2008;466(3): 677–83.

37. Murphy SB, Ganz R, Müller ME. The prognosis in untreated dysplasia of the hip. J Bone Joint Surg Am 1995;77:985–9.

38. Leunig M, Beck M, Kalhor M, et al. Fibrocystic changes at anterosuperior femoral neck: prevalence in hips with femoroacetabular impingement. Radiology 2005;236(1):237–46.

39. Kassarjian A, Yoon LS, Belzile E, et al. Triad of MR arthrographic findings in patients with cam-type femoroacetabular impingement. Radiology 2005; 236(2):588–92.

40. Pfirrmann CW, Duc SR, Zanetti M, et al. MR arthrography of acetabular cartilage delamination in femoroacetabular cam impingement. Radiology 2008; 249(1):236–41.

41. Martinez AE, Li SM, Ganz R, et al. Os acetabuli in femoro-acetabular impingement: stress fracture or unfused secondary ossification centre of the acetabular rim? Hip Int 2006;16(4):281–6.

42. Bredella MA, Ulbrich EJ, Stoller D, et al. Femoroacetabular impingement. Magn Reson Clin North Am 2013;21(1):45–64.

43. Pfirrmann CW, Mengiardi B, Dora C, et al. Cam and pincer femoroacetabular impingement: characteristic MR arthrographic findings in 50 patients. Radiology 2006;240(3):778–85.

44. Sutter R, Dietrich TJ, Zingg PO, et al. How useful is the alpha angle for discriminating between symptomatic patients with cam-type femoroacetabular impingement and asymptomatic volunteers? Radiology 2012;264(2):514–21.

45. Murphy SB, Simon SR, Kijewski PK, et al. Femoral Anteversion. J Bone Joint Surg Am 1987;69:1169–76.

46. Pollard TCB, McNally EG, Wilson DC, et al. Localised cartilage assessment with three-dimensional dGEMRIC in symptomatic hips with normal morphology and cam deformity. J Bone Joint Surg Am 2010;92: 2557–69.

47. Bittersohl B, Steppacher S, Haamberg T, et al. Cartilage damage in femoroacetabular impingement (FAI): preliminary results on comparison of standard diagnostic vs delayed gadolinium-enhanced magnetic resonance imaging of cartilage (dGEMRIC). Osteoarthritis Cartilage 2009;17:1297–306.

48. Jessel RH, Zilkens C, Tiderius C, et al. Assessment of osteoarthritis in hips with femoroacetabular impingement in hips using delayed gadolinium enhanced MRI of cartilage. J Magn Reson Imaging 2009;30:1110–5.

49. Notzli HP, Wyss TF, Stoecklin CH, et al. The contour of the femoral head-neck junction as a predictor for the risk of anterior impingement. J Bone Joint Surg Br 2002;84(4):556–60.

50. Fadul DA, Carrino JA. Imaging of femoroacetabular impingement. J Bone Joint Surg Am 2009; 91(Suppl 1):138–43.

51. Kassarjian A, Brisson M, Palmer WE. Femoroacetabular impingement. Eur J Radiol 2007;63(1): 29–35.

52. Tannast M, Langlotz U, Siebenrock KA, et al. Anatomic referencing of cup orientation in total hip arthroplasty. Clin Orthop Relat Res 2005;436: 144–50.

53. Walker JA, Pagnotto M, Trousdale RT, et al. Preliminary pain and function after labral reconstruction during femoroacetabular impingement surgery. Clin Orthop Relat Res 2012;470(12):3414–20.

54. Botser IB, Smith TW Jr, Nasser R, et al. Open surgical dislocation versus arthroscopy for femoroacetabular impingement: a comparison of clinical outcomes. Arthroscopy 2011;27(2):270–8.

55. Standaert CJ, Manner PA, Herring SA. Expert opinion and controversies in musculoskeletal and sports medicine: femoroacetabular impingement. Arch Phys Med Rehabil 2008;89(5):890–3.

Imaging of Soft Tissue Abnormalities About the Hip

Judong Pan, MD, PhD, Miriam A. Bredella, MD*

KEYWORDS

- Hip • Joint capsule • Tendons • Plica • Capsule • Myotendinous strain
- Ischiofemoral impingement

KEY POINTS

- Selection of appropriate imaging modalities and solid knowledge-base of imaging anatomy and functional roles of various soft tissue structures are essential for radiologists to make accurate diagnosis of soft tissue abnormalities about the hip.
- Identification of the intra-articular or extra-articular location is a critical first step in the evaluation of soft tissue abnormalities about the hip.
- Common intra-articular pathologic conditions about the hip include synovial plicae, and inflammatory and proliferative disorders of the synovium; common extra-articular abnormalities include bursitis and muscular or tendinous pathologic conditions, which can be further categorized according to the mechanism of injury and the anatomic or functional compartments affected.

IMAGING TECHNIQUES

Radiography

Plain radiography remains an important imaging modality for the initial assessment of soft tissue abnormalities of the adult hip in many cases. At the authors' institution, the standard views include anteroposterior and frog-leg lateral views of the symptomatic hip. An elongated femoral neck view is included when femoroacetabular impingement is the clinical question. In addition, an anteroposterior view of the pelvis is often included to assist in assessment of hip pain. The presence of intra-articular osteocartilaginous bodies, mineralization within the soft tissue abnormality, and associated periosteal reaction or bony destruction can be visualized. The presence of a joint effusion can be inferred from displacement of fat pads about the hip, including the gluteus, iliopsoas, and obturator internus fat pads, although bulging of a fat pad is recognized as an insensitive secondary sign of joint effusion.[1]

Ultrasonography

As a cost-effective and readily available technique, ultrasonography (US) allows real time cross-sectional interrogation of soft tissue structures about the hip. Usually, targeted US examination in the area of the patient's symptoms or palpable abnormality is performed. The size, location, and echotexture of the abnormalities can be characterized, and vascularity can be evaluated with color Doppler. US can also be used to detect hip joint effusion and guide various soft tissue interventions. Because there is no ionizing radiation involved, US is a particularly valuable tool in the evaluation of soft tissue abnormalities in the pediatric population. In addition, US allows dynamic evaluation of soft tissue structures and is, therefore, the modality of choice in the evaluation of suspected snapping hip syndrome.[2]

CT

The leading indication for performing CT in patients with hip pain is trauma. Owing to its

Disclosure: The authors have nothing to disclose.
Division of Musculoskeletal Imaging and Intervention, Department of Radiology, Massachusetts General Hospital and Harvard Medical School, 55 Fruit Street, YAW-6E, Boston, MA 02114, USA
* Corresponding author.
E-mail address: mbredella@partners.org

Radiol Clin N Am 51 (2013) 353–369
http://dx.doi.org/10.1016/j.rcl.2012.10.003
0033-8389/13/$ – see front matter © 2013 Elsevier Inc. All rights reserved.

cross-sectional capability, and high-quality multi-planar and volumetric reformations, CT is also helpful in the further delineation of soft tissue abnormalities and associated mineralization, and secondary osseous changes initially detected on plain radiographs. CT is the preferred imaging modality in the evaluation of soft tissue pathology in patients who have contraindications to MR imaging or who have surgical hardware in the region of clinical concern.

MR Imaging

MR imaging of the hip and the pelvis is commonly performed in patients who present with hip pain. Dedicated imaging of the symptomatic hip is preferred in most cases because it provides better spatial resolution and higher signal-to-noise ratio, due to the small field of view and the use of a dedicated surface coil. When patients have bilateral symptoms or the clinical entity is a systemic process or metastatic disease, imaging of the pelvis including both hips can be performed.

At the authors' institution, when performing hip MR imaging, we first survey the pelvis using a coronal short tau inversion recovery (STIR) sequence. Higher resolution MR images of the hip can be then obtained by placing a local surface coil (eg, body matrix coil, dedicated hip coil) over the symptomatic hip and using a small field of view (16–20 cm). Four imaging planes are routinely used and different types of sequences are included: coronal T2 fat-saturated fast spin echo, coronal T1 fast spin echo, sagittal proton density (PD) fast spin echo, axial PD fast spin echo, and oblique axial fat-saturated PD fast spin echo, prescribed along the long axis of the femoral neck (**Table 1**). When the patient presents with a palpable abnormality, or when there is clinical concern for a neoplastic or infectious process, we use a specific protocol that requires the technologist to place a skin marker over the area of palpable abnormality or clinical symptoms, and center the scan accordingly. The sequences that we routinely use in this protocol include fast spin echo coronal and axial T1, fast spin echo sagittal T2 with fat saturation, axial fast spin echo T2 with fat saturation, and postgadolinium axial and coronal or sagittal fast spin echo T1-weighted fat-saturated sequence if there is concern for a neoplasm.

For magnetic resonance (MR) examinations of the pelvis, we use the following sequences: coronal T1-weighted fast spin echo, coronal STIR, axial PD fast spin echo, and axial and sagittal T2 fat-suppressed fast spin echo sequences. The acetabulum, proximal femora, and pelvic structures should always be adequately covered.

In cases of suspected intracapsular or capsular abnormalities, direct MR arthrography is the modality of choice. For direct MR arthrography, we use diluted MR contrast agent, created by adding 0.8 mL of gadopentetate dimeglumine to 100 mL of normal saline. Ten mL of this solution is mixed with 5 mL of nonionic iodinated contrast and 5 mL of lidocaine 1% (final dilution ratio of 1:250) within a 20-mL syringe. A 22-gauge needle is placed within the hip joint and approximately 10 to 12 mL of solution is injected to achieve capsular distension. The use of iodinated contrast enables fluoroscopic confirmation of intra-articular needle placement, as well as detection of extracapsular contrast extravasation. A surface coil is positioned over the hip to decrease the field of view and improve spatial resolution. Our protocol for MR

Table 1
Routine hip MR imaging protocol

Sequence	FOV (mm)	Matrix	TR (ms)	TE (ms)	TI (ms)	Bandwidth (kHz)	Echo Train Length
Coronal STIR (pelvis)	360	320 × 192	4060	48	200	200	7
Axial PD FSE	200	256 × 256	2730	9	–	300	5
Coronal T1 FSE	200	384 × 307	650	15	–	303	5
Coronal T2 FSE FS	200	256 × 256	3070	60	–	250	11
Sagittal PD FSE	200	384 × 307	3500	43	–	303	7
Oblique axial PD FSE FS	160	384 × 257	3640	48	–	303	5
Axial T2 FSE FS	200	256 × 154	4000	69	–	250	11

Routine hip MR imaging protocol is performed with a local surface coil (body matrix coil or dedicated hip coil) on a 3 Tesla MR scanner.
Abbreviations: FOV, field of view; FS, fat saturation; FSE, fast spin echo; TE, echo time; TR, repetition time.

arthrography includes the same coronal, sagittal, axial, and oblique axial imaging planes as used in a conventional MR imaging of the hip. Sequences include fat-saturated T1 fast spin echo, T1 fast spin echo, and fat-saturated PD fast spin echo (**Table 2**).

INTRACAPSULAR AND CAPSULAR SOFT TISSUE ABNORMALITIES
Joint Capsule and Synovium

The joint capsule attaches proximally to the acetabular rim, labrum, and transverse ligament, and distally to the base of the trochanters. The capsule has several thickenings, also known as capsular ligaments, which serve to reinforce the joint.[3,4] These thickenings include the pubofemoral, iliofemoral, and ischiofemoral ligaments, which are composed of superficial, longitudinally oriented fibers. A deep layer of circularly oriented fibers known as the zona orbicularis encircles the capsule at the base of the femoral neck.[5]

The synovium represents a layer of specialized mesenchymal tissue found between the joint capsule and the joint cavity that is essential for the function of the locomotor apparatus.[6] It consists of an outer layer of fibrofatty or loose areolar tissue (subintima), and an inner intima of two to three thin sheets of specialized cells called synoviocytes. In large joints, such as the hip, a well developed vascular network and relatively abundant mature adipose tissue exist just beneath the intima, to provide nutrients to the synovium and the avascular articular cartilage.[6]

Synovial Plica

Synovial plicae represent remnants of synovial membranes from the mesenchymal tissue or synovial reflections formed during embryonic development. There have been extensive studies of the role of synovial plicae in knee pain.[7] Synovial plicae in the hip are increasingly recognized as a cause of hip pain. In a cadaveric study, Fu and colleagues[8] described two forms of morphology in synovial plicae in the hip: flat and villous. In addition, they also described three types of hip synovial plicae by their anatomic location. The ligamental plica (**Fig.** 1A, B) is located at the acetabular notch adjacent to the ligamentum teres. The neck plica (see **Fig.** 1C, D) is a synovial reflection located between the joint capsule and the inferomedial aspect of the femoral neck. The labral plica (see **Fig.** 1E, F) is interposed between the anterosuperior labrum and the overlying joint capsule. Among the three types of plicae, the labral plicae appear larger than the ligamental or neck plicae, and carry an increased risk of impingement between the articular surface of the femoral head and the lower part of the acetabulum during medial rotation of the thigh. Subsequently, there have been several reports of symptomatic hip plicae, with improvement of symptoms after arthroscopy and resection of the plicae.[9,10] A recent study by Bencardino and colleagues[11] showed a high prevalence of synovial plicae in symptomatic patients using MR arthrography. However, their study did not show a statistically significant association between the presence of synovial plicae and hip pathologic conditions, such as femoroacetabular impingement, labral abnormalities, or osteoarthritis.

The pectinofoveal fold, described by Blankenbaker and colleagues[12] as a potential mimicker of synovial plicae, represents a band-like synovial fold that arises from the medial aspect of the femoral neck and extends inferiorly to attach to the joint capsule or less commonly the proximal femur. The fold has a high prevalence (up to 95%) and demonstrates variable imaging appearance and attachment sites.

Table 2
Routine hip MR arthrogram protocol

Sequence	FOV (mm)	Matrix	TR (ms)	TE (ms)	Bandwidth (kHz)	Echo Train Length
Coronal T1 FSE	160	448 × 269	610	15	302	3
Coronal T1 FSE FS	160	384 × 230	570	15	237	3
Oblique axial T1 FSE	160	384 × 230	650	14	237	3
Axial T2 FSE FS	160	384 × 230	3500	82	237	11
Coronal T2 FSE FS	160	384 × 230	3960	82	210	11
Sagittal T1 FSE FS	160	448 × 318	640	13	211	3

Routine hip MR arthrogram protocol is performed with a local surface coil (body matrix coil or dedicated hip coil) on a 3 Tesla MR scanner.
Abbreviations: FOV, field of view; FS, fat saturation; FSE, fast spin echo; TR, repetition time; TE, echo time.

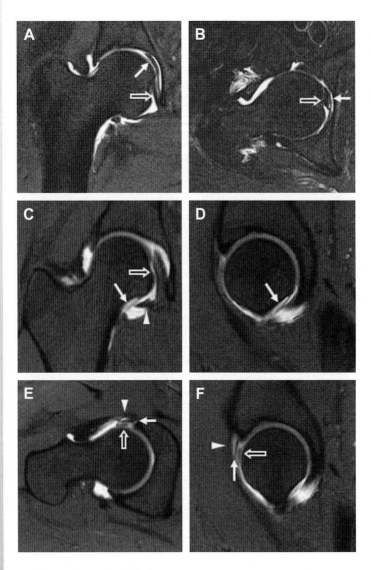

Fig. 1. Synovial plicae. (*A, B*) Coronal T1 fast spin echo (FSE) with fat saturation (FS) and axial T2 FSE FS MR arthrographic oblique images of the right hip show a ligamental plica (*white arrow*) adjacent to the ligamentum teres (*open arrow*). (*C, D*) Coronal and sagittal T1 FSE FS MR arthrographic images demonstrate a neck plica (*white arrow*), which represents a synovial reflection along the inferomedial aspect of the femoral neck. Adjacent structures include the transverse ligament (*arrowhead*) and the ligamentum teres (*open arrow*). (*E, F*) Oblique axial and sagittal T1 FSE FS MR arthrographic images demonstrate a labral plica (*white arrow*) interposed between the joint capsule (*arrowhead*) and the anterosuperior labrum, where there is a bucket handle tear (*open arrow*).

INFLAMMATORY AND PROLIFERATIVE DISEASE OF THE SYNOVIUM
Rheumatoid Arthritis

Rheumatoid arthritis (RA) is characterized by inflammatory proliferation of the synovial lining of the joint capsule. Secondary marginal erosions, diffuse cartilage loss, and joint effusion are frequently present as well. All synovial lined structures can be affected, including bursae and tendon sheaths. RA is a systemic disease that typically has a bilateral, symmetric distribution. Therefore, simultaneous imaging of both hips using at least one fluid-sensitive sequence of the pelvis is indicated.

On plain radiographs, concentric or superomedial joint space narrowing can be seen secondary to diffuse cartilage loss, compared with the typical superolateral joint space narrowing seen in osteoarthritis. Bony erosions may be present as well. On MR images, synovial proliferation or pannus is typically present, which demonstrates low signal on T1-weighted images and high signal on T2-weighted or STIR sequences (**Fig. 2**).[2,13] In the acute or active phase of the disease, the pannus demonstrates strong enhancement after administration of intravenous contrast. Pannus may subsequently become fibrotic and show low signal intensity on all sequences, and no enhancement in chronic disease. The MR signal characteristic of pannus can vary depending on the presence or absence of fibrotic change and hemorrhage. When the fibrotic portion of the pannus detaches from the synovium, rice bodies can be visualized as low signal intensity filling defects in the presence of a joint effusion. Diffuse cartilage loss and

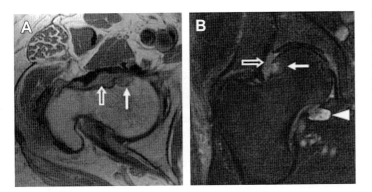

Fig. 2. RA. (*A*) Oblique axial proton density (PD) FSE image shows a marginal erosion of the femoral neck anteriorly (*white arrow*) and synovial thickening (*open arrow*) in a patient with known history of RA. (*B*) Coronal T2 FSE FS image shows that the proliferative synovial tissue (*open arrow*) is hyperintense to skeletal muscle. A marginal erosion (*white arrow*) is evident, as well as a small joint effusion (*arrowhead*).

cortical erosions are other common MR imaging findings in RA.

Synovial Chondromatosis

Synovial chondromatosis represents a benign proliferative disorder of the synovium, characterized by formation of cartilaginous or osteocartilaginous bodies. Two distinct forms of synovial chondromatosis exist. Primary synovial chondromatosis is characterized by benign neoplastic proliferation of the synovial membrane, with formation of multiple cartilaginous or osteocartilaginous bodies of relatively uniform size within synovial-lined structures such as the joint capsules, bursae, or tendon sheaths. The hip is third most commonly affected joint, after the knee and the elbow.[14] In secondary synovial chondromatosis, there are preexisting conditions that lead to secondary proliferation of synovium. These conditions include trauma, osteoarthritis, osteonecrosis, and neuropathic arthropathy. In secondary synovial chondromatosis, there are fewer intra-articular bodies and the bodies are less uniform and larger in size compared with the primary form.[14]

On plain radiographs, the characteristic imaging finding is the presence of multiple ossified or calcified intra-articular bodies (Fig. 3A). Bone erosions are frequently visible. In secondary synovial chondromatosis, findings related to underlying conditions such as osteoarthritis and osteonecrosis are often evident. On MR images, intra-articular bodies can have variable signal intensity. Mineralized bodies may demonstrate a low signal intensity rim with internal T1 hyperintense signal similar to the signal of dense cortical bone and fatty marrow respectively (see Fig. 3B, C). Alternatively, the bodies may demonstrate diffuse low signal on T1-weighted and fluid sensitive sequences. Nonmineralized bodies show signal characteristics similar to hyaline cartilage. Other common imaging features include synovial thickening, bone erosions, and synovial herniation.[15]

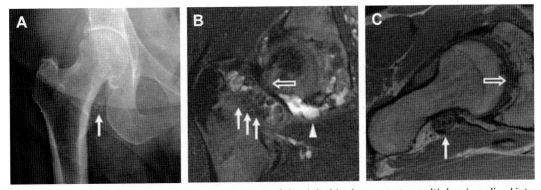

Fig. 3. Synovial chondromatosis. (*A*) Frontal radiograph of the right hip demonstrates multiple mineralized intra-articular bodies (*white arrow*) and evidence of mild osteoarthritis. (*B*) Coronal T2 FSE FS image of a different patient shows numerous intra-articular osteocartilaginous bodies (*white arrows*), most of which are T2 and T1 hypointense, suggestive of mineralization. A linear low-signal band (*open arrow*) represents the zona orbicularis. A joint effusion is present (*arrowhead*). (*C*) Oblique axial T1 FSE image in the same patient shows several osteocartilaginous bodies (*white arrow*) in the posterior recess of the joint. There is evidence of osteoarthritis with cartilage loss and remodeling of the medial acetabulum (*open arrow*).

Pigmented Villonodular Synovitis

Pigmented villonodular synovitis (PVNS) is characterized by benign hemorrhagic proliferation of the synovium. Malignant transformation has been reported, but is extremely rare.[16] PVNS most commonly affects the knee, and the second most commonly affected joint is the hip.[14] Synovial proliferation can be diffuse or focal. Plain radiographs may show multiple juxta-articular erosions that are similar to other inflammatory arthropathies. Osteoarthritic changes can also be observed.[17] On MR images, the hemorrhagic proliferative synovial tissue manifests as synovial-based nodules or masses with low signal on both T1- weighted and T2-weighted fast spin echo or STIR sequences with associated cortical erosions (**Fig. 4**). Classically, "blooming" artifact can be detected on gradient echo sequences due to the presence of hemosiderin deposits. Scattered foci of increased signal intensity on T1-weighted images may be seen and are thought to be related to the presence of lipid-laden macrophages.[18]

EXTRACAPSULAR SOFT TISSUE PATHOLOGIC CONDITIONS
Bursae and Bursitis

There are three main bursal groups about the hip.[1] These are the trochanteric bursa, the ischial or ischiogluteal bursa, and the iliopsoas bursa.

The trochanteric bursa has three discrete components: the subgluteus maximus bursa, the subgluteus medius bursa, and the subgluteus minimus bursa. The subgluteus maximus bursa is located between the posterior facet of the greater trochanter of the femur and the gluteus maximus muscle.[19] The subgluteus medius bursa is located underneath the gluteus medius tendon, and overlies the lateral facet of the greater trochanter.[19] The subgluteus minimus bursa is located deep to the gluteus minimus tendon, and superficial to the anterior facet of the greater trochanter.[19] Chronic excessive friction by the overlying iliotibial band and gluteal tendons may lead to trochanteric bursitis.[20] On MR images, bursal fluid is typically hypointense on T1-weighted images and hyperintense on fluid-sensitive sequences (**Fig. 5**). Synovial thickening, internal debris, septations, and fluid-fluid levels are other common findings suggesting the presence of inflammation and/or hemorrhage.

The iliopsoas bursa lies between the iliopsoas musculotendinous unit and the anterior hip joint capsule. It is the largest synovial bursa in humans[21,22] and, in 10% to 15% of adult hips, there is communication between the bursa and the hip joint.[23] The most common cause of iliopsoas bursitis is chronic friction of the iliopsoas tendon against the anterior hip joint. Other common causes include systemic disease such as rheumatoid arthritis or infection.[20] MR imaging features of iliopsoas bursitis are similar to those of trochanteric bursitis (**Fig. 6A, B**). When the fluid collection is large and complex, it can have a mass-like appearance (see **Fig. 6C, D**). In that scenario, knowing its location anterior to the hip joint and investigation of its relation to the iliopsoas tendon is important for making an accurate diagnosis.

Ischial or ischiogluteal bursitis is an uncommon cause of buttock pain and often overlooked clinically. It commonly occurs after sports-related injuries or occupation-related repetitive stress involving the ischial tuberosity. It can be diagnosed by US or MR imaging by both its characteristic

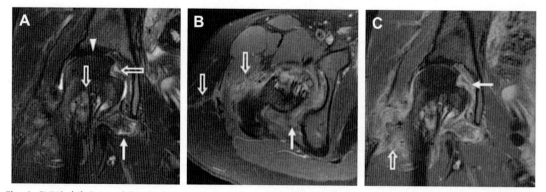

Fig. 4. PVNS. (*A*) Coronal T2 FSE FS image of a 17 year-old female who is status post synovectomy for PVNS presenting with recurrent disease. There is proliferation of the low-signal intensity synovium (*white arrow*) with extensive erosion of the inferomedial femoral neck, as well as the fovea capitis (*open arrows*). There is substantial osteoarthritis with predominantly superolateral cartilage loss (*arrowhead*). (*B, C*) Axial and coronal T1 postgadolinium FSE FS images show avid enhancement of the synovial tissues (*white arrows*). Prior surgical scars in the subcutaneous soft tissue and lateral thigh musculature are also noted to be enhancing (*open arrows*).

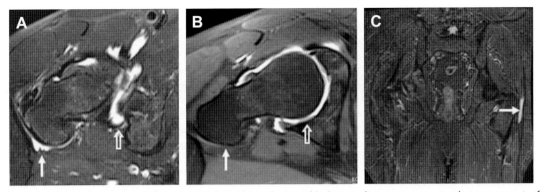

Fig. 5. Trochanteric bursitis. (*A*) Axial T2 FSE FS MR arthrographic image demonstrates a moderate amount of high T2 fluid in the subgluteus maximus bursa (*white arrow*) overlying the posterior facet of the greater trochanter. Intra-articular contrast (*open arrow*) is also T2 bright. (*B*) Oblique axial T1 FSE FS MR arthrographic image shows T1 bright intra-articular contrast (*open arrow*) but no contrast within the trochanteric bursa (*white arrow*). (*C*) STIR image of the pelvis in a different patient shows a fluid collection between the left greater trochanter and gluteus maximus (*arrow*), consistent with trochanteric bursitis.

location adjacent to the inferomedial aspect of the ischial tuberosity and by its cystic appearance.[24,25]

Muscles and Tendons

Abnormalities of the muscles and tendons of the pelvis and hips can be assessed according to their mechanisms of injury or their anatomic or functional compartment.

There are three main categories of injuries to the musculotendinous unit based on the mechanism of injury and the site of involvement.[1] These comprise tendinous avulsion, muscle contusion, and myotendinous strain, which can involve the tendinous attachment, muscle belly, or myotendinous junction, respectively.

Tendinous avulsion

The major mechanisms of acute avulsion injury at the tendon attachment sites include excessive eccentric muscle contraction or passive lengthening.[26] In the hip and pelvis, avulsion

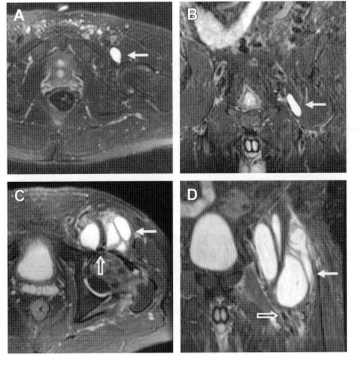

Fig. 6. Iliopsoas bursitis. (*A, B*) Axial and coronal T2 FSE FS images show T2 hyperintense fluid within the iliopsoas bursa anterior to the hip joint (*white arrows*). (*C, D*) Axial and coronal T2 FSE FS images of a patient with rheumatoid arthritis show a large multiloculated fluid collection (*white arrows*) with multiple internal septations anterior to the left hip joint. The iliopsoas tendon (*open arrows*) is immediately adjacent to the mass-like fluid collection, consistent with iliopsoas bursitis.

injuries occur frequently at the ischial tuberosity, anterior superior iliac spine, anterior inferior iliac spine, greater trochanter, lesser trochanter, and pubic bone. Avulsion fractures are readily diagnosed by plain radiography, which shows avulsed osseous fragments with variable degree of displacement.[27] MR imaging is the preferred imaging modality for evaluation of tendinous avulsions. In cases of acute avulsion injury, the torn remnant of the tendon can be visualized and the degree of tendon retraction can be measured (Fig. 7). Frequently, an adjacent hematoma, periosteal stripping and bone marrow edema may be evident at the tendinous attachment site.[1] In chronic avulsion injury, soft tissue scarring, fatty infiltration, and atrophy of affected muscles may be present.

Other tendinous injuries

There is a wide spectrum of tendon abnormalities. Tendinopathy or tendinosis may develop from repetitive microtrauma, intrasubstance degeneration, or weakening from other underlying systemic conditions such as gout, diabetes, and collagen vascular disease.[1] Strong deceleration and acute tensile overload can cause acute partial or complete tendon rupture.[1] See later discussion of abnormalities involving individual tendons described according to their anatomic or functional compartments.

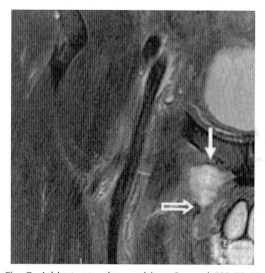

Fig. 7. Adductor tendon avulsion. Coronal FSE T2 FS image shows increased T2 signal in the region of the adductor tendon origin from the right pubis, which may represent an area of hemorrhage (*white arrow*). The adductor longus tendon (*open arrow*) is torn and retracted inferolaterally by approximately 2 cm from its origin.

Myotendinous strain

Unlike tendon avulsion, in which injury occurs at the tendinous attachment to an osseous structure, myotendinous strain involves the myotendinous junction. Myotendinous strain can be classified on MR imaging based on the degree of disruption.[28] In a grade 1 myotendinous strain, there is only minor disruption of fibers at the myotendinous junction. This leads to interstitial edema and hemorrhage, which extends into the adjacent muscle fascicles and produces a feathery MR pattern (Fig. 8A).[28,29] A grade 2 strain manifests as partial tearing of the myotendinous unit without significant associated retraction (see Fig. 8B). Hematomas at the myotendinous junction and perifascial fluid collections are often present. In a grade 3 myotendinous strain, there is complete rupture of the myotendinous unit. Frank retraction may be evident in these injuries and can be readily assessed by MR imaging for preoperative planning purpose (see Fig. 8C).

Muscle contusion

Muscle contusions are usually related to blunt trauma. The most commonly affected muscle group is the gluteal musculature. Based on the severity of the lesion, the MR appearance varies.[1] In mild muscle contusion, diffuse edematous changes of the muscle fibers are present and are characterized by a feathery appearance on fluid-sensitive sequences, similar to that seen in grade 1 myotendinous strains. However, in muscle contusion, the edema mainly involves the muscle belly, compared with the myotendinous junction with myotendinous strains (Fig. 9A). With more severe trauma, intramuscular hematomas can develop and cause increased girth of the muscle belly. The MR signal characteristics of an intramuscular hematoma can be variable, depending on multiple factors, including the age of the hematoma, the degree of hemoglobin oxidation, and the field strength of the MR imaging system[1] Typically, intramuscular hematomas present as heterogeneous collections on both T1-weighted and fluid-sensitive sequences (see Fig. 9B, C, from a different patient than shown in A). Clinically, it is often important to differentiate an intramuscular hematoma from a soft tissue sarcoma. MR imaging findings that suggest a soft tissue sarcoma include a homogeneous signal intensity, high signal intensity on T2-weighted sequences, presence of solid-enhancing components, and interval growth in size.[30,31] MR imaging features that favor intramuscular hematoma include high-signal intensity on T1-weighted sequences, lack of enhancement, and the presence of a low-signal intensity hemosiderin rim (see Fig. 9B, C).[30,32]

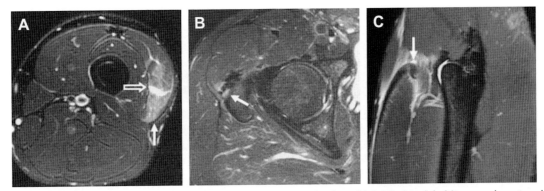

Fig. 8. Myotendinous strain. (*A*) Axial FSE T2 FS image shows feathery high T2 signal (*white arrow*) centered within the posterolateral aspect of the vastus lateralis, in the region of the myotendinous junction, consistent with a grade 1 myotendinous strain. A very small hematoma (*open arrow*) is present, but there is no evidence of tendon tear. (*B*) Axial T2 FSE FS image shows a small partial thickness tear of the gluteus minimus tendon (*white arrow*) at its greater trochanteric attachment, with minimal muscle edema at the myotendinous junction consistent with grade 2 myotendinous strain. (*C*) Sagittal T2 FSE FS image of a patient with a grade 3 strain demonstrates complete rupture of the myotendinous unit of rectus femoris (*white arrow*), approximately 3 cm distal to the anterior inferior iliac spine, with surrounding edema or hemorrhage and significant distal tendon retraction.

However, the imaging characteristics of soft tissue sarcomas are highly variable and overlap with those of intramuscular hematomas. Therefore, when there is any clinical suspicious for a soft tissue sarcoma, particularly when a history of significant trauma is lacking, intramuscular masses should be followed with clinical examination or imaging to resolution, or biopsied for a definitive diagnosis.

Myositis ossificans

Myositis ossificans is a benign, self-limiting process characterized by heterotopic ossification within skeletal muscle. The pathogenesis of myositis ossificans is unknown, although activation of osteoprogenitor cells in the perimysial tissue may be involved. It is frequently associated with traumatic injury such as muscle contusion,[33] but sometimes history of trauma may not be apparent. Because myositis ossificans may appear mass-like, it is often important to differentiate it from a soft tissue sarcoma. The typical appearance of myositis ossificans includes a peripheral rim of ossification and progressive ossification in a centripetal fashion (**Fig. 10**A). On MR imaging, however, the signal intensity can be quite variable and the typical peripheral mineralization may be difficult to appreciate (see **Fig. 10**B, C).

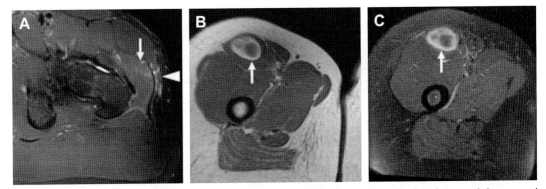

Fig. 9. Muscle contusion. (*A*) Axial T2 FSE FS image shows mild feathery edema in the gluteus minimus muscle (*white arrow*), predominantly located along the superficial surface of the muscle, with relative sparing of the myotendinous junction. There is overlying subcutaneous soft tissue swelling (*arrowhead*), which is suggestive of associated superficial soft tissue contusion. (*B*) Pregadolinium T1 FSE FS weighted image in a different patient shows a heterogeneous mass within the rectus femoris (*white arrow*), which demonstrates high T1 signal in the periphery of the mass and low T1 signal centrally. Increased T1 signal is likely related to blood products. (*C*) Post-gadolinium T1 FSE FS image of the same patient (*B*) shows increased signal in the peripheral aspect of the mass (*white arrow*), but no definite enhancement is seen.

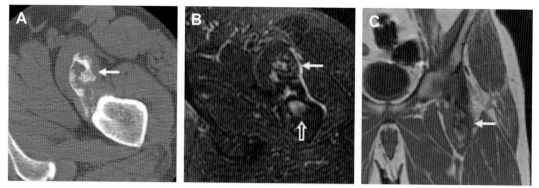

Fig. 10. Myositis ossificans. (*A*) Axial CT image of the left hip shows heterotopic ossification (*white arrow*) in the iliopsoas muscle, with a peripheral sclerotic rim and a central area of low attenuation. (*B*) Axial T2 FSE FS image demonstrates an area of focal signal abnormality in the iliopsoas muscle (*white arrow*). A peripheral rim of low T2 signal is suggestive of mineralization. Centrally, there is patchy high T2 signal intensity. Bone marrow edema (*open arrow*) is present in the adjacent lesser trochanter. (*C*) Coronal T1 FSE image again shows the focal area of signal abnormality with a peripheral low signal intensity rim (*white arrow*). Areas of high T1 signal are suggestive of ossification.

COMPARTMENTS OF THE HIP AND THIGH

Muscle and tendon abnormalities of the hips and pelvis can also be evaluated based on the anatomic or functional compartment. The muscles and tendons of the pelvis and hip can be divided into four compartments based on their anatomic location and functional roles.[34] The anterior compartment consists of the hip flexors. The posterior compartment includes the hip extensors and external rotators. Hip adductors constitute the medial compartment and the lateral compartment contains hip abductors and internal rotators.

Anterior Compartment

The anterior compartment muscles include the psoas major and minor, which form the iliopsoas, the sartorius, and the quadriceps. Only pathologic conditions of the iliopsoas and quadriceps muscles are discussed because lesions of these two muscle groups are the most commonly encountered in the anterior compartment.

Iliopsoas

The iliopsoas tendon has a complex anatomy.[35,36] As the iliacus descends down the pelvis, some of its fibers cross medially and join the psoas major tendon to form the iliopsoas tendon, which inserts onto the lesser trochanter. In some patients, the crossing fibers terminate at the level of the femoral neck, and below this level there is a thin intramuscular tendon in the medial aspect of the iliacus muscle, separated from the parallel iliopsoas tendon by a fatty fascial cleft. The remaining iliacus muscle fibers directly attach to the proximal femoral diaphysis. In some patients a fatty fascial cleft is seen on T1-weighted MR sequences as

a thin T1 bright longitudinal band, and this should not be confused with a longitudinal split tear of the iliopsoas tendon.[36] The iliopsoas tendon lies in a groove between the anterior inferior iliac spine laterally and the iliopectineal eminence medially.

Iliopsoas tendinopathy and tendon tears

The severity of iliopsoas tendon injuries increases with age. In patients 65 years and younger, the most common injuries are muscle strains and partial tears, which are usually related to sports injuries and other traumatic events. In patients older than 65 years, complete tears are more commonly seen. In this age group, tendon abnormalities are most commonly the result of nonathletic injuries, such as chronic systemic disease, corticosteroid use, and complications from total hip arthroplasty.[37–40] Occasionally, tendon injuries are spontaneous in origin.

On MR imaging, tendinopathy is manifested as thickening or increased intrasubstance signal intensity of the tendon along its course or at the insertion.[34] Associated findings include high T2 signal intensity within the peritendinous soft tissues and fluid in the iliopsoas bursa. Partial tendon tears are characterized on MR imaging by focal fluid signal within the tendon that may or may not extend into the tendon surface, or discontinuity of some of the tendon fibers. The most common locations of the tears are the iliopsoas tendon attachment, either adjacent to or at the level of the lesser trochanter.[37,38] Complete tendon rupture presents as complete discontinuity of tendon fibers, with or without significant retraction of the torn tendinous remnants (**Fig. 11**A, B). Intramuscular hematoma may be observed in partial or complete tendon tears and

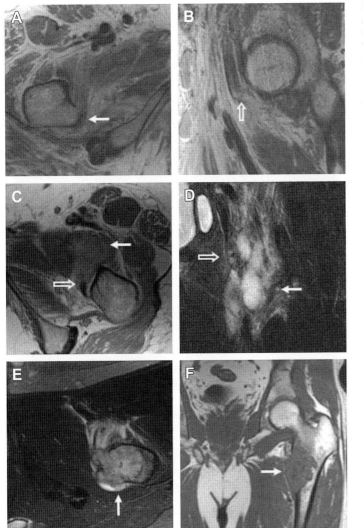

Fig. 11. Iliopsoas tendon tears. (*A*) Axial PD FSE image shows absence of the normal iliopsoas tendon at the lesser trochanteric attachment (*white arrow*). (*B*) Sagittal PD FSE image shows a torn and retracted iliopsoas tendon (*open arrow*). (*C, D*) Axial PD FSE and coronal T2 FSE FS images show a heterogeneous mass (*white arrows*) within the iliopsoas muscle, compatible with an intramuscular hematoma resulting from an iliopsoas tendon tear (*open arrows*). (*E, F*) Axial PD FSE and coronal T1 FSE images demonstrate a destructive mass (*white arrows*) centered on the lesser trochanter, with an associated iliopsoas tendon tear. Biopsy showed metastatic renal cell cancer.

demonstrates variable MR signal characteristics (see **Fig. 11**C, D).

In skeletally immature patients, avulsion of the iliopsoas tendon with detachment of the lesser trochanter is more common because of the relative weakness of the apophysis-bone interface.[34,40] In contrast, underlying metastatic disease must be excluded in older adults with atraumatic or spontaneous avulsion injuries of the lesser trochanter (see **Fig. 11**E, F).

Snapping hip

Snapping hip syndrome is characterized by sudden, painful, audible snapping of the hip.[34,41] It is typically seen in young athletic adults. Painful symptoms are reproduced with specific movements, which most frequently involve moving the hip from a frog-leg position to a neutral position. Snapping hip syndrome can have extra-articular

or intra-articular causes. Extra-articular causes are further divided into external and internal types.[34,41]

The external type involves lateral structures such as the iliotibial band and the gluteus maximus muscle. Snapping occurs as these structures moves over the greater trochanter during hip flexion and extension. External snapping is usually a clinical diagnosis and seldom requires imaging.

Internal snapping related to the iliopsoas tendon is suggested as the most common type of snapping hip syndrome.[42] The iliopsoas tendon most commonly snaps at two locations: the iliopectineal eminence and the lesser trochanter. US is the preferred imaging modality for evaluation of the iliopsoas tendon in snapping hip syndrome because it not only allows dynamic evaluation of the tendon during snapping but also enables static assessment of the tendon for associated tendon pathologic conditions and bursitis.[42–44] Snapping can usually be induced when a flexed, abducted and externally rotated hip returns to a full extension position and is seen on US as a sudden rapid lateral-to-medial movement of the tendon as it passes over the iliopectineal eminence or the lesser trochanter.[42–44] US can also be used to guide diagnostic and/or therapeutic injection of corticosteroid and local anesthetics into the iliopsoas bursa.[45,46] In addition to US, dynamic MR imaging using fast gradient-echo sequences can also be used to demonstrate abnormal motion of the iliopsoas tendon. Dynamic MR imaging can be performed using open-configuration magnets or, if the patients are small in size, conventional large-bore magnets.[34] On MR imaging, the location and quality of the iliopsoas tendon can be readily assessed and fluid within the bursa can be identified (**Fig. 12**).

The causes for intra-articular snapping hip syndrome include labral tears, intra-articular bodies, synovial chondromatosis, synovial folds, and fracture fragments.[34,41] In these cases, the intra-articular conditions are commonly evaluated with MR arthrography.

Quadriceps

The quadriceps muscle group includes the rectus femoris, vastus lateralis, vastus intermedius, and vastus medialis. Among these muscles, rectus femoris tendon injuries are the most common. Injuries to the rectus femoris typically occur when the hip is hyperextended and the knee is flexed during athletic activities.[34,47] The origin of the rectus femoris origin has two components: the straight head attaches to the anterior inferior iliac spine, and the reflected head attaches more posterolaterally to the acetabulum.[34,47] Avulsion injures to the straight head are more common. Partial or complete tears of the straight head can be delineated with MR imaging and are often accompanied by bone marrow edema in the anterior inferior iliac spine and peritendinous soft tissue

edema (**Fig. 13**A, B). The reflected head of the rectus femoris is less commonly injured and may demonstrate similar imaging findings except that the location of findings is more posterior and lateral to the anterior inferior iliac spine (see **Fig. 13**C, D).

Posterior Compartment: the Hamstring Muscle Complex

The posterior compartment contains muscles that serve as hip extensors and external rotators.[34,47] Injuries most commonly involve the hamstrings, which are composed of the semimembranosus, biceps femoris, and semitendinosus muscles.

The hamstring muscle complex serves as both hip extensors and knee flexors because it spans two joints.[48] The long head of the biceps femoris and the semitendinosus share a common origin from the medial facet of the ischial tuberosity. The short head of the biceps tendon arises from the lateral linea aspera, lateral supracondylar line, and intermuscular septum, and is considered by some not to be a true hamstring because it does not span two joints. The biceps femoris attaches distally onto the fibular head, whereas the semitendinosus attaches onto the proximal aspect of medial tibia. The origin of the semimembranosus tendon is the superolateral facet of the ischial tuberosity, which is anterior and lateral to the common origin of the biceps femoris and semitendinosus. Distally, it has multiple insertions by way of five tendon arms that attach onto the posterior aspect of the medial tibial condyle.[34,49] The hamstrings also play a role in the stabilization of the sacroiliac joints. In up to the 50% of individuals, the fibers at the origin of the long head of the biceps femoris are directly continuous with the lower border of the sacrotuberous ligament.[50]

The primary function of the hamstring complex is eccentric contraction, which occurs when the muscles are passively stretched. Injuries to the hamstring tendons, therefore, occur mostly during

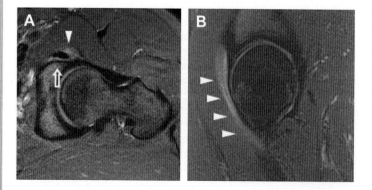

Fig. 12. Snapping hip syndrome, internal type. (*A*) Oblique axial T2 FSE FS image shows edema and inflammation (*arrowhead*) of the iliopsoas tendon where it crosses over the iliopectineal eminence (*open arrow*). (*B*) Sagittal T2 FSE FS image again shows peritendinous soft tissue edema (*arrowheads*).

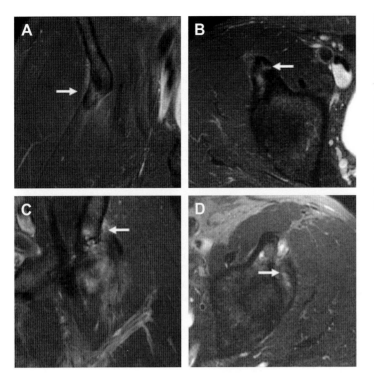

Fig. 13. Rectus femoris tendon tears. (*A*, *B*) Coronal and axial T2 FSE FS images show a partial thickness tear of the direct head of rectus femoris (*white arrows*) at its attachment to the anterior inferior iliac spine, with associated mild peritendinous edema. (*C*, *D*) Coronal and axial T2 FSE FS images show a partial thickness tear (*white arrows*) of the reflected head of the rectus femoris at its attachment posterior and lateral to the anterior inferior iliac spine, with associated soft tissue and bone marrow edema.

passive stretching when the hip is flexed and the knee is extended,[51] and range from low-grade muscle strains, to complete tear or avulsion (**Fig. 14**). Hamstring muscle injuries typically occur in the region of the myotendinous junction, although avulsive stress injuries adjacent to the hamstring origin are not infrequently seen. In mild hamstring strains, edema can be seen around

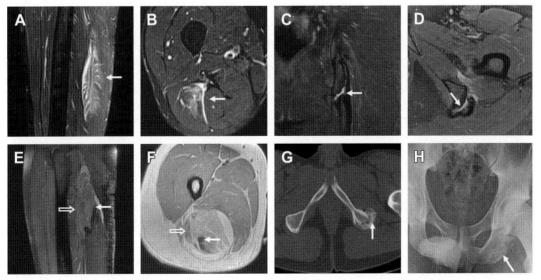

Fig. 14. Hamstring tendon injuries. (*A*, *B*) Sagittal and axial T2 FSE FS images show feathery edema (*white arrows*) along the myotendinous junction of the biceps femoris, consistent with a grade 1 myotendinous strain. (*C*, *D*) Coronal and axial T2 FSE FS images show a partial thickness tear (*white arrows*) of the conjoined tendon of the biceps femoris and semitendinosus at the ischial tuberosity attachment. (*E*, *F*) Coronal T2 FSE FS and axial T1 images of the right thigh show an acute avulsion injury of the hamstring tendon with complete tendon rupture, significant distal tendon retraction (*white arrows*) and a large heterogeneous adjacent hematoma (*open arrows*). (*G*, *H*) Axial CT image and frontal radiograph of the pelvis show an old avulsion injury of the left hamstring tendon, with bony proliferative change and remodeling of the left ischial tuberosity (*white arrows*).

the myotendinous junction, without frank disruption of fibers (see **Fig. 14**A, B). In more severe injuries with partial (see **Fig. 14**C, D) or full thickness (see **Fig. 14**E, F) tendon tears, discontinuity of a portion of the tendon or the entire tendon may occur, either at the myotendinous junction or at the tendon origin.[34] Avulsive ischial stress injuries may occur in the absence of visible tendon abnormality. In this scenario, MR imaging is helpful in detecting bone marrow edema at the ischial tuberosity using fluid-sensitive sequences. In cases of chronic injuries, bony proliferative changes of the ischial tuberosity can develop (see **Fig. 14**G, H).

Medial Compartment: the Adductors

The adductors serve to adduct and flex the thigh, and include the adductor longus, magnus, and brevis, as well as the obturator externus and quadratus femoris. The adductor longus originates from the anterior pubis, and inserts onto the linea aspera of the femur. The adductor brevis originates from the inferior pubic ramus, and also inserts onto the linea aspera. The adductor magnus originates from the ischial tuberosity and pubis, and attaches onto the linea aspera, supracondylar femur, and adductor tubercle in the medial distal femur.

Similar to tendons in the other compartments of the hip, the adductor tendons are subject to various injuries including tendinopathy, partial or full thickness tears, and calcific tendinitis.

Adductor insertion avulsion syndrome
Adductor insertion avulsion syndrome, also known as thigh splints, represents a painful condition affecting the proximal to midfemur at the insertion of the adductor muscles.[52,53] When the condition is longstanding, radiographs may show foci of calcifications along the posterior aspect of the proximal thigh, which occurs secondary to chronic inflammatory change. Radionuclide bone scintigraphy may show focal increased radiotracer uptake in the same location. On MR imaging, there may be thickening and signal abnormality of the adductor tendons, and edema in the soft tissues surrounding the adductor attachment may also be evident.[52,53]

Quadratus femoris and ischiofemoral impingement
The quadratus femoris muscle originates from the inferolateral margin of the ischium, just anterior to the origin of the hamstring tendons.[54] It inserts into the posterior medial aspect of the proximal femur, along the quadrate tubercle of the posterior intertrochanteric ridge. The quadratus femoris is bordered anteriorly by the obturator externus muscle, and posteriorly by fat and the sciatic nerve.

Injuries to the quadratus femoris include myotendinous strains, partial tears, or impingement.[55–57] Ischiofemoral impingement, or impingement of the quadratus femoris muscle is increasingly recognized as a cause of hip pain. This abnormality is best assessed on axial MR imaging images.[56,57] The presence of ischiofemoral impingement can be associated with developmental or acquired narrowing of the osseous space (ischiofemoral space) between the lesser trochanter and ischial tuberosity of less than or equal to 17 mm (**Fig. 15**A), or the soft tissue space (quadratus femoris space) between the hamstring tendon origin and iliopsoas tendon insertion of less than or equal to 8 mm (see **Fig. 15**A), that allows passage of the quadratus femoris muscle. In cases of ischiofemoral impingement, abnormalities of the quadratus femoris muscle include muscular edema, partial tear, and fatty infiltration (see **Fig. 15**B, C). Associated hamstring tendon abnormalities such as edema or partial tears may also be observed.

Lateral Compartment: the Gluteal Muscles

The gluteal muscles are strong hip abductors that are analogous to the rotator cuff of the shoulder in terms of their function. The greater trochanter is the main attachment site for the abductor tendons. The greater trochanter has four facets; the anterior, lateral, posterior superior, and posterior. Each facet has a specific tendinous attachment and specific nearby bursa.[19,20] The gluteus medius attachment can be divided into three parts.[19,20] The main tendon attaches onto the posterior superior facet, the lateral tendon fibers attach onto the lateral facet, and the anterior portion of the tendon attaches onto the gluteus minimus tendon. The gluteus minimus attachment consists of two parts.[19,20] The main tendon attaches onto the anterior facet, and some tendon fibers insert into the ventral and superior capsule of the hip joint. The gluteus maximus is not a hip abductor and is, therefore, not discussed in this article.

Greater trochanteric pain syndrome
Greater trochanteric pain syndrome is a clinical condition characterized by pain in the lateral hip and tenderness over the greater trochanter. It is commonly associated with trochanteric bursitis (see **Fig. 5**) and gluteal tendon abnormalities.[58–60] On MR imaging, a spectrum of tendon abnormalities, including peritendinitis, tendinopathy, and partial and complete tears, can be observed (**Fig. 16**). Secondary findings include bursitis,

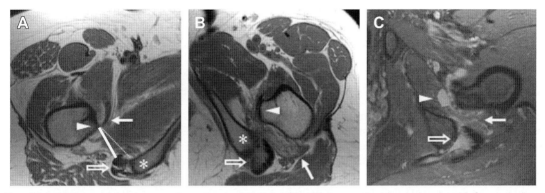

Fig. 15. Ischiofemoral impingement syndrome. (*A*) Axial T1 FSE image shows a normal ischiofemoral space (*dotted white line*), which is the distance between the lesser trochanter (*arrowhead*) and ischial tuberosity (*asterisks*), and a normal quadratus femoris space (*solid white line*). which is the distance between the iliopsoas tendon insertion (*white arrow*) and hamstring tendon origin (*open arrow*). (*B*) Axial T1 FSE image in a different patient shows narrowing of the ischiofemoral space between the lesser trochanter (*arrowhead*) and ischial tuberosity (*asterisks*). There is fatty infiltration of the quadratus femoris muscle (*white arrow*), with hamstring tendinopathy and partial tearing (*open arrow*). (*C*) Axial T2 FSE FS image of a different patient with ischiofemoral impingement shows intramuscular edema (*white arrow*) and adventitial bursa formation (*arrowhead*) in the quadratus femoris. A partial tear of the hamstring tendon (*open arrow*) is also present.

bony changes, and fatty atrophy. Increased peritrochanteric T2 signal is always present in patients with trochanteric pain syndrome. However, it has a poor specificity in predicting trochanteric pain syndrome because it is also present in many asymptomatic individuals.[58] Calcific tendinitis of the gluteal tendons, or hydroxyapatite deposition disorder, can also cause greater trochanteric pain syndrome, and manifests as amorphous calcifications along the gluteal tendons near the greater trochanter. Trochanteric pain syndrome can also be seen in patients who undergo total

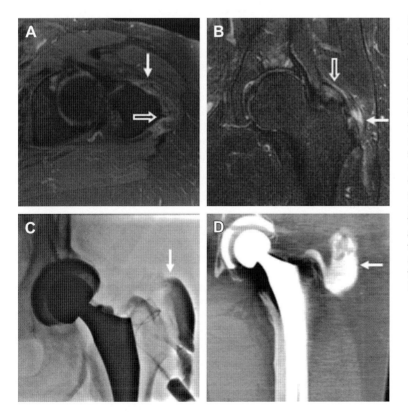

Fig. 16. Gluteal tendon tears. (*A, B*) Oblique axial and coronal T2 FSE FS images show partial tearing of the gluteus minimus (*white arrows*) and gluteus medius (*open arrows*) tendons at their attachment to the anterior facet and posterior superior facet of the greater trochanter, respectively, with peritendinous soft tissue edema or hemorrhage. (*C, D*) Fluoroscopic and coronal reformatted CT arthrographic images of a different patient demonstrate extravasation of contrast material (*white arrows*) through full-thickness tears of the gluteus minimus and medius, extending into the soft tissues overlying the lateral hip.

hip arthroplasty (see **Fig. 16**C, D). MR imaging findings are similar to patients with native hips and include gluteal tendon tears, fatty atrophy of the gluteus muscles, and bursitis.[61]

SUMMARY

Hip pain is a common clinical problem and, in many patients is the result of soft tissue pathologic conditions. Diagnostic imaging plays an increasingly important role in the clinical management of these patients. Understanding the anatomy and functional roles of various soft tissue structures about the hip is essential for evaluation of soft tissue abnormalities. The intra-articular or extra-articular location of a lesion can be determined by selecting the most appropriate imaging modality. Careful evaluation of soft tissue structures using a systematic approach can allow the radiologist to make an accurate diagnosis of various soft tissue abnormalities around the hip.

REFERENCES

1. Bencardino JT, Kassarjian A, Palmer WE. Magnetic resonance imaging of the hip: sports-related injuries. Top Magn Reson Imaging 2003;14:145–60.
2. Mengiardi B, Pfirrmann CW, Hodler J. Hip pain in adults: MR imaging appearance of common causes. Eur Radiol 2007;17:1746–62.
3. Martin HD, Savage A, Braly BA, et al. The function of the hip capsular ligaments: a quantitative report. Arthroscopy 2008;24:188–95.
4. Wagner FV, Negrao JR, Campos J, et al. Capsular ligaments of the hip: anatomic, histologic, and positional study in cadaveric specimens with MR arthrography. Radiology 2012;263:189–98.
5. Ito H, Song Y, Lindsey DP, et al. The proximal hip joint capsule and the zona orbicularis contribute to hip joint stability in distraction. J Orthop Res 2009; 27:989–95.
6. O'Connell JX. Pathology of the synovium. Am J Clin Pathol 2000;114:773–84.
7. Garcia-Valtuille R, Abascal F, Cerezal L, et al. Anatomy and MR imaging appearances of synovial plicae of the knee. Radiographics 2002;22:775–84.
8. Fu Z, Peng M, Peng Q. Anatomical study of the synovial plicae of the hip joint. Clin Anat 1997;10: 235–8.
9. Atlihan D, Jones DC, Guanche CA. Arthroscopic treatment of a symptomatic hip plica. Clin Orthop Relat Res 2003;411:174–7.
10. Katz LD, Haims A, Medvecky M, et al. Symptomatic hip plica: MR arthrographic and arthroscopic correlation. Skeletal Radiol 2010;39:1255–8.
11. Bencardino JT, Kassarjian A, Vieira RL, et al. Synovial plicae of the hip: evaluation using MR

12. Blankenbaker DG, Davis KW, De Smet AA, et al. MRI appearance of the pectinofoveal fold. AJR Am J Roentgenol 2009;192:93–5.
13. Koulouris G, Morrison WB. MR imaging of hip infection and inflammation. Magn Reson Imaging Clin N Am 2005;13:743–55.
14. Llauger J, Palmer J, Roson N, et al. Nonseptic monoarthritis: imaging features with clinical and histopathologic correlation. Radiographics 2000; 20(Spec No):S263–78.
15. Kim SH, Hong SJ, Park JS, et al. Idiopathic synovial osteochondromatosis of the hip: radiographic and MR appearances in 15 patients. Korean J Radiol 2002;3:254–9.
16. Kalil RK, Unni KK. Malignancy in pigmented villonodular synovitis. Skeletal Radiol 1998;27:392–5.
17. Cotten A, Flipo RM, Chastanet P, et al. Pigmented villonodular synovitis of the hip: review of radiographic features in 58 patients. Skeletal Radiol 1995;24:1–6.
18. Bancroft LW, Peterson JJ, Kransdorf MJ. MR imaging of tumors and tumor-like lesions of the hip. Magn Reson Imaging Clin N Am 2005;13:757–74.
19. Pfirrmann CW, Chung CB, Theumann NH, et al. Greater trochanter of the hip: attachment of the abductor mechanism and a complex of three bursae—MR imaging and MR bursography in cadavers and MR imaging in asymptomatic volunteers. Radiology 2001;221:469–77.
20. Blankenbaker DG, Tuite MJ. The painful hip: new concepts. Skeletal Radiol 2006;35:352–70.
21. Armstrong P, Saxton H. Ilio-psoas bursa. Br J Radiol 1972;45:493–5.
22. Harper MC, Schaberg JE, Allen WC. Primary iliopsoas bursography in the diagnosis of disorders of the hip. Clin Orthop Relat Res 1987;221:238–41.
23. Steinbach LS, Schneider R, Goldman AB, et al. Bursae and abscess cavities communicating with the hip. Diagnosis using arthrography and CT. Radiology 1985;156:303–7.
24. Cho KH, Lee SM, Lee YH, et al. Non-infectious ischiogluteal bursitis: MRI findings. Korean J Radiol 2004;5: 280–6.
25. Kim SM, Shin MJ, Kim KS, et al. Imaging features of ischial bursitis with an emphasis on ultrasonography. Skeletal Radiol 2002;31:631–6.
26. Stevens MA, El-Khoury GY, Kathol MH, et al. Imaging features of avulsion injuries. Radiographics 1999;19:655–72.
27. Manaster BJ. From the RSNA Refresher Courses. Radiological Society of North America. Adult chronic hip pain: radiographic evaluation. Radiographics 2000;20(Spec No):S3–25.
28. Palmer WE, Kuong SJ, Elmadbouh HM. MR imaging of myotendinous strain. AJR Am J Roentgenol 1999; 173:703–9.

29. Steinbach LS, Fleckenstein JL, Mink JH. Magnetic resonance imaging of muscle injuries. Orthopedics 1994;17:991–9.

30. Gomez P, Morcuende J. High-grade sarcomas mimicking traumatic intramuscular hematomas: a report of three cases. Iowa Orthop J 2004;24:106–10.

31. Imaizumi S, Morita T, Ogose A, et al. Soft tissue sarcoma mimicking chronic hematoma: value of magnetic resonance imaging in differential diagnosis. J Orthop Sci 2002;7:33–7.

32. Lee YS, Kwon ST, Kim JO, et al. Serial MR imaging of intramuscular hematoma: experimental study in a rat model with the pathologic correlation. Korean J Radiol 2011;12:66–77.

33. Kneeland JB. MR imaging of sports injuries of the hip. Magn Reson Imaging Clin N Am 1999;7: 105–15, viii.

34. Bancroft LW, Blankenbaker DG. Imaging of the tendons about the pelvis. AJR Am J Roentgenol 2010;195:605–17.

35. Blankenbaker DG, Tuite MJ. Iliopsoas musculotendinous unit. Semin Musculoskelet Radiol 2008;12:13–27.

36. Polster JM, Elgabaly M, Lee H, et al. MRI and gross anatomy of the iliopsoas tendon complex. Skeletal Radiol 2008;37:55–8.

37. Bui KL, Ilaslan H, Recht M, et al. Iliopsoas injury: an MRI study of patterns and prevalence correlated with clinical findings. Skeletal Radiol 2008;37:245–9.

38. Bui KL, Sundaram M. Radiologic case study: iliopsoas tendon rupture. Orthopedics 2008;10:31. doi: pii: orthosupersite.com/view.asp?rID=32083.

39. Lecouvet FE, Demondion X, Leemrijse T, et al. Spontaneous rupture of the distal iliopsoas tendon: clinical and imaging findings, with anatomic correlations. Eur Radiol 2005;15:2341–6.

40. Shabshin N, Rosenberg ZS, Cavalcanti CF. MR imaging of iliopsoas musculotendinous injuries. Magn Reson Imaging Clin N Am 2005;13:705–16.

41. Deslandes M, Guillin R, Cardinal E, et al. The snapping iliopsoas tendon: new mechanisms using dynamic sonography. AJR Am J Roentgenol 2008; 190:576–81.

42. Pelsser V, Cardinal E, Hobden R, et al. Extraarticular snapping hip: sonographic findings. AJR Am J Roentgenol 2001;176:67–73.

43. Cardinal E, Buckwalter KA, Capello WN, et al. US of the snapping iliopsoas tendon. Radiology 1996;198: 521–2.

44. Vaccaro JP, Sauser DD, Beals RK. Iliopsoas bursa imaging: efficacy in depicting abnormal iliopsoas tendon motion in patients with internal snapping hip syndrome. Radiology 1995;197:853–6.

45. Idjadi J, Meislin R. Symptomatic snapping hip: targeted treatment for maximum pain relief. Phys Sportsmed 2004;32:25–31.

46. Wahl CJ, Warren RF, Adler RS, et al. Internal coxa saltans (snapping hip) as a result of overtraining: a report of 3 cases in professional athletes with a review of causes and the role of ultrasound in early diagnosis and management. Am J Sports Med 2004;32:1302–9.

47. Chatha DS, Arora R. MR imaging of the normal hip. Magn Reson Imaging Clin N Am 2005;13:605–15.

48. Miller JP, Croce RV. Analyses of isokinetic and closed chain movements for hamstring reciprocal coactivation. J Sport Rehabil 2007;16:319–25.

49. Koulouris G, Connell D. Hamstring muscle complex: an imaging review. Radiographics 2005;25: 571–86.

50. van Wingerden JP, Vleeming A, Snijders CJ, et al. A functional-anatomical approach to the spine-pelvis mechanism: interaction between the biceps femoris muscle and the sacrotuberous ligament. Eur Spine J 1993;2:140–4.

51. LaBan MM, McNeary L. An avulsion of the semitendinosus and biceps femoris conjoined tendons. Am J Phys Med Rehabil 2008;87:168.

52. Anderson MW, Kaplan PA, Dussault RG. Adductor insertion avulsion syndrome (thigh splints): spectrum of MR imaging features. AJR Am J Roentgenol 2001;177:673–5.

53. Tshering-Vogel D, Waldherr C, Schindera ST, et al. Adductor insertion avulsion syndrome, "thigh splints": relevance of radiological follow-up. Skeletal Radiol 2005;34:355–8.

54. Kassarjian A, Tomas X, Cerezal L, et al. MRI of the quadratus femoris muscle: anatomic considerations and pathologic lesions. AJR Am J Roentgenol 2011; 197:170–4.

55. O'Brien SD, Bui-Mansfield LT. MRI of quadratus femoris muscle tear: another cause of hip pain. AJR Am J Roentgenol 2007;189:1185–9.

56. Patti JW, Ouellette H, Bredella MA, et al. Impingement of lesser trochanter on ischium as a potential cause for hip pain. Skeletal Radiol 2008;37:939–41.

57. Torriani M, Souto SC, Thomas BJ, et al. Ischiofemoral impingement syndrome: an entity with hip pain and abnormalities of the quadratus femoris muscle. AJR Am J Roentgenol 2009;193:186–90.

58. Blankenbaker DG, Ullrick SR, Davis KW, et al. Correlation of MRI findings with clinical findings of trochanteric pain syndrome. Skeletal Radiol 2008; 37:903–9.

59. Cvitanic O, Henzie G, Skezas N, et al. MRI diagnosis of tears of the hip abductor tendons (gluteus medius and gluteus minimus). AJR Am J Roentgenol 2004; 182:137–43.

60. Kong A, Van der Vliet A, Zadow S. MRI and US of gluteal tendinopathy in greater trochanteric pain syndrome. Eur Radiol 2007;17:1772–83.

61. Pfirrmann CW, Notzli HP, Dora C, et al. Abductor tendons and muscles assessed at MR imaging after total hip arthroplasty in asymptomatic and symptomatic patients. Radiology 2005;235:969–76.

Meniscal Injuries and Imaging the Postoperative Meniscus

Brendan R. Barber, MBChB, MRCS, FRCR*,
Eugene G. McNally, MB Bch, BAO, FRCPI, FRCR

KEYWORDS

- Meniscal anatomy and pathology • 3T MRI • Diagnostic pitfalls • Meniscal surgery
- Postoperative imaging

KEY POINTS

- Knowledge of meniscal anatomy is key to understanding the important role the meniscus plays in the structure and function of the knee and the various pathologic changes, such as mucoid degeneration, meniscal tears, chondrocalcinosis, and ossification (meniscal stone).
- 3T magnetic resonance imaging provides improved resolution; however, there are several diagnostic pitfalls to be aware of.
- Meniscus-preserving surgery, such as meniscal repair and transplantation, is becoming more frequent; the diagnosis of postoperative meniscal pathologic conditions is particularly challenging.

INTRODUCTION

Meniscal injuries are common. Magnetic resonance (MR) imaging is considered the imaging modality of choice in diagnosing meniscal pathology in the nonoperative knee. The information gained from MR imaging plays a central role in determining the need for surgical intervention.

The increasing awareness of the importance of the meniscus in maintaining the structure and function of the knee has resulted in an emphasis on meniscus-preserving surgery. Meniscal repair and transplantation are becoming more frequent, with a resultant increase in postoperative imaging. A good knowledge of the anatomy, pathologic conditions, surgery performed, and possible imaging options is required for accurate interpretation.

This article aims to review the anatomy, pathology, and diagnostic pitfalls related to meniscal injury and the challenges faced with postoperative imaging.

ANATOMY

The menisci are C-shaped fibrocartilaginous structures that lie between the femoral condyles and tibial plateau. They perform several important functions in the knee joint: (1) increase stabilization of the knee by deepening the contact between the femoral condyles and tibial plateau, (2) distribute hoop forces evenly across the articular contact surface, (3) aid proprioception because of their nerve fibers in the anterior and posterior thirds, and (4) aid lubrication.[1,2]

Structurally, the menisci are comprised of thick collagen fibers predominantly arranged in a circumferential pattern, supported by radially oriented tie fibers. This arrangement provides the meniscus with good tensile strength and

Funding sources: Nil.
Conflicts of interest: Nil.
Department of Radiology, Nuffield Orthopaedic Centre, Oxford University Hospitals NHS Trust, Windmill Road, Headington, Oxford OX3 7HE, UK
* Corresponding author.
E-mail address: brendan.barber@nhs.net

Radiol Clin N Am 51 (2013) 371–391
http://dx.doi.org/10.1016/j.rcl.2012.10.008
0033-8389/13/$ – see front matter

aids the even distribution of force.[2] Disruption of the meniscus leads to uneven loading of the cartilage and early osteoarthrosis.[3] The meniscal roots are the sites at which the menisci are directly attached to the central tibial plateau by fibers extending out from the anterior and posterior thirds. They help to resist hoop stress and the outward displacement of the menisci during axial loading.[4] Descriptively, each meniscus is divided longitudinally into 3 segments: the anterior third, the body (middle third), and the posterior third (Fig. 1).

The meniscal blood supply is derived from the medial and lateral geniculate arteries. In adults, the peripheral 20% to 30% of the meniscus is vascularized (the red zone), whereas the inner two-thirds are relatively avascular (the white zone).[5] A mixed vascularity pink zone is occasionally described between the two.

Medial Meniscus

The medial meniscus covers approximately 50% of the medial tibial plateau[3] and is more tightly adherent to the joint capsule than the lateral meniscus. The anterior third is smaller, approximately one-third to one-half of the size of the posterior third, and is attached to the medial tibial spine just anterior to the anterior cruciate ligament (ACL) insertion (see Fig. 1). The posterior third attaches anterior to the tibial insertion of the posterior cruciate ligament (PCL). The medial meniscus is attached to the femoral condyle and tibial plateau by the coronary ligaments, which form the deep portion of the medial collateral ligament (MCL).[6]

Lateral Meniscus

The lateral meniscus is smaller than the medial meniscus and covers approximately 70% of the lateral surface of the tibial plateau.[3] The anterior and posterior thirds are of equal size (see Fig. 1). The anterior third of the meniscus attaches anterior to the tibial spine and shares some fibers with the anterior cruciate ligament. The posterior third attaches just posterior to the tibial spine. The lateral meniscus is loosely attached to the joint capsule, particularly in the posterolateral corner where the posterior third attaches to the capsule via the popliteomeniscal fascicles.[6] The popliteus tendon passes between these fascicles posterior to the lateral meniscus (Fig. 2).

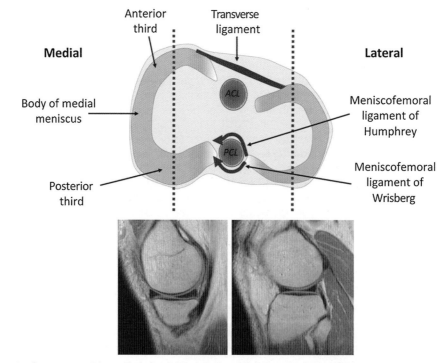

Fig. 1. Meniscal anatomy with sagittal slices through the menisci at the level of the dotted lines. Note the larger posterior third compared with the anterior third of the medial meniscus, whereas the anterior and posterior horn of the lateral meniscus are the same size. ACL, anterior cruciate ligament; PCL, posterior cruciate ligament. (*Courtesy of* Kathryn Stevens, MD, Stanford, California.)

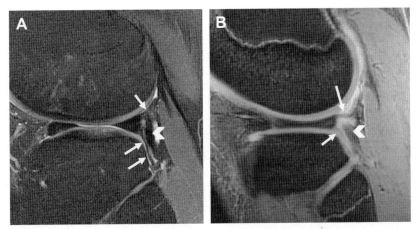

Fig. 2. (*A, B*) Sagittal proton-density fat-saturated images from 2 different patients demonstrating the postero-superior and anteroinferior popliteomeniscal fascicles (*arrows*) and the popliteus tendon passing between them (*arrowhead*).

Related Anatomy

The meniscofemoral ligaments (MFLs) attach the posterior third of the lateral meniscus to the lateral margin of the posterior medial femoral condyle. They pass on either side of the PCL and help to stabilize the posterior third of the meniscus.[7] The anterior limb of the MFL is called the ligament of Humphrey and the posterior the ligament of Wrisberg (**Fig. 3**).

The transverse (anterior) ligament runs between the anterior thirds of the menisci through the posterior aspect of the Hoffa fat pad[8] and functions to stabilize the anterior third of the medial meniscus (**Fig. 4**).[9] A posterior intermeniscal ligament is also described but is rarely visualized on routine MR imaging.

The oblique meniscomeniscal ligament runs between the posterior third of one meniscus to the anterior third of the other meniscus and is named according to its anterior attachment.[10] Both oblique meniscomeniscal ligaments run through the intercondylar notch passing between the ACL and PCL and have no known function.[10]

Anatomic Variants

Discoid meniscus

The discoid meniscus is a developmental variant in which the meniscus has a thickened disklike shape (**Fig. 5**). They are more common on the lateral side. Three types are described: partial, complete, and the Wrisberg variant.[11] The partial and complete variants are determined by the amount of coverage of the tibial plateau. Both have normal tibial attachments and are stable. The rare Wrisberg variant has no posterior capsular attachment and no attachment to the tibia. The only attachment to the posterior horn is

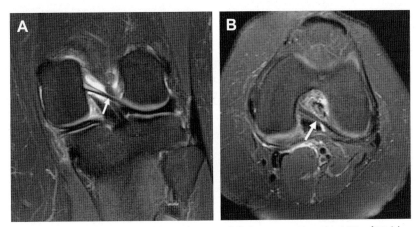

Fig. 3. Coronal proton-density fat-saturated (PD FS) image (*A*) demonstrating the MFL of Wrisberg (*arrow*) and (*B*) axial PD FS image demonstrating the MFL of Humphrey (*arrow*) passing anterior to the PCL.

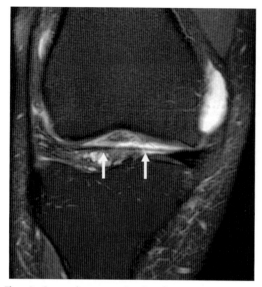

Fig. 4. Coronal proton-density fat-saturated image demonstrating the anterior transverse ligament running between the anterior thirds of the medial and lateral menisci (*arrows*).

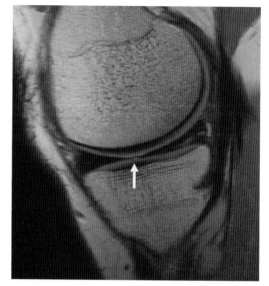

Fig. 6. Sagittal proton-density image of the medial meniscus demonstrating meniscal flounce. The meniscus appears buckled (*arrow*), which is a normal finding and should not be confused with a tear.

the MFL of Wrisberg[12]; therefore, the meniscus is unstable and hypermobile.[13]

Meniscal flounce

Meniscal flounce is a buckled meniscus, which occurs most commonly on the medial side (**Fig. 6**). This appearance was thought to be

a transient appearance related to valgus stress on the knee secondary to ligamentous injuries[14] and is not associated with a meniscal tear. A more recent article has shown that meniscal flounce can occur in the absence of internal derangement and is related to the position of the meniscus on the tibial plateau. The appearance

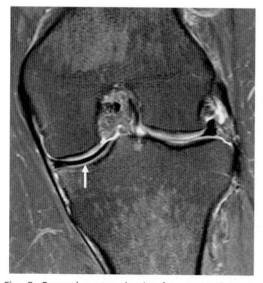

Fig. 5. Coronal proton-density fat-saturated image demonstrating a discoid medial meniscus (*arrow*), very rare compared with the more common lateral discoid meniscus.

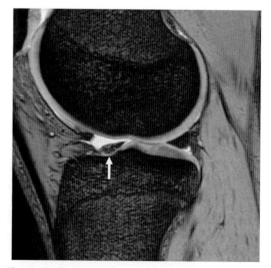

Fig. 7. Sagittal gradient echo image demonstrating the speckled appearance of the anterior third of the lateral meniscus (*arrow*), which can be mistaken for a meniscal tear.

of the buckled meniscus can be altered by changing the position of the knee and should not be mistaken for a meniscal tear.[15]

Speckled appearance of anterior third of lateral meniscus

The anterior third of the lateral meniscus frequently has a speckled appearance (**Fig. 7**) and is caused by the fibers of the ACL inserting into the meniscus. This appearance is usually seen on the medial sagittal images[16] and should not be confused with a tear.

Normal Meniscal MR Imaging Appearances

The menisci are predominantly of low signal on all but ultrashort echo time (TE) sequences because of their fibrocartilaginous composition. In children and young adults, intermediate to high signal intensity is often noted in the posterior third, representing normal vascularity or tie fibers. This appearance should not be misinterpreted as a tear (**Fig. 8**).[17] The menisci of elderly patients may also show high signal because of mucoid degeneration.

The average size of the meniscus varies with the population under study. The most common measurement used is the size of the central third in the coronal plane. If coronal images are not available, the appearance of the meniscus in the sagittal plane may be used to assess meniscal size. On peripheral sagittal images, the middle thirds of the menisci appear as a bow tie, whereas more centrally the anterior and posterior thirds appear as triangular structures.

Diagnostic MR Imaging Sequences

Several sequences have been advocated for imaging of meniscal tears; however, a short TE is required for optimizing the detection of tears.[18] A short TE results in reduced scan time, decreased flow, and susceptibility artifacts. The most commonly used sequences include spin echo, fast spin echo, gradient echo, and proton density with or without fat saturation.[19]

The 3T MR imaging now produces images of a higher resolution with thinner slices at a greater speed compared with 1.5T imaging, which is caused by the higher signal-to-noise ratio that can be achieved with the higher magnetic field.[20] Adjustments need to be made to ensure optimal tissue contrast because imaging at 3T increases the T1 relaxation time and shortens the T2 relaxation time.[21] Images are also more prone to susceptibility and chemical shift artifact.[21] The improved resolution and thinner slices allow more accurate and definitive diagnosis of meniscal tears compared with 1.5T imaging.[22] The use of 3T imaging also allows the application of fat suppression sequences, which improves perception of fine anatomic detail.[23]

A range of sensitivity and specificity of 3T MR in the detection of meniscal tears has been reported in the literature. Magee and Williams[22] reported a sensitivity and specificity of 96% and 97%, respectively, compared with arthroscopy. Sampson and colleagues[24] reported a sensitivity and specificity of 84% and 93%, respectively, compared with arthroscopy. Von Engelhardt and colleagues[25] reported a sensitivity and specificity of 79% and 95% for both menisci. The latter 2 studies both reported deceased sensitivity for the detection of meniscal tears in the lateral meniscus compared with the medial meniscus. Some of this may be caused by overinterpretation of the anterior horn variation described earlier.

The 3T imaging has also advanced the development of 3-dimensional (3D) imaging techniques. Isotropic voxels allow reconstructions in multiple planes with varying slice thickness. A more recent study by Ristow and colleagues[26] showed that 3D fast spin echo sequences had only minor limitations in diagnostic performance compared with standard 2D sequences; however, meniscal lesions were not well demonstrated.

PATHOLOGY

Pathologic changes within the meniscus include mucoid degeneration, meniscal tears and

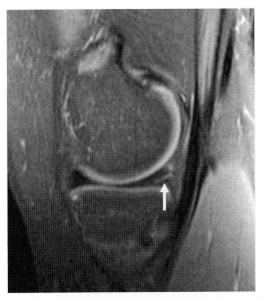

Fig. 8. Sagittal proton-density fat-saturated image of the lateral meniscus of an adolescent patient. Note the increased signal in the posterior third of the meniscus (*arrow*), which is a normal finding and can be mistaken for a tear.

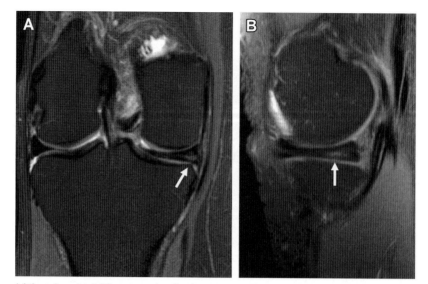

Fig. 9. Coronal (*A*) and sagittal (*B*) proton-density fat-saturated images demonstrating increased signal (*arrow*) within the body of the medial meniscus consistent with mucoid degeneration.

associated cysts, chondrocalcinosis, and ossification (meniscal stone). Meniscal tears may be simple or complex. Simple tears are divided into those with a vertical, horizontal, or radial orientation. Traumatic tears tend to be vertical in nature, whereas tears related to degenerative change tend to be horizontal.[27] Mixed patterns are termed complex tears, and these may be associated with displaced fragments.

Meniscal Degeneration

Meniscal degeneration results in increased signal intensity within the substance of the meniscus that does not reach the articular surface (**Fig. 9**).

Histologically, the high signal corresponds to areas of mucoid degeneration and eosinophilic degeneration within the meniscus.[28] Increased signal intensity can also be seen acutely following exercise.[29] In view of the variable causes and occasional transient nature of these nonspecific signal changes, overuse of the term *meniscal degeneration* is to be avoided and its use has little impact on patient management.

Meniscal Tears: Pathologic Appearances on MR Imaging

Simple meniscal tears

A simple meniscal tear is defined as linear increased signal intensity within a meniscus that

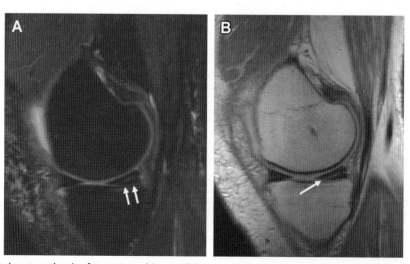

Fig. 10. Sagittal proton-density fat-saturated image (*A*) and sagittal proton-density image (*B*) depicting areas of abnormal signal (*arrows*) where it is difficult to determine whether the signal actually reaches the surface.

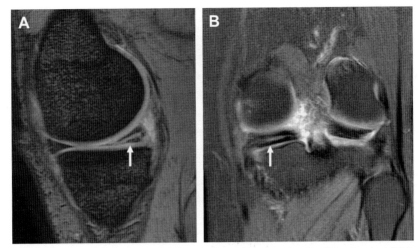

Fig. 11. Sagittal proton-density fat-saturated (*A*) and coronal proton-density fat-saturated (*B*) images demonstrate a horizontal cleavage tear in the posterior third of the medial meniscus (*arrows*).

reaches an articular surface. Meniscal grading[30] has been used in the past but is now largely obsolete. In up to 10% of cases, it can be difficult to determine whether the increased signal actually reaches the meniscal surface (**Fig. 10**).[31] It is important to appreciate that it is not always possible to be definitive, and equivocal situations do occur. The 2-slice-touch rule has been shown to increase the positive predictive value of diagnosing meniscal tears in the lateral meniscus with fewer false positives in the medial meniscus.[32] A meniscus is considered torn if there are 2 or more MR images with abnormal findings and possibly torn if there is only one image with an abnormal finding. Several indirect signs of meniscal tears, such as bone marrow edema, have also been described by Bergin and colleagues[33] that may improve diagnostic confidence; however, this study was limited by the lack of a control group. Improved resolution with 3T imaging should reduce the frequency of uncertainty.[22]

Types of simple tears

An accurate description of the meniscal tear is important because this will have a direct impact on management.[6] The description should include the site (which third), size, orientation (radial, vertical vs horizontal), and whether the tear is peripheral (red zone) or central (white zone) in location.[34]

Horizontal cleavage tears Horizontal tears run parallel to the tibial plateau, separating the meniscus into superior and inferior fragments.[35] These tears are commonly degenerate in nature.[27]

Horizontal tears appear as a line of increased signal intensity within the meniscus that usually

extends to the articular surface (**Fig. 11**). They may be asymptomatic in older individuals and can be associated with parameniscal cysts.

Radial tears Radial tears are oriented perpendicular to the long axis of the meniscus and perpendicular to the tibial plateau in the so-called z axis.[36] These tears disrupt the circumferential collagen bundles responsible for the generation of hoop stresses, which results in poor distribution of axial load.[6]

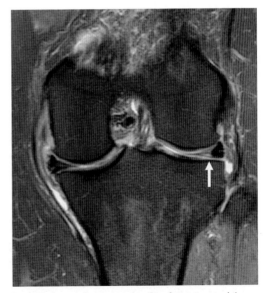

Fig. 12. Coronal proton-density fat-saturated image of a radial tear with a truncated inner meniscal margin in the middle third of a lateral meniscus (*arrow*).

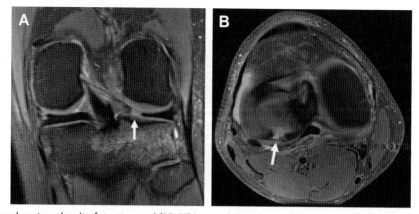

Fig. 13. Coronal proton-density fat-saturated (PD FS) image (*A*) and axial PD FS image (*B*) demonstrating the cleft sign of a radial tear with linear vertical high signal in the posterior third of the lateral meniscus (*arrow*).

Four signs have been described for the diagnosis of a radial tear[37]:

- Truncated triangle sign whereby there is an abrupt end to the normal triangular contour of the meniscus (**Fig. 12**)
- Cleft sign whereby the slice is perpendicular to the tear and a high signal line passes through the meniscus (**Fig. 13**)
- Marching cleft sign, similar to the cleft sign with the high signal line appearing to move position on sequential images
- Ghost meniscus whereby the slice is parallel to a complete radial tear and partial volume artifact creates an intermediate or gray signal (**Fig. 14**)

Two types of radial tears have characteristic appearances and merit specific mention. These tears are parrot-beak tears and radial tears of the meniscal root.

Parrot-beak tears Parrot-beak tears are radial tears that have a more oblique orientation than simple radial tears, running at an angle to the true perpendicular to the longitudinal axis of the meniscus, and producing the marching cleft sign on MR imaging (**Fig. 15**). Parrot-beak tears often result in a flap of unstable tissue[6]; even though the flap itself may be small, these tears can be relatively symptomatic. Fortunately, parrot-beak tears are relatively easy to treat with arthroscopic trimming.

Meniscal root tears The meniscal roots are the sites of attachment of the medial and lateral menisci to the central tibial plateau. Tears of the posterior meniscal roots can be easily overlooked on MR imaging and arthroscopically.[38,39] The characteristic sign is the ghost meniscus sign on sagittal images (**Fig. 16**); on coronal images, a cleft of high T2 signal is visualized between the posterior meniscus and distal PCL (see **Fig. 16**).

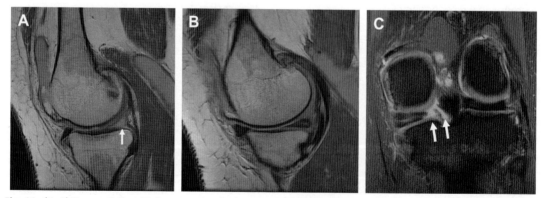

Fig. 14. (*A, B*) Sequential sagittal proton-density images: (*A*) The ghost meniscus sign (*arrow*) of a radial tear. The meniscus is normal on the adjacent slice (*B*). (*C*) The corresponding coronal proton-density fat-saturated image demonstrates a large radial tear of the posterior medial meniscal root (*arrows*).

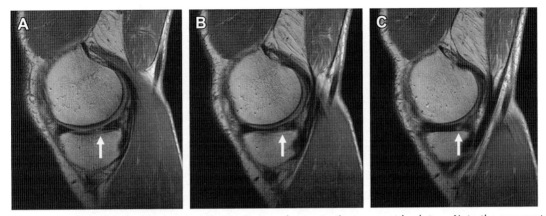

Fig. 15. (A–C) Sequential sagittal proton-density images demonstrating a parrot-beak tear. Note the apparent change in position of the high signal (arrows) consistent with the marching cleft sign.

Posterior root tears are important tears to document because they can result in extrusion of the meniscus and early development of osteoarthritis.[40] Extrusion of the meniscus also results in altered load bearing across the joint, increasing the risk of developing a subchondral insufficiency fracture, most commonly seen in the medial femoral condyle (Fig. 17).

Vertical tears Vertical tears are longitudinal tears that run parallel to the long axis of the meniscus and perpendicular to the tibial plateau.[6] A pure vertical tear runs at a constant distance to the margin of the meniscus. Oblique variants are also not uncommon and these too demonstrate a type of marching cleft sign. Vertical tears manifest as increased signal intensity within the meniscus (Fig. 18). If the tear is long enough, the inner fragment may become displaced, and these tears are easily missed.[6] Many vertical tears are located in the peripheral third of the meniscus, within the vascularized red zone. This finding is important and should be noted in the MR report, along with the length of the tear. Tears in the red zone may heal spontaneously or may be amenable to meniscal repair.

Meniscocapsular separation Vertical peripheral tears in the red zone behave differently to white-zone tears. Vertical tears that lie just outside the meniscus essentially behave like soft tissue injuries and can lead to meniscal instability. These injuries are also referred to as meniscocapsular separation, when the meniscus separates from the capsule. Meniscocapsular separation is more common medially and can occur at the coronary ligaments, the meniscocapsular junction, or within the peripheral portion of the meniscus.[41] Like red-zone tears, there is a stronger propensity to heal spontaneously. On the lateral side, meniscal tears

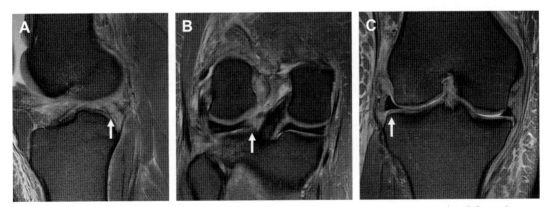

Fig. 16. Sagittal proton-density fat-saturated (PD FS) image (A) and coronal PD FS images (B, C) from the same patient demonstrating a lateral meniscal root tear and extrusion of the meniscus. Note the ghost sign (A) (arrow), cleft of high signal (B) (arrow), and meniscal extrusion (C) (arrow).

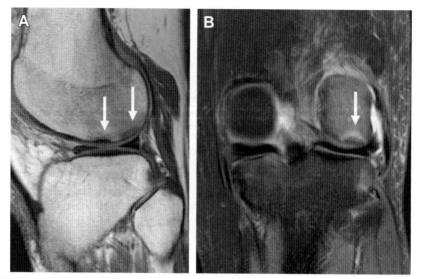

Fig. 17. Sagittal proton-density (PD) image (*A*) and coronal PD fat-saturated image (*B*) of the same patient demonstrate subchondral insufficiency fractures of the lateral femoral condyle (*arrows*), with associated bone marrow edema.

involve the posterolateral corner and the popliteomeniscal fascicles and can be difficult to diagnose.[42]

Signs of medial meniscocapsular separation include meniscal displacement relative to the tibia, fluid between the meniscus and capsule, a tear within the peripheral portion of the meniscus, and an irregular meniscal margin (**Fig. 19**).[41]

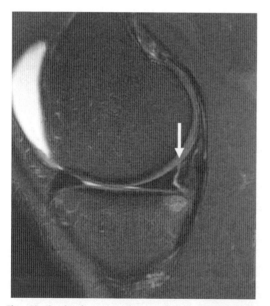

Fig. 18. Sagittal proton-density fat-saturated image demonstrating a peripheral vertical tear of the posterior third of the medial meniscus (*arrow*), with focal bone marrow edema in the adjacent medial tibial plateau.

Lateral signs of meniscocapsular separation include meniscal displacement relative to the tibia and disruption of the popliteomeniscal fascicles.[42]

Complex meniscal tears

Tears that have components in more than one plane or tears associated with displaced fragments are termed complex.[34] Complex tears with displaced fragments are among the most recognizable in knee MR imaging but are also among the most underdiagnosed. Complex tears result in abnormal morphology and may manifest as focal defects, irregular margins, or truncation of the meniscus.[6] The classic is the buckethandle tear, but a large number of variants also occur.

Bucket-handle tears A bucket-handle tear is a longitudinal tear whereby the inner fragment has become displaced. This fragment is most commonly found in the intercondylar notch.[43] Several signs have been described for the diagnosis of a bucket-handle tear, the first two being the most common[44]:

- Absent bow-tie sign: On sagittal images, the body of the meniscus is reminiscent of a bow tie and should be seen on at least 2 consecutive sagittal images, depending on the slice thickness and interslice gap. The meniscus is considered abnormal when the bow tie appears on only one image.
- Fragment in the notch sign: The meniscal fragment is displaced into the intercondylar notch adjacent to the tibial spine.

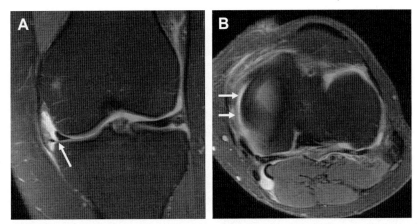

Fig. 19. Coronal proton-density fat-saturated (PS FS) image (*A*) and axial PD FS (*B*) demonstrating fluid between the medial meniscus and joint capsule (*arrows*) consistent with meniscocapsular separation.

- Double PCL sign: The fragment is displaced and lies anterior and parallel to the PCL (**Fig. 20**).
- Truncated meniscus: There is a loss of the normal triangular contour.

Other signs of flap tears

- Double anterior horn or flipped meniscal sign: The displaced posterior meniscal fragment lies adjacent to the anterior horn (**Fig. 21**).
- Disproportionate posterior horn sign: The posterior displaced meniscal fragment flips medially to lie adjacent to the meniscal root, which gives the appearance of an enlarged posterior meniscus adjacent to the meniscal attachment compared with the more peripheral portion of the meniscus, which seems disproportionately small.

- Flipped medial meniscus: The meniscal fragment flips into the adjacent synovial recess (see below).
- Floating meniscus: The meniscus is avulsed from the tibia and is completely surrounded by joint fluid.

Flipped medial meniscus A flipped medial meniscus is a horizontal tear of the medial meniscus in which the inferior fragment of the meniscus flips into the adjacent synovial recess, usually deep to the MCL (**Fig. 22**).[45] This diagnosis should be considered when the meniscus seems thinner than normal or seems to have a fragment missing. It is important to document the displaced fragment because these can be easily missed at surgery with a resultant poor outcome.[46] Unstable meniscal tears are also more prone to cause hyaline cartilage damage when compared with horizontal cleavage tears.[47]

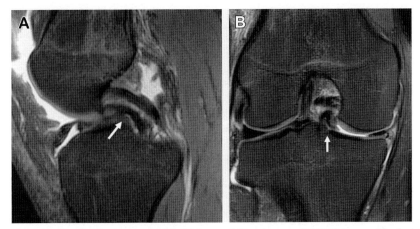

Fig. 20. Sagittal proton-density fat-saturated (PD FS) image (*A*) and coronal PDS FS image (*B*) of a bucket-handle tear in the same patient, with the displaced fragment lying adjacent to the PCL and forming the double-PCL sign (*arrows*).

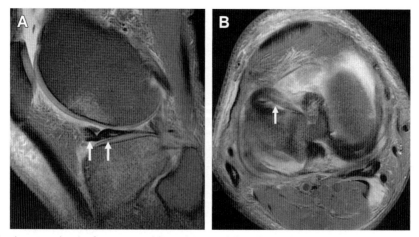

Fig. 21. Sagittal proton-density fat-saturated (PD FS) image (*A*) and axial PD FS image (*B*) of a bucket-handle tear demonstrating the double anterior horn sign (*arrows*).

Discoid meniscal tears As previously described, the discoid meniscus is a developmental variant in which the meniscus has a thickened disklike shape. Because of their abnormal shape, discoid menisci are more prone to tears compared with normal menisci (**Fig. 23**).[48] Multiple tears within the same meniscus are not uncommon, and the tear type is related to the type of discoid meniscus. Complete discoid menisci tend to develop simple horizontal tears, whereas partial develop radial, degenerate, and complex tears.[49]

Meniscal Cysts

Meniscal cysts arise from within (intrameniscal) or adjacent (parameniscal) to the meniscus and are commonly but not always associated with a meniscal tear.[50] There are numerous theories as to the cause of meniscal cysts. One widely held belief is that synovial fluid is extruded through a meniscal tear (**Fig. 24**).[51] In the absence of a tear, meniscal cyst formation may be caused by cystic degeneration.[51]

Intrameniscal cysts appear as increased signal within an enlarged meniscus. Parameniscal cysts appear as lobulated lesions with increased signal adjacent to the meniscus.[50] Parameniscal cysts may also extend along tissue planes. Medial cysts may extend anteriorly to lie superficial to the MCL (**Fig. 25**). Lateral cysts may extent anteriorly to lie deep to the iliotibial band and posterolaterally to lie deep to the LCL.[52]

Anterior third meniscal cysts may be difficult to differentiate from other cysts that occur in the

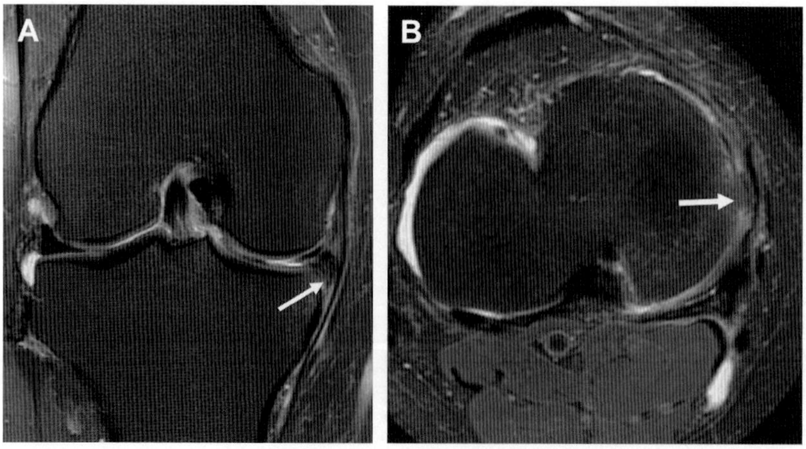

Fig. 22. Coronal proton-density fat-saturated (PD FS) image (*A*) and axial PD FS image (*B*) showing a horizontal tear of the middle third of the medial meniscus with a fragment of the meniscus that has displaced into the medial gutter (*arrow*).

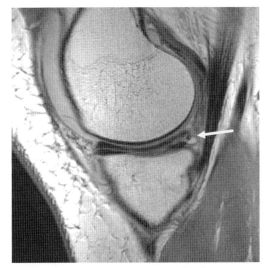

Fig. 23. Sagittal proton-density image of a discoid medial meniscus with a horizontal cleavage tear and parameniscal cyst (*arrow*).

anterior joint space. Ganglion cysts arising from the ACL and less often the anterior intermeniscal ligament may also extend into Hoffa fat pad.[53,54]

Chondrocalcinosis

Chondrocalcinosis is caused by calcium salt deposition in the meniscus, which can result in increased signal intensity on T1-weighted, proton density, and inversion recovery sequences (**Fig. 26**).[55] The sensitivity and specificity of diagnosing meniscal tears is reduced because the high signal caused by chondrocalcinosis can simulate or mask a meniscal tear.[55]

Ossification (Meniscal Stone)

Meniscal ossicles are rare intrameniscal bone fragments that are most commonly seen in the posterior

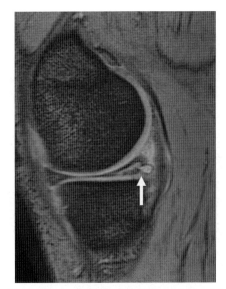

Fig. 24. Sagittal gradient echo of the posterior third of a medial meniscus demonstrating a parameniscal cyst (*arrow*) arising from a horizontal tear of the meniscus.

third of the medial meniscus.[56] They consist of corticated bone marrow covered by synovial cartilage and demonstrate high signal on T1 and proton-density sequences, and low signal on T2 (**Fig. 27**). It is important to differentiate meniscal ossicles from loose bodies because this will affect management.[57]

Pitfalls

Although MR imaging is accurate in the diagnosis of meniscal injury, there are several pitfalls that can lead to a false-positive diagnosis of a meniscal tear.

False positive caused by abnormal signal

- Magic angle phenomenon: This phenomenon is increased signal intensity in the

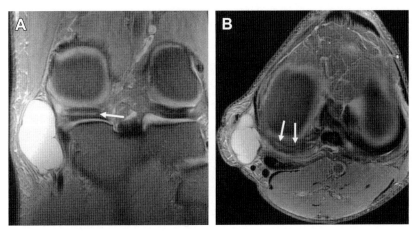

Fig. 25. Coronal proton-density fat-saturated (PD FS) image (*A*) and axial PD FS image (*B*) of a posterior medial meniscal tear (*arrows*) and a large meniscal cyst that lies superficial to the medial capsule.

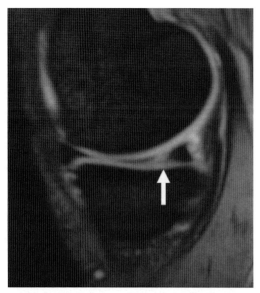

Fig. 26. Sagittal proton-density fat-saturated image demonstrating increased signal (*arrow*) within the posterior third of the medial meniscus consistent with chondrocalcinosis of the meniscus.

inner portion of the posterior third of the lateral meniscus caused by its up sloping orientation.[58]

- Speckled anterior horn lateral meniscus: This variant is a normal variant whereby the fibers of the ACL inserting into the meniscus simulate a torn meniscus (**Fig. 7**).[16]
- Edge artifact: A horizontal line of increased signal intensity can be seen on the most peripheral sagittal image because of the concave outer margin of the meniscus.[59]
- Chondrocalcinosis: Susceptibility artifact caused by calcium deposition may mimic or conceal a meniscal tear.[55]

- Pulsation artifact from popliteal artery: Pulsation artifact from the popliteal artery can extend through the posterior horn of the lateral meniscus mimicking a tear.[6]

False positive caused by anatomic variation

- Transverse (anterior) ligament: The attachment of this ligament to the meniscus may mimic a meniscal tear (**Fig. 28**).[59]
- Meniscofemoral ligaments: The attachment of the ligaments of Humphrey and Wrisberg to the posterior third of the lateral meniscus may mimic a tear.[60]
- Meniscomeniscal ligaments: The attachments of the ligaments to the menisci may mimic a tear.[10]
- Popliteus tendon: The popliteus tendon passes between the posterior horn of the lateral meniscus and the capsule, which gives the appearance of a vertical tear within the meniscus (**Fig. 29**).[59]

POSTOPERATIVE IMAGING

There is a well-established correlation between the amount of meniscal tissue removed and the onset of osteoarthritis,[61,62] so the emphasis is now placed on meniscal preserving surgery.

Partial Meniscectomy

In a partial meniscectomy, the surgeon attempts to preserve the outer third of the meniscus because this is the predominant load-bearing surface.[63] A circumferential meniscectomy involves a resection of the inner aspect of the meniscus (**Fig. 30**). A segmental resection involves a focal resection of almost the complete width of the meniscus with the loss of a portion of the outer third.[64]

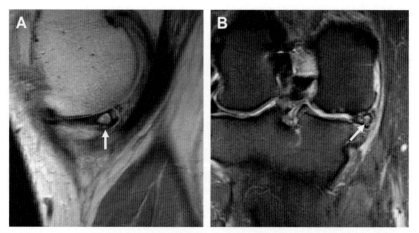

Fig. 27. Sagittal proton-density (PD) image (*A*) and coronal PD fat-saturated image (*B*) through the body of the medial meniscus. There is an area of high signal within the meniscus in keeping with an intrameniscal ossicle (*arrow*).

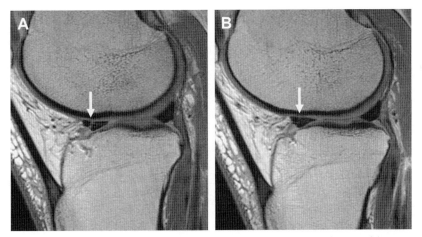

Fig. 28. (*A, B*) Sequential sagittal proton-density images showing the transverse (anterior) ligament arising from the anterior horn of the lateral meniscus mimicking a tear (*arrow*).

Stable horizontal tears can be treated conservatively. Unstable tears can be treated with partial resection of the unstable portion only, which leaves a residual tear evident on MR imaging.[65]

Meniscal Repair

A meniscal repair of a tear is ideally performed when (1) the tear is within the peripheral or red zone of the meniscus, (2) the tear is longitudinal in orientation, and (3) is greater than 1 cm in

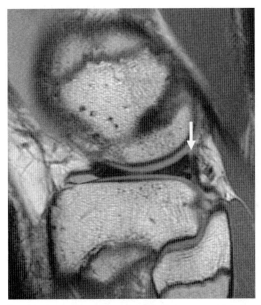

Fig. 29. Sagittal proton-density fat-saturated image of the posterior third of a lateral meniscus. High signal is noted (*arrow*) between the meniscus and the popliteus tendon, which can be mistaken for a meniscal tear.

length.[66] The fragments can be fixed using a variety of sutures, bioabsorbable arrows, tacks, and darts. Healing of the meniscus takes approximately 4 months (**Fig. 31**). Healed or partially healed repairs are usually asymptomatic, whereas failed repairs are usually symptomatic.[65]

Meniscal tears that are less than 1 cm in length and are within the peripheral or red zone of the meniscus have been shown to heal spontaneously[67]

Meniscal Transplantation

Meniscal transplantation can be performed with allograft or collagen-based meniscal replacement. The technique is usually reserved for young patients who have symptomatic irreparable tears or who have undergone previous meniscectomy.[65] The anterior and posterior meniscal anchors are fixed using bone plugs and sutures with the margin of the meniscus sutured to the capsule. This procedure can be performed arthroscopically or as an open procedure.[68]

Imaging of Postoperative Menisci

The role of imaging of the postoperative knee is to assess the stability or recurrence of a tear on the meniscal remnant, identify tears in another area of the meniscus, and identify other causes of postoperative knee pain. Various imaging options are available.

Conventional MR imaging

The sequences used with conventional MR in the evaluation of the postoperative meniscus are broadly similar to those applied to preoperative knees.[69] As previously discussed, 3T scanning provides higher resolution at thinner slices, which

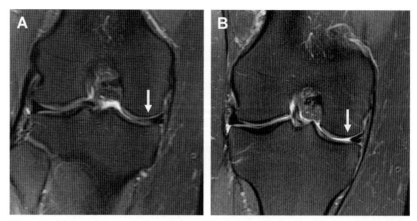

Fig. 30. Coronal proton-density fat-saturated preoperative (*A*) and postoperative (*B*) imaging of the middle third of the medial meniscus. (*A*) A meniscal tear (*arrow*) and (*B*) the truncated appearance (*arrow*) following a partial circumferential meniscectomy of less than 25%.

is an advantage in postoperative imaging. However, images are more prone to susceptibility and chemical shift artifact.[21]

Indirect MR arthrography
Indirect MR arthrography involves intravenous injection of contrast with subsequent synovial excretion of contrast. Imaging is then performed 10 to 20 minutes after injection and following exercise of the joint.[65]

Direct MR arthrography
Direct MR arthrography involves an injection of gadolinium contrast into the joint. This technique has 3 advantages over conventional MR: (1) distension of the joint making fluid more likely to extend into

a tear, (2) the lower viscosity of gadolinium compared with synovial fluid making it more likely extend into a tear, and (3) the higher signal-to-noise ratio of T1-weighted images.[70]

Computed tomography arthrography
Computed tomography (CT) arthrography involves an injection of iodine contrast into the joint. Imaging is then performed 10 to 20 minutes after injection and following exercise of the joint.[65]

Pathologic Appearances on MR Imaging

Assessment of postoperative menisci on MR imaging is difficult. The most important aid to diagnosis is a clear understanding of the nature and location of the surgery performed. Unfortunately,

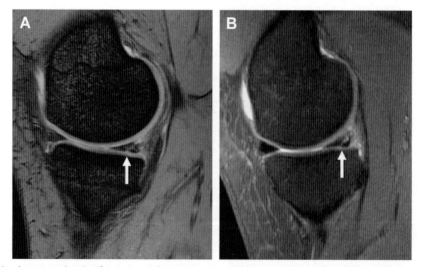

Fig. 31. Sagittal proton-density fat-saturated preoperative (*A*) and postoperative (*B*) imaging of the posterior third of the medial meniscus. (*A*) A peripheral tear (*arrow*). (*B*) Image obtained 4 months after meniscal repair. Note the persistent high signal within the postoperative meniscus (*arrow*), which was a normal postoperative appearance.

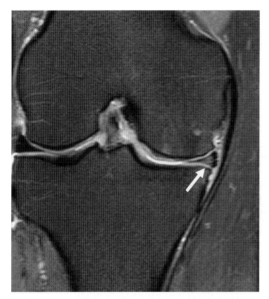

Fig. 32. Coronal proton-density fat-saturated image of the middle third of the medial meniscus that shows increased signal (*arrow*) in the meniscus but no recurrent tear.

this information is not always available. Comparison with previous preoperative imaging can also help locate the previous tear because the standard criteria of abnormal signal and abnormal morphology can be applied to the diagnosis of tears distant from the surgical site.

Postoperative menisci may have increased signal intensity because of preexisting meniscal degenerative change or healing of the meniscus, which can mimic a tear. Increased signal may persist for up to 1 year following a successful meniscal repair or meniscal healing (**Fig. 32**).[71] The morphology of the postoperative meniscus will also be altered depending on the procedure performed and the appearance of the initial tear.[71]

In conventional MR imaging, the criteria of abnormal signal and morphology still apply but are less accurate for meniscal tears at the site of surgery compared with the preoperative knee. Useful signs suggestive of a retear are frank fluid within the line extending to the meniscal surface, a displaced meniscal fragment, or a definite change in configuration compared with the previous tear (**Fig. 33**).[72,73] The appearance (or failure to resolve) of a meniscal cyst is also a feature suspicious of an active tear. Conventional MR imaging has a reported accuracy of up to 90% in patients who have undergone a meniscal resection of less than 25%.[74] Accuracy decreases as the amount of meniscus resected increases.[69]

Arthrography is helpful in patients who have had a meniscal repair and those with more than 25% of the meniscus resected in the absence of osteoarthritis, chondral injury, and osteonecrosis.[75] A recurrent tear at the surgical site is diagnosed by visualizing extension of contrast into the substance of the meniscus.[75] The contrast between iodinated contrast and the meniscus on CT is greater than intra-articular gadolinium and the meniscus on MR imaging. Consequently, CT arthrography is used by the authors in preference (**Fig. 34**).

MR imaging following meniscal transplantation can provide information about the status of the graft and the capsular attachment. However, there is poor correlation between MR imaging and clinical findings.[76]

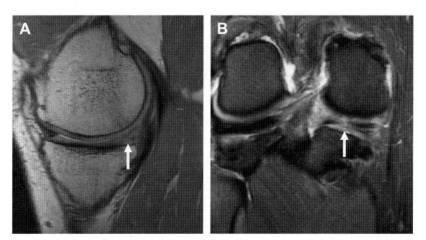

Fig. 33. Sagittal proton-density (PD) image (*A*) and coronal PD fat-saturated image (*B*), which demonstrates increased signal (*arrow*) within the posterior third of the meniscus in keeping with a new radial tear of a postoperative meniscus.

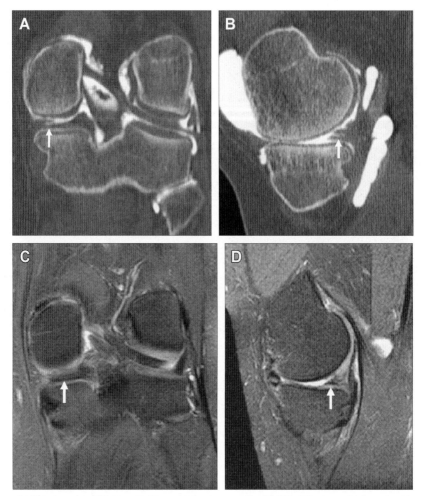

Fig. 34. Coronal (*A*) and sagittal (*B*) images from a CT arthrography (CTA) with coronal (*C*) and sagittal (*D*) proton-density fat-saturated images from MR imaging of the same patient obtained following meniscal repair. On the CTA images, note the contrast in the repaired meniscus (*arrow*) consistent with a new tear. This tear cannot be identified on the MR images (*arrows* indicating the position of the tear).

SUMMARY

The aim of any radiologist is to provide an accurate report to assist the clinicians in instituting the correct patient management. Although conventional MR imaging is well established in diagnosing meniscal pathologic conditions in the nonoperative knee, the diagnosis of postoperative meniscal pathologic conditions presents more of a challenge. Accurate reporting in both scenarios requires an understanding of the basic anatomy, pathology, diagnostic pitfalls, and surgical procedures involved with meniscal pathologic conditions.

ACKNOWLEDGMENTS

Thank you to Dr Kathryn Stevens for providing some of the images included in this review article.

REFERENCES

1. Bessette GC. The meniscus. Orthopedics 1992; 15(1):35–42.
2. Fithian DC, Kelly MA, Mow VC. Material properties and structure-function relationships in the menisci. Clin Orthop Relat Res 1990;(252):19–31.
3. Rath E, Richmond JC. The menisci: basic science and advances in treatment. Br J Sports Med 2000; 34(4):252–7.
4. Brody JM, Hulstyn MJ, Fleming BC, et al. The meniscal roots: gross anatomic correlation with 3-T MRI findings. AJR Am J Roentgenol 2007;188(5):W446–50.
5. Arnoczky SP, Warren RF. Microvasculature of the human meniscus. Am J Sports Med 1982;10(2): 90–5.
6. Anderson MW. MR imaging of the meniscus. Radiol Clin North Am 2002;40(5):1081–94.

7. Lee BY, Jee WH, Kim JM, et al. Incidence and significance of demonstrating the meniscofemoral ligament on MRI. Br J Radiol 2000;73(867):271–4.

8. de Abreu MR, Chung CB, Trudell D, et al. Anterior transverse ligament of the knee: MR imaging and anatomic study using clinical and cadaveric material with emphasis on its contribution to meniscal tears. Clin Imaging 2007;31(3):194–201.

9. Muhle C, Thompson WO, Sciulli R, et al. Transverse ligament and its effect on meniscal motion. Correlation of kinematic MR imaging and anatomic sections. Invest Radiol 1999;34(9):558–65.

10. Sanders TG, Linares RC, Lawhorn KW, et al. Oblique meniscomeniscal ligament: another potential pitfall for a meniscal tear–anatomic description and appearance at MR imaging in three cases. Radiology 1999; 213(1):213–6.

11. Samoto N, Kozuma M, Tokuhisa T, et al. Diagnosis of discoid lateral meniscus of the knee on MR imaging. Magn Reson Imaging 2002;20(1):59–64.

12. Kim YG, Ihn JC, Park SK, et al. An arthroscopic analysis of lateral meniscal variants and a comparison with MRI findings. Knee Surg Sports Traumatol Arthrosc 2006;14(1):20–6.

13. Singh K, Helms CA, Jacobs MT, et al. MRI appearance of Wrisberg variant of discoid lateral meniscus. AJR Am J Roentgenol 2006;187(2):384–7.

14. Kim BH, Seol HY, Jung HS, et al. Meniscal flounce on MR: correlation with arthroscopic or surgical findings. Yonsei Med J 2000;41(4):507–11.

15. Park JS, Ryu KN, Yoon KH. Meniscal flounce on knee MRI: correlation with meniscal locations after positional changes. AJR Am J Roentgenol 2006; 187(2):364–70.

16. Shankman S, Beltran J, Melamed E, et al. Anterior horn of the lateral meniscus: another potential pitfall in MR imaging of the knee. Radiology 1997;204(1): 181–4.

17. Takeda Y, Ikata T, Yoshida S, et al. MRI high-signal intensity in the menisci of asymptomatic children. J Bone Joint Surg Br 1998;80(3):463–7.

18. Rubin DA, Paletta GA Jr. Current concepts and controversies in meniscal imaging. Magn Reson Imaging Clin N Am 2000;8(2):243–70.

19. Helms CA. The meniscus: recent advances in MR imaging of the knee. AJR Am J Roentgenol 2002; 179(5):1115–22.

20. Gold GE, Han E, Stainsby J, et al. Musculoskeletal MRI at 3.0 T: relaxation times and image contrast. AJR Am J Roentgenol 2004;183(2):343–51.

21. Gold GE, Suh B, Sawyer-Glover A, et al. Musculoskeletal MRI at 3.0 T: initial clinical experience. AJR Am J Roentgenol 2004;183(5):1479–86.

22. Magee T, Williams D. 3.0-T MRI of meniscal tears. AJR Am J Roentgenol 2006;187(2):371–5.

23. Lee SY, Jee WH, Kim SK, et al. Proton density-weighted MR imaging of the knee: fat suppression versus without fat suppression. Skeletal Radiol 2011;40(2):189–95.

24. Sampson MJ, Jackson MP, Moran CJ, et al. Three Tesla MRI for the diagnosis of meniscal and anterior cruciate ligament pathology: a comparison to arthroscopic findings. Clin Radiol 2008;63(10):1106–11.

25. von Engelhardt LV, Schmitz A, Pennekamp PH, et al. Diagnostics of degenerative meniscal tears at 3-Tesla MRI compared to arthroscopy as reference standard. Arch Orthop Trauma Surg 2008;128(5):451–6.

26. Ristow O, Steinbach L, Sabo G, et al. Isotropic 3D fast spin-echo imaging versus standard 2D imaging at 3.0 T of the knee–image quality and diagnostic performance. Eur Radiol 2009;19(5):1263–72.

27. Hough AJ Jr, Webber RJ. Pathology of the meniscus. Clin Orthop Relat Res 1990;(252):32–40.

28. Hodler J, Haghighi P, Pathria MN, et al. Meniscal changes in the elderly: correlation of MR imaging and histologic findings. Radiology 1992;184(1): 221–5.

29. Kursunoglu-Brahme S, Schwaighofer B, Gundry C, et al. Jogging causes acute changes in the knee joint: an MR study in normal volunteers. AJR Am J Roentgenol 1990;154(6):1233–5.

30. Stoller DW, Martin C, Crues JV 3rd, et al. Meniscal tears: pathologic correlation with MR imaging. Radiology 1987;163(3):731–5.

31. Helms CA, Major NM, Anderson MW, et al. Musculoskeletal MRI. 2nd edition. Philadelphia: Saunders Elsevier; 2009.

32. De Smet AA, Tuite MJ. Use of the "two-slice-touch" rule for the MRI diagnosis of meniscal tears. AJR Am J Roentgenol 2006;187(4):911–4.

33. Bergin D, Hochberg H, Zoga AC, et al. Indirect soft-tissue and osseous signs on knee MRI of surgically proven meniscal tears. AJR Am J Roentgenol 2008; 191(1):86–92.

34. Fox MG. MR imaging of the meniscus: review, current trends, and clinical implications. Radiol Clin North Am 2007;45(6):1033–53, vii.

35. Jee WH, McCauley TR, Kim JM, et al. Meniscal tear configurations: categorization with MR imaging. AJR Am J Roentgenol 2003;180(1):93–7.

36. Magee T, Shapiro M, Williams D. MR accuracy and arthroscopic incidence of meniscal radial tears. Skeletal Radiol 2002;31(12):686–9.

37. Harper KW, Helms CA, Lambert HS 3rd, et al. Radial meniscal tears: significance, incidence, and MR appearance. AJR Am J Roentgenol 2005;185(6): 1429–34.

38. Jones AO, Houang MT, Low RS, et al. Medial meniscus posterior root attachment injury and degeneration: MRI findings. Australas Radiol 2006; 50(4):306–13.

39. Lee SY, Jee WH, Kim JM. Radial tear of the medial meniscal root: reliability and accuracy of MRI for diagnosis. AJR Am J Roentgenol 2008;191(1):81–5.

40. Lerer DB, Umans HR, Hu MX, et al. The role of meniscal root pathology and radial meniscal tear in medial meniscal extrusion. Skeletal Radiol 2004; 33(10):569–74.

41. De Maeseneer M, Shahabpour M, Vanderdood K, et al. Medial meniscocapsular separation: MR imaging criteria and diagnostic pitfalls. Eur J Radiol 2002;41(3):242–52.

42. LaPrade RF, Konowalchuk BK. Popliteomeniscal fascicle tears causing symptomatic lateral compartment knee pain: diagnosis by the figure-4 test and treatment by open repair. Am J Sports Med 2005; 33(8):1231–6.

43. Magee TH, Hinson GW. MRI of meniscal bucket-handle tears. Skeletal Radiol 1998;27(9):495–9.

44. Aydingoz U, Firat AK, Atay OA, et al. MR imaging of meniscal bucket-handle tears: a review of signs and their relation to arthroscopic classification. Eur Radiol 2003;13(3):618–25.

45. Lecas LK, Helms CA, Kosarek FJ, et al. Inferiorly displaced flap tears of the medial meniscus: MR appearance and clinical significance. AJR Am J Roentgenol 2000;174(1):161–4.

46. Vande Berg BC, Malghem J, Poilvache P, et al. Meniscal tears with fragments displaced in notch and recesses of knee: MR imaging with arthroscopic comparison. Radiology 2005;234(3):842–50.

47. Zamber RW, Teitz CC, McGuire DA, et al. Articular cartilage lesions of the knee. Arthroscopy 1989; 5(4):258–68.

48. Rohren EM, Kosarek FJ, Helms CA. Discoid lateral meniscus and the frequency of meniscal tears. Skeletal Radiol 2001;30(6):316–20.

49. Bin SI, Kim JC, Kim JM, et al. Correlation between type of discoid lateral menisci and tear pattern. Knee Surg Sports Traumatol Arthrosc 2002;10(4):218–22.

50. Anderson JJ, Connor GF, Helms CA. New observations on meniscal cysts. Skeletal Radiol 2010; 39(12):1187–91.

51. Campbell SE, Sanders TG, Morrison WB. MR imaging of meniscal cysts: incidence, location, and clinical significance. AJR Am J Roentgenol 2001; 177(2):409–13.

52. De Maeseneer M, Shahabpour M, Vanderdood K, et al. MR imaging of meniscal cysts: evaluation of location and extension using a three-layer approach. Eur J Radiol 2001;39(2):117–24.

53. Saddik D, McNally EG, Richardson M. MRI of Hoffa's fat pad. Skeletal Radiol 2004;33(8):433–44.

54. Lektrakul N, Skaf A, Yeh L, et al. Pericruciate meniscal cysts arising from tears of the posterior horn of the medial meniscus: MR imaging features that simulate posterior cruciate ganglion cysts. AJR Am J Roentgenol 1999;172(6):1575–9.

55. Kaushik S, Erickson JK, Palmer WE, et al. Effect of chondrocalcinosis on the MR imaging of knee menisci. AJR Am J Roentgenol 2001;177(4):905–9.

56. Schnarkowski P, Tirman PF, Fuchigami KD, et al. Meniscal ossicle: radiographic and MR imaging findings. Radiology 1995;196(1):47–50.

57. Tyler P, Datir A, Saifuddin A. Magnetic resonance imaging of anatomical variations in the knee. Part 2: miscellaneous. Skeletal Radiol 2010;39(12): 1175–86.

58. Peterfy CG, Janzen DL, Tirman PF, et al. "Magic-angle" phenomenon: a cause of increased signal in the normal lateral meniscus on short-TE MR images of the knee. AJR Am J Roentgenol 1994; 163(1):149–54.

59. Herman LJ, Beltran J. Pitfalls in MR imaging of the knee. Radiology 1988;167(3):775–81.

60. Vahey TN, Bennett HT, Arrington LE, et al. MR imaging of the knee: pseudotear of the lateral meniscus caused by the meniscofemoral ligament. AJR Am J Roentgenol 1990;154(6):1237–9.

61. Henning CE, Lynch MA. Current concepts of meniscal function and pathology. Clin Sports Med 1985; 4(2):259–65.

62. Steenbrugge F, Verdonk R, Verstraete K. Long-term assessment of arthroscopic meniscus repair: a 13-year follow-up study. Knee 2002;9(3):181–7.

63. Radin EL, de Lamotte F, Maquet P. Role of the menisci in the distribution of stress in the knee. Clin Orthop Relat Res 1984;(185):290–4.

64. Newman AP, Daniels AU, Burks RT. Principles and decision making in meniscal surgery. Arthroscopy 1993;9(1):33–51.

65. Toms AP, White LM, Marshall TJ, et al. Imaging the post-operative meniscus. Eur J Radiol 2005;54(2): 189–98.

66. DeHaven KE. Decision-making factors in the treatment of meniscus lesions. Clin Orthop Relat Res 1990;(252):49–54.

67. Weiss CB, Lundberg M, Hamberg P, et al. Non-operative treatment of meniscal tears. J Bone Joint Surg Am 1989;71(6):811–22.

68. Sgaglione NA, Steadman JR, Shaffer B, et al. Current concepts in meniscus surgery: resection to replacement. Arthroscopy 2003;19(Suppl 1): 161–88.

69. Recht MP, Kramer J. MR imaging of the postoperative knee: a pictorial essay. Radiographics 2002; 22(4):765–74.

70. Sciulli RL, Boutin RD, Brown RR, et al. Evaluation of the postoperative meniscus of the knee: a study comparing conventional arthrography, conventional MR imaging, MR arthrography with iodinated contrast material, and MR arthrography with gadolinium-based contrast material. Skeletal Radiol 1999;28(9): 508–14.

71. White LM, Kramer J, Recht MP. MR imaging evaluation of the postoperative knee: ligaments, menisci, and articular cartilage. Skeletal Radiol 2005;34(8): 431–52.

72. McCauley TR. MR imaging evaluation of the postoperative knee. Radiology 2005;234(1):53–61.
73. Lim PS, Schweitzer ME, Bhatia M, et al. Repeat tear of postoperative meniscus: potential MR imaging signs. Radiology 1999;210(1):183–8.
74. Applegate GR, Flannigan BD, Tolin BS, et al. MR diagnosis of recurrent tears in the knee: value of intraarticular contrast material. AJR Am J Roentgenol 1993;161(4):821–5.
75. Magee T, Shapiro M, Rodriguez J, et al. MR arthrography of postoperative knee: for which patients is it useful? Radiology 2003;229(1): 159–63.
76. Verdonk PC, Verstraete KL, Almqvist KF, et al. Meniscal allograft transplantation: long-term clinical results with radiological and magnetic resonance imaging correlations. Knee Surg Sports Traumatol Arthrosc 2006;14(8):694–706.

The Extensor Mechanism of the Knee

Simon Ostlere, FRCR

KEYWORDS

- Knee extensor mechanism • Anterior knee pain • Patellofemoral instability
- Magnetic resonance imaging • Ultrasound

KEY POINTS

- Anterior knee pain is an exceedingly common symptom that is usually managed conservatively without resorting to imaging. Imaging is helpful in a minority of cases with persistent or atypical symptoms.
- Focal symptoms related to the patellar or quadriceps tendon can be adequately assessed on ultrasound. Percutaneous therapies for tendinosis can be performed under ultrasound guidance.
- Static and dynamic MR imaging can be used to assess the degree of patellofemoral dysplasia and subluxation in patients with suspected patellofemoral instability.
- Radiographs, occasionally supplemented by CT, are usually adequate for imaging fractures. MR imaging is often performed in cases of patellar dislocation and when osteochondral fractures are suspected.

INTRODUCTION

The extensor mechanism of the knee consists of the extensor muscles, the quadriceps tendon, the patellofemoral joint, the patellar tendon, and the tibial tubercle. Patients with disorders of the extensor mechanism can present following an acute traumatic event or with persistent anterior knee pain. In many cases a confident diagnosis can be made on clinical grounds. Imaging is generally reserved for cases where symptoms are relatively nonspecific, when symptoms do not improve, or when surgery is being considered. Achieving a specific diagnosis in the younger patient may be elusive, because anterior knee pain without any identifiable pathology is common. The principle acute traumatic lesions are patellar fracture or dislocation, tibial tubercle fracture, and quadriceps or patellar tendon rupture. Extensor mechanism pathology resulting in more chronic symptoms can be broadly divided into tendinopathy, articular surface lesions, and patellofemoral maltracking.

Radiographs, MR imaging, and ultrasound are the main imaging techniques used for assessing the extensor mechanism. Radiographs are the mainstay in acute trauma, although MR imaging is useful for diagnosing acute patellar dislocation. Ultrasound is the optimum method for diagnosing isolated tendon abnormalities. In the older age group, pain related to the patellofemoral joint is usually due to osteoarthritis, which can be diagnosed on radiographs. Static and dynamic MR imaging is often used for an assessment of symptoms related to the patellofemoral joint in the younger age group, particularly in patients with suspected patellofemoral dysplasia and instability.

ANATOMY

The extensor mechanism of the knee consists of the quadriceps tendon and its associated muscles, the patellofemoral joint, the patellar tendon, and the tibial tubercle. The quadriceps tendon is formed by the confluence of tendons

Department of Radiology, Nuffield Orthopaedic Centre, Oxford University Hospitals, Windmill Road, Oxford OX3 7LD, UK
E-mail address: simon.ostlere@ouh.nhs.uk

Radiol Clin N Am 51 (2013) 393–411
http://dx.doi.org/10.1016/j.rcl.2012.11.006
0033-8389/13/$ – see front matter © 2013 Elsevier Inc. All rights reserved.

from the 3 vastus muscles and the rectus femoris. The distal end of vastus medialis muscle inserts on the medial side of the quadriceps tendon and lies close to the superior pole of the patella. The patella is a sesamoid bone lying within the quadriceps/patellar tendon and has 2 main articular facets, usually a substantial lateral facet and a smaller, more sagittally orientated, medial facet. The patella narrows inferiorly to form the inferior pole of the patella. The patella is supported by complex medial and lateral retinacula. The medial retinaculum includes the medial patellofemoral ligament, the most important stabilizer of the patella, which arises from the medial margin of the patella and inserts into the medial femoral epicondyle.[1] The patella articulates with the trochlear of the distal femur, and the proximal portion of the trochlear is where the groove is shallowest. With the knee in the flexed position, the patella articulates with the distal and deeper part of the trochlear groove. In extension the patella articulates with the shallower proximal portion of the trochlear. Instability of the patellofemoral joint therefore occurs when the knee is approaching full extension. There are synovial recesses both medially and laterally. These recesses lie deep to the retinacula and communicate with the suprapatellar pouch, which itself lies deep to the quadriceps tendon. The patellar tendon is a straplike structure extending from the inferior margin of the patella to the tibial tubercle and is 5 times wider than it is thick. The relative lateral position of the tibial tubercle means the patellar tendon has an oblique orientation in the coronal plane. The degree of angulation of the tendon in the coronal plane is an important factor in patellofemoral maltracking. The relative position of the tubercle can be estimated clinically, as the angle between a line drawn from the anterosuperior iliac spine to the center of the patella and a line from the center of the patella to the tibial tubercle, forming the so-called Q angle. The normal angle is quoted as being between 15° and 20°. As a measure of potential patellofemoral instability, the Q angle has the disadvantage of being dependant on the patellar position, so that paradoxically the more medial the patella is positioned the greater the Q angle.[2] Lying immediately deep to the patellar tendon is Hoffa's fat pad, usually referred to as the infrapatellar fat pad in orthopedic literature. The 3 bursae related to the extensor mechanism are the prepatellar bursa overlying the patella, the superficial infrapatellar bursa lying superficial to the distal half of the patellar tendon, and the deep infrapatellar bursa interposed between the distal patellar tendon and tibial tubercle.

IMAGING TECHNIQUES

Radiographs, MR imaging, and ultrasound are the main techniques used for assessing patients with pathologic related to the extensor mechanism. Radiographs are inevitably performed in acute trauma, but their value in chronic anterior knee pain is limited. MR imaging may be useful in some cases of acute trauma, particularly when radiographs are negative. The method used for imaging patients with chronic anterior knee pain varies according to local preferences and expertise. If simple confirmation of a suspected soft tissue problem, such as proximal patellar tendinosis, is required, then ultrasound is appropriate. MR imaging is more appropriate in patients with more global symptoms or suspected patellofemoral joint pathology. Patients with typical clinical signs of Osgood Schlatter disease rarely require imaging. Occasionally a radiograph or ultrasound is performed to reassure the patient, the patient's parents, and the referring clinician that there is no sinister pathology. Various features of patellofemoral dysplasia may be identified on radiographs, but MR imaging is vastly superior for the assessment of knee joint morphology. Skyline views (Merchant views) of the patellofemoral joint taken with the knee in around 30° of flexion may be misleading, because subluxation often only occurs as the knee approaches full extension. The degree of patellar subluxation can be assessed with tracking studies using MR imaging or CT. True dynamic studies have a theoretical advantage over methods using multiple static images, as dynamic studies more closely simulate normal daily activity.

Routine MR imaging protocols are sufficient for most pathology related to the extensor mechanism. The proton density fat suppression sequence, which is universally included in routine knee protocols, is sensitive for tendon, bone, and articular cartilage pathology. The sagittal and axial planes are the most useful for assessing patellofemoral dysplasia. Several methods of performing dynamic MR imaging of the patellofemoral joint have been described in the literature, including the acquisition of multiple static images, the acquisition of images during active controlled knee extension, real-time MR imaging, and a weight-bearing technique using an upright MR imaging scanner. The use of a weight-bearing upright technique should simulate the biomechanics of the knee joint better while performing everyday activities. Recent research shows that supine non-weight-bearing techniques tend to be more sensitive, and possibly oversensitive, for subluxation in early degrees of flexion compared

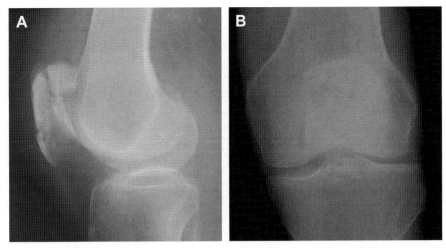

Fig. 1. (*A*) Lateral and (*B*) frontal radiographs showing a stellate fracture of the patella.

with a weight-bearing technique in a small cohort of patients with anterior knee pain. The degree of patellar tilt was the same for both techniques.[3] The technique used in the author's institution involves the acquisition of multiple axial slices through the center of the patella during control extension of the knee from 30° of flexion to full extension.[4] To ensure controlled extension, the patient slowly deflates a beach ball placed between the patient's shins and the roof of the magnet. The patient can control the rate of deflation via a connecting valve. During this maneuver, multiple series of axial images are continuously obtained through the patella. For each series an image through the center of the patella is chosen. These images are then displayed on a cine-loop.

IMAGING FINDINGS
Acute Injury

The commonest acute injuries are fracture and dislocation of the patella. Fractures of the tibial tubercle, and rupture of the quadriceps or patellar tendon, are much rarer injuries. A direct blow to the patella may result in a hemorrhage into the prepatellar bursa or a shearing injury of the prepatellar fat, the latter being equivalent to the Morel-Lavallée lesion of the thigh.[5]

Patellar fracture
Fractures of the patella may be transverse, vertical, or stellate. Transverse fractures are often associated with a distraction of the proximal fragment. Treatment is either surgical or conservative depending on the fracture patterns and degree of displacement. The common transverse and stellate type of patellar fracture are usually well

demonstrated on radiographs and no further imaging is required (**Figs. 1** and **2**). Sagitally orientated vertical fractures are more of a challenge and may only be obvious on the skyline or Merchant view, a projection that is not routinely performed in trauma cases. In practice CT is the easiest method of identifying this fracture. Avulsion of the inferior pole of the patella is a fracture seen predominately in the immature skeleton and is often termed a "sleeve fracture," because a sleeve of unossified cartilage and bone is stripped off the lower pole of the patella (**Fig. 3**).[6]

Tibial tubercle fracture
Avulsion of the tibial tubercle is an injury of the immature skeleton. Lesions range from a non-displaced minor fracture at the patellar tendon insertion to more extensive lesions involving the tibial articular surface. Small non-displaced fractures may be treated conservatively, whereas

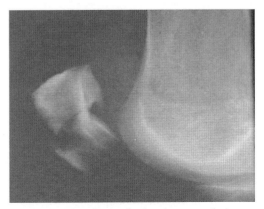

Fig. 2. Lateral radiograph showing a typical transverse intra-articular fracture with minor displacement.

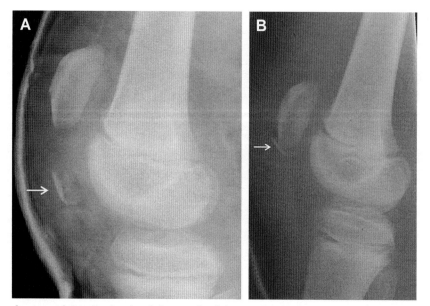

Fig. 3. Sleeve fracture of the distal pole of the patella. (*A*) Lateral radiograph in cast showing displaced sleeve fracture (*arrow*). (*B*) Radiograph following surgical reduction of the displaced fragment (*arrow*).

displaced or extensive fractures require fixation. The tibial tubercle apophysis is in continuity with the proximal tibial epiphysis, and avulsion fractures may therefore involve the articular surface of the tibiofemoral joint (**Fig. 4**).[7]

Dislocation

Patellar dislocation is very common and may occur following relatively trivial injury. Because

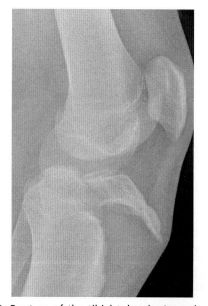

Fig. 4. Fracture of the tibial tubercle. Lateral radiograph of the knee demonstrates a displaced avulsion fracture of the tibial tubercle involving the tibiofemoral articular surface.

the injury often involves an osteochondral fracture, there is usually a large hemarthrosis, which hampers clinical assessment. Patellar dislocation is usually associated with a dysplastic patellofemoral joint (seelater discussion).

Acute patellar dislocation may be difficult to differentiate from other acute knee injuries on clinical grounds. The history of a twisting injury with clinical evidence of a large joint effusion and tenderness over the medial patellar retinaculum is typical. Radiographic features include a large effusion or lipohemarthrosis, an osteochondral fracture, and features of patellofemoral dysplasia. An osteochondral fragment arising from the femur is sometimes seen just anterior to the femoral condyles on the lateral radiograph, resulting in the so-called "sliver sign" (**Fig. 5**).[8] Often no bony injury can be detected on radiographs, and MR imaging is required to make the diagnosis. Dislocation of the patella results in an impaction injury of the medial edge of the patella against the anterolateral surface of the lateral femoral condyle and is usually associated with a tear of the medial retinacular complex.[9] More often than not there is a chondral or osteochondral fracture of either the medial aspect of the patella or the lateral femoral condyle resulting in a loose body. The most consistent features seen on MR imaging are subcortical edemalike signal representing trabecular microfractures, with or without an osteochondral or chondral defect from the anterolateral femoral condyle and/or medial aspect of the patella, and disruption of the medial retinaculum (**Figs. 5–8**). The medial retinacular

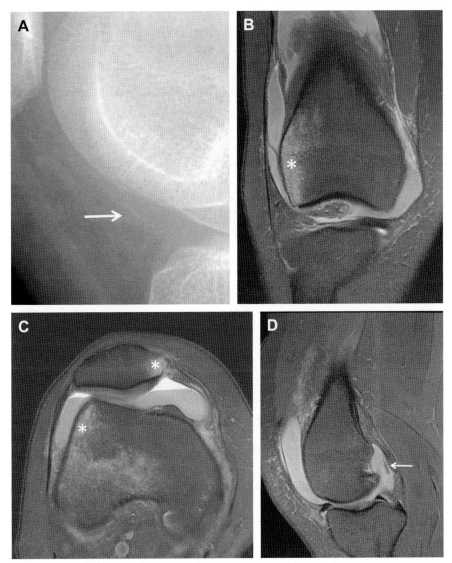

Fig. 5. Acute patellar dislocation. (*A*) Lateral radiograph showing prominent joint effusion and a small sliver of bone lying in the anterior joint space (*arrow*). (*B*) Coronal, (*C*) axial, and (*D*) sagittal proton density with fat suppression (PD FS) MR images showing subcortical high signal involving the lateral femoral condyle and medial patella (*asterisks*). On the sagittal view the small osteochondral fragment is now seen to lie in the posterior joint space (*arrow*). The axial view demonstrates a fluid-fluid level indicating hemarthrosis.

complex can be disrupted at the patellar or femoral attachments or in the midsubstance and may involve the medial patellofemoral ligament, which is an important stabilizer of the patella (**Fig. 9**).[10] With recurrent dislocation in patients with patellofemoral dysplasia, the medial retinaculum is less likely to tear. Subtle signs of patellar dislocation on MR imaging and radiographs, such as bony irregularity at the medial aspect of the patella and an osteochondral defect of the lateral femoral condyle, may become permanent markers of previous patellar dislocation (**Fig. 10**).

Acute chondral injury

Acute articular cartilage defects in the absence of dislocation are unusual and require MR imaging for diagnosis. The trochlear side of the joint is usually involved. Typical appearances are of a well-defined, full-thickness, or large partial thickness defect with acutely angled margins, and an intra-articular loose body corresponding to the displaced fragment (**Fig. 11**).[11] A shearing-type injury may result in delamination of articular cartilage, with fluid signal seen between the cartilage and the subchondral bone plate on MR imaging. The extent of the injury may be

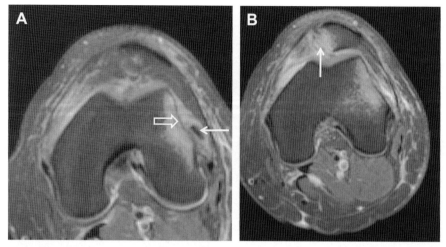

Fig. 6. Acute patellar dislocation. Axial PD FS images showing (*A*) a bony defect at the medial margin of the patella (*arrow*) and (*B*) associated osteochondral fragment at the site of impaction injury (*arrow*) with a depressed fracture of the lateral femoral condyle (*open arrow*).

understated if this lesion is not appreciated on the MR imaging.[12]

Patellar and quadriceps tendon tears

Acute rupture of the patellar or quadriceps tendon is relatively rare and inevitably occurs in compromised tendons affected by a systemic metabolic disorder or severe degenerative tendinosis. The diagnosis may be suspected on the radiograph when the tendon appears widened and indistinct, and when there is either displacement of the patella or avulsion fractures. The diagnosis can be confirmed with ultrasound or MR imaging (**Figs. 12** and **13**). Quadriceps rupture is sometimes associated with avulsion fragments originating from the superior pole of the patella, which can be readily identified on a radiograph (**Fig. 14**). Several cases of spontaneous bilateral rupture of the quadriceps tendon have occurred in patients with renal failure.[13]

Anterior soft tissue injury

Lying directly superficial to the patella is the prepatellar bursa, which may be involved by direct trauma. Hemorrhagic bursitis can be suspected on radiographs performed for possible patellar fracture when soft tissue swelling is seen anterior to the patella. Prepatellar bursal effusion can be readily diagnosed on both ultrasound and MR imaging. The Morel-Lavallée lesion is a shearing injury of the prepatellar soft tissues that results in linear signal abnormality on MR imaging and must be differentiated from the prepatellar bursa. With the Morel-Lavallée lesion, the abnormality is seen to extend beyond the normal bounds of the prepatellar bursa (**Fig. 15**).

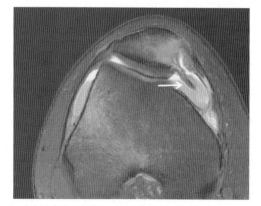

Fig. 7. Acute patellar dislocation. Axial PD FS image showing partial detachment of the articular cartilage of the medial facet of the patella (*arrow*).

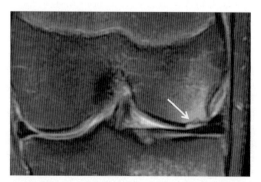

Fig. 8. Recent patellar dislocation. Coronal PD FS image showing a typical small peripheral osteochondral lesion of the lateral femoral condyle (*arrow*).

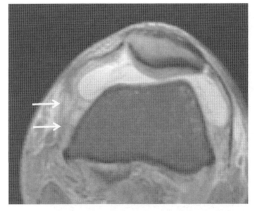

Fig. 9. Acute patellar dislocation. Axial PD FS image demonstrating a tear of the medial retinaculum at its femoral attachment (*arrows*).

Anterior Knee Pain

Anterior knee pain is common and usually settles with conservative management without resorting to imaging. When imaging is performed, the commonest conditions encountered are patellofemoral maltracking, articular surface abnormalities, and patellar tendon overuse lesions. Arriving at a specific diagnosis is often elusive in the younger individual, particularly in the adolescent age group, in which the prevalence of anterior knee pain has been reported as being as high as 18%.[14] Anterior knee pain syndrome and patellofemoral pain syndrome are general terms used to describe the presence of anterior knee pain in the young adult or adolescent with no specific clinical or imaging findings.[15] The typical case is a young woman with pain exacerbated by repetitive knee flexion, particularly while descending stairs, or by a prolonged period of sitting with the knees flexed. The term chondromalacia is more specific and implies that there are some pathologic changes within the retropatellar cartilage.

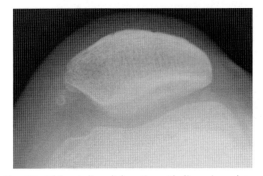

Fig. 10. Old patellar dislocation. Skyline view shows an established avulsion fracture at the origin of the medial retinaculum. The trochlear groove is shallow.

Tendinosis and traction-type lesions of the patellar tendon are common in adolescents and young adults and present as activity-related pain centered on the proximal or distal ends of the tendon.

Patellofemoral maltracking

Maltracking of the patella during flexion and extension is a common cause of anterior knee pain. A shallow proximal portion of the trochlear groove, an excessive laterally positioned tibial tubercle, and a high riding patella (patella alta) are anomalies frequently encountered in patients with patellofemoral maltracking.[16]

The degree of maltracking ranges from minor lateral subluxation and/or tilt of the patella to frank dislocation. The typical patient is an adolescent or young woman. Lateral patellar compression syndrome is a type of maltracking where there is lateral tilt of the patella without substantial subluxation, resulting in excessive pressure being exerted on the articular surfaces of the lateral facet of the patellofemoral joint. A laterally positioned tibial tubercle and tight lateral retinaculum contribute to the syndrome. The treatment of patellofemoral maltracking is overwhelmingly conservative. Surgical options include medialization of the tibial tubercle, trochleoplasty, medial patellofemoral ligament repair, and lateral retinacular release.

The lateral radiograph or sagittally oriented MR imaging can give an accurate assessment of patella alta. The ratio of the length of the posterior surface of the patellar tendon to the length of the patella should normally be less than 1.3 (Fig. 16).[16] An excessively flat or convex proximal portion of the trochlear can be diagnosed on the lateral radiograph by analyzing the relationship of the line representing the trough of the trochlear groove, and a line representing the anterior limit of the medial or lateral condyles. Crossing of these lines indicates a loss of the normal groove. A visible bump just superior to this indicates a convex configuration to the trochlear at this point (Fig. 17).[17] Although radiographs may give some indication of patellofemoral dysplasia, the morphology of the patellofemoral joint is best demonstrated on MR imaging. Patella alta, the depth of the trochlear groove, the degree of inclination of the lateral facet of the trochlea, and the position of the tibial tubercle can all be easily analyzed.[18–20] The relative position of the tibial tubercle is estimated by measuring the tibial tuberosity-trochlear groove (TT-TG) distance. The TT-TG value is obtained by measuring the distance between parallel lines (perpendicular to a line connecting the posterior articular surfaces

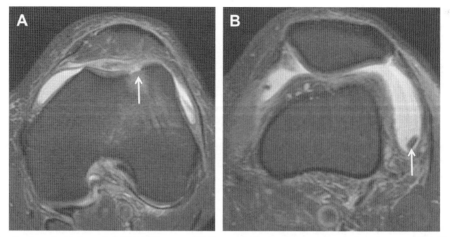

Fig. 11. Acute chondral injury. Axial PD FS images (*A*) through the trochlear groove showing a well-defined chondral defect involving the lateral facet of the trochlear groove (*arrow*). (*B*) The fragment is seen lying in the lateral synovial recess (*arrow*). The linear low signal component indicates involvement of the subchondral bone plate.

of the femoral condyles) drawn through the deepest point of the trochlear groove and the tibial tubercle on superimposed axial images. All cases with a TT-TG over 20 mm will demonstrate instability on dynamic tracking studies.[4] It is generally accepted that a measurement less than 15 mm can be considered normal and that values between 15 mm and 20 mm are equivocal (**Fig. 18**).

Patellofemoral dysplasia leads to lateral tilting and subluxation of the patella. Maltracking occurs when the patella begins to disengage from the proximal portion of the trochlear groove as the knee approaches full extension. Radiographic skyline views are obtained with the knee in approximately 30% of flexion and are therefore insensitive for patellar subluxation and for determining the configuration of the important proximal portion of the trochlear groove (**Fig. 19**). On static MR imaging pathologic changes associated with subluxation may be identified. The TT-TG distance, patella alta, the distance between the lower extent of the vastus medialis muscle to the patella, and an excessively shallow proximal portion of the trochlear groove correlate with patellofemoral maltracking. There is a strong inverse

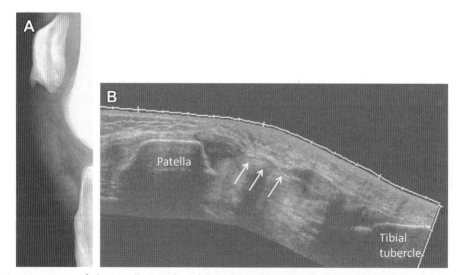

Fig. 12. Acute rupture of the patellar tendon. (*A*) Radiograph showing a widened patellar tendon with ill-defined margins, and there is cranial displacement of the patella. (*B*) Extended field-of-view longitudinal ultrasound showing a tear of the patellar tendon with a 2-cm gap (*arrows*).

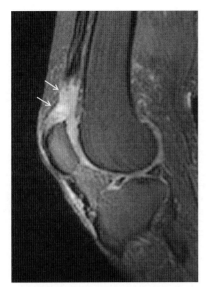

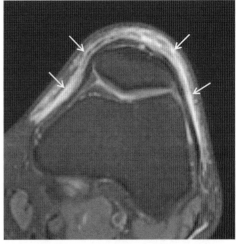

Fig. 13. Acute quadriceps tendon rupture. Sagittal PD FS image showing rupture of the distal end of the tendon (*arrows*).

Fig. 15. Morel-Lavallée lesion. Axial PD FS image showing a linear high-signal lesion in the anterior subcutaneous fat extending beyond the expected margins of the prepatellar bursa both medially and laterally (*arrows*).

relationship between the degree of patellar engagement (the percentage of patellar cartilage overlapping with trochlear cartilage) and patellar maltracking.[18] The angle of inclination of the lateral facet of the trochlear using the posterior intercondylar line as a baseline is associated with instability, with an angle of less than 11° being abnormal.[20] Lateral subluxation may be obvious on static axial MR imaging with the knee in full

extension but lesser degrees of subluxation may be difficult to diagnose. Dynamic patellofemoral tracking studies are probably the best way of demonstrating patellofemoral instability. When interpreting the images, the radiologist must take into account the internal rotation of the femur that occurs naturally during extension. The degree of subluxation correlates with symptoms. Grade I, representing minimal subluxation, is seen in

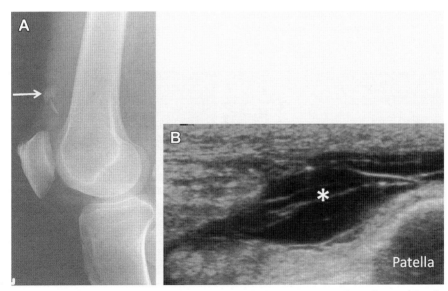

Fig. 14. Acute quadriceps rupture. (*A*) Lateral knee radiograph showing retracted patellar avulsion fracture fragments (*arrow*). (*B*) Longitudinal ultrasound shows rupture of the quadriceps tendon with a fluid filled gap (*asterisk*).

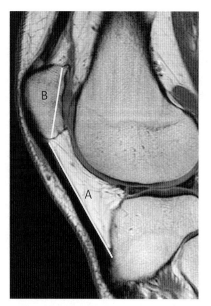

Fig. 16. Patella alta. Sagittal T1-weighted image showing an excessive patellar tendon to patella ratio (A/B).

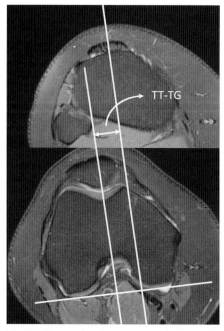

Fig. 18. TT-TG measurement. On axial PD FS images the TT-TG measurement represents the distance between parallel lines through the trochlear groove and center of the tibial tubercle, using the posterior margins of the femoral condyles as a baseline.

one-third of the asymptomatic population. Grade II, representing moderate subluxation, is seen in 9% of the asymptomatic population. Grade III, representing marked subluxation, is only seen in symptomatic individuals (**Fig. 20**).[4] In most cases subluxation can be adequately assessed clinically and dynamic imaging is only required in a minority of cases.

Articular surface pathology
Articular cartilage defects in the older age group are invariably a manifestation of osteoarthritis.

Imaging beyond the radiograph is not required. Severe osteoarthritis of the patellofemoral joint with relative sparing of the tibiofemoral compartments and chondrocalcinosis is typical of calcium pyrophosphate dihydrate deposition disease (**Fig. 21**). Osteoarthritis may affect either the medial or the lateral facets of the patellofemoral joint. An unusual but well-described appearance

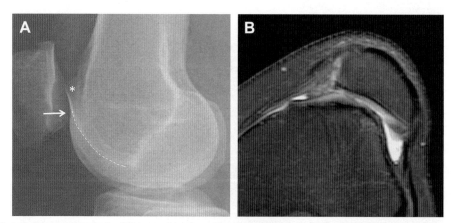

Fig. 17. Patellofemoral dysplasia. (*A*) Lateral knee radiographs showing the line representing the deepest point of the trochlear groove (*dashed line*) crossing the ventral margins of the femoral condyles (*arrow*) with a bony prominence just cranial to this (*asterisk*). (*B*) Axial PD FS image of the same patient showing a convex configuration to the trochlear articular surface with lateral subluxation of the patella.

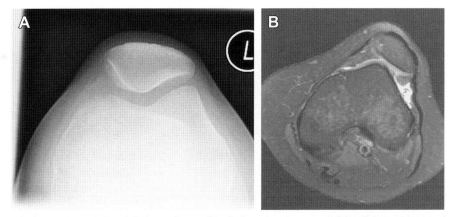

Fig. 19. Patellofemoral instability. (A) The radiographic skyline view is normal. (B) Axial PD FS image through the proximal portion of the trochlear with the knee in the fully extended position demonstrates a shallow trochlear groove and lateral subluxation of the patella.

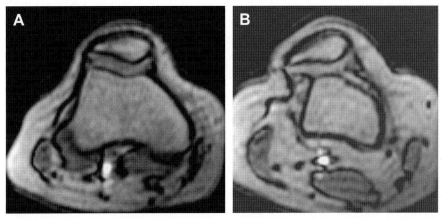

Fig. 20. Dynamic study for patellofemoral maltracking. Selected images from a series of axial scans obtained during gradual knee extension. (A) Image obtained with the knee in approximately 20° of flexion showing a normal relationship of the patella to the trochlear groove. (B) Image obtained with the knee approaching full extension. There is lateral subluxation of the patella. There is internal rotation of the femur, which, if not appreciated, may result in an underestimation of the degree of subluxation.

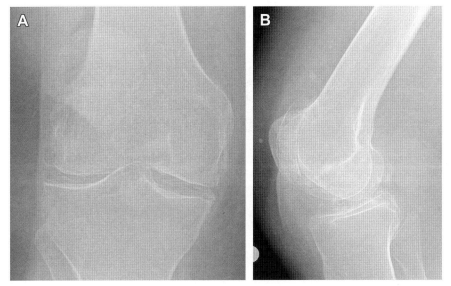

Fig. 21. Chronic calcium pyrophosphate dihydrate deposition disease. (A) Frontal radiograph showing relative sparing of the tibiofemoral joint and chondrocalcinosis. (B) Lateral radiograph showing severe patellofemoral osteoarthritis.

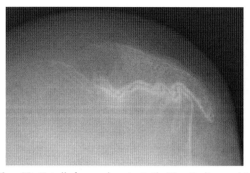

Fig. 22. Patellofemoral osteoarthritis. Radiographic skyline shows the unusual sawlike appearance.

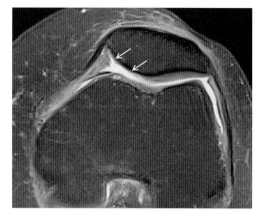

Fig. 23. Patellofemoral osteoarthritis. Axial PD FS image showing diffuse full-thickness cartilage loss over the medial articular facet of the patella (arrow).

is an erosion of the patellar articular surfaces resembling the edge of a saw (Fig. 22).[21] Osteoarthritis is an extremely common finding on routine MR imaging of middle-aged and elderly patients. Superficial and full-thickness articular cartilage defects, usually with sloping margins, fissuring, and fibrillation, are all features that may be seen on MR imaging (Fig. 23). The full-thickness defects are usually accompanied by subchondral bony marrow edema and/or cysts. There is poor correlation between grades of articular cartilage defects and symptoms.[22]

In the younger patient MR imaging is the investigation tool of choice for patients with chronic pain arising from the patellofemoral joint. A minor degree of articular cartilage damage seen in the younger age group is often termed chondromalacia and may be associated with knee pain. Swelling, fraying, and fissuring of the articular cartilage are well demonstrated on high-resolution MR imaging. Simple signal change without macroscopic abnormality may also be encountered (Fig. 24).

Another condition that is seen primarily in the younger age group is osteochondritis dissecans. The underlying pathology in this condition is focal necrosis of subchondral bone, probably as a result of chronic repetitive microtrauma. The lesions may be unstable when secondary defects in the articular cartilage frequently occur. Common sites for the lesion in the knee are the lateral aspect of the medial femoral condyle and the weight-bearing surface of the lateral femoral condyle. Involvement of the patellofemoral joint is much rarer. Patellofemoral lesions are most commonly located at the apex of the patella. Occasionally the lesion is encountered on the femoral side of the joint, with the lateral facet of the trochlear being favored.[23] The lesion may be identified on radiographs but MR imaging is more sensitive. On MR imaging a subchondral bony fragment can usually be identified, with or without disruption of the overlying articular cartilage (Fig. 25). This bony fragment is

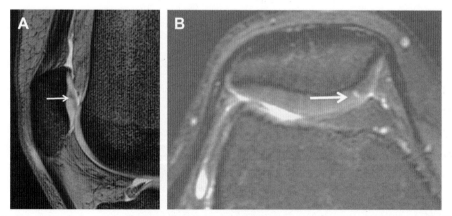

Fig. 24. Chondromalacia in young adults. (A) Sagittal T2-weighted gradient echo image demonstrating minor signal change within the retropatellar cartilage (arrow). (B) Axial PD FS image showing a minor fissure of the retropatellar cartilage (arrow).

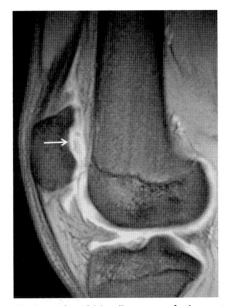

Fig. 25. Osteochondritis dissecans of the patella. Sagittal T2-weighted gradient echo image demonstrates a defect in the apex of the patella containing a small osteochondral fragment (*arrow*).

necrotic and usually shows low signal intensity on T1-weighted images. Surrounding bone edema and cystic change may be present. The lesion is deemed unstable when fluid signal or cystic change is seen deep to the fragment or when a defect of the articular cartilage is detected. Occasionally the osteochondral fragment becomes detached, resulting in an intra-articular loose body.

A bipartite patella is a common anomaly whereby the superolateral portion of the patella forms a separate ossicle. Although this can be considered to be a normal variant, there is evidence that the lesion may be associated with pain, particularly when there is edema related to the lesion seen on MR imaging (**Fig. 26**).[24]

There are several recognized rudimentary folds, or plicae, of the knee synovium. The medial patellar plica lies close to the medial aspect of the patellofemoral joint and when prominent may become entrapped within the joint. This entrapment has been implicated as a cause of anterior knee pain. The reported clinical features include pain and crepitus over the medial edge of the patella.[25] Although there is considerable uncertainty as to its clinical significance, an association between the degree of medial extension of the plica and pain has been reported (**Fig. 27**).[26] However, correlation between the MR imaging and surgical findings has been reported as poor.[27,28]

Patellar and quadriceps tendon

The commonest disorder of the patellar tendon is proximal patellar tendinosis (jumper's knee), which primarily affects the adolescent and younger adult. This condition is usually sports related and in extreme cases may be highly disabling. The pathology in this condition is typically located in the deep portion of the tendon immediately adjacent to the inferior pole of the patella. On ultrasound the tendon is seen to be focally widened, hypoechoic, and hypervascular (**Fig. 28**). Calcification may be identified in more chronic cases. On MR imaging this focal pathology is seen as high signal on fluid-sensitive sequences (**Fig. 29**). In addition there is often ill-defined edema within the surrounding soft tissues, and bone marrow edema within the adjacent inferior pole of the patella. The condition

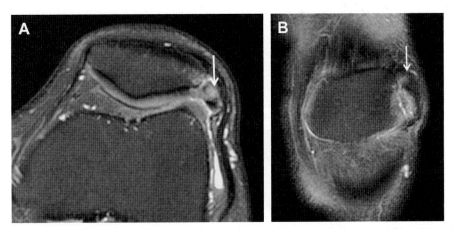

Fig. 26. Bipartite patella. (*A*) axial and (*B*) coronal PD FS images demonstrating a typical bipartite patella with considerable bony edema (*arrows*).

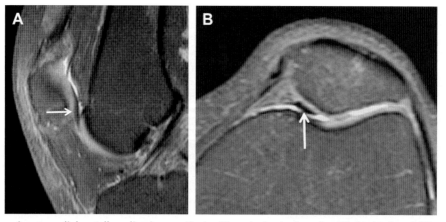

Fig. 27. Prominent medial patellar plica in a patient with anterior knee pain. (*A*) Sagittal and (*B*) axial PD FS images demonstrating a slightly thickened plica extending into the medial portion of the patellofemoral joint (*arrows*).

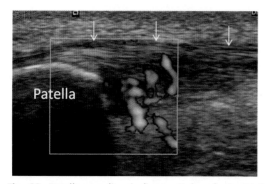

Fig. 28. Patellar tendinosis (jumper's knee). Sagittal ultrasound demonstrating a hypoechoic, hypervascular lesion within the deep portion of the tendon adjacent to the inferior pole of the patella. The superficial fibers of the tendon appear normal (*arrows*).

is usually self-limiting. There is a popular trend for percutaneous treatment of this condition including dry needling and injection of platelet-rich plasma or autologous blood.[29,30]

Another common condition is lateral patellar tendon impingement, the underlying cause of which is a reduced distance between the patellar tendon and the lateral femoral condyle. This entity is frequently identified on MR imaging but is rarely associated with symptoms. On MR imaging high T2 signal is seen at the most lateral aspect of Hoffa's fat pad between the lateral portion of the proximal patellar tendon and the lateral femoral condyle (**Fig. 30**). The condition is associated with a high riding patella, a laterally positioned tibial tubercle, and patellar maltracking.[31,32] The abnormality is more likely to be associated with

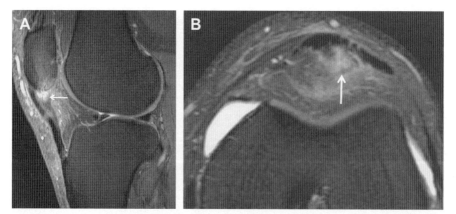

Fig. 29. Patellar tendinosis (jumper's knee). (*A*) Sagittal and (*B*) axial PD FS images demonstrating high T2 signal in the deep portion of the patellar tendon (*arrows*). There is also reactive bone marrow edema within the inferior pole of the patella. The axial image demonstrates the focal nature of the lesion.

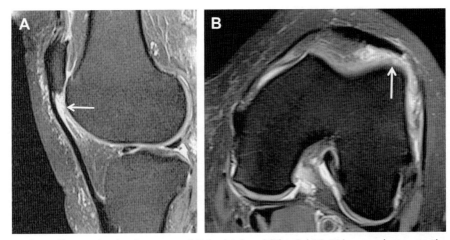

Fig. 30. Lateral patellar tendon impingement. (*A*) Sagittal and (*B*) axial PD FS images demonstrating impingement of the patellar tendon on the lateral femoral condyle with edema in the intervening soft tissues (*arrows*).

pain if there are signs of focal tendinosis within the patellar tendon at the site of impingement.[31] Because this abnormality is commonly seen on MR imaging in patients with no symptoms related to this area, the significance of this finding should be interpreted with caution.

In the child, overuse injury of the proximal patellar tendon (Sinding-Larsen–Johansson syndrome) is a rare self-limiting condition. The chronic traction at the inferior pole of the patella results in the formation of heterotopic ossification, giving a typical imaging appearance. The diagnosis can be readily made on radiographs, ultrasound, or MR imaging (**Fig. 31**).

Osgood Schlatter disease is a similar overuse traction injury at the insertion of the patellar tendon into the tibial tubercle. The condition is usually self-limiting but may sometimes persist

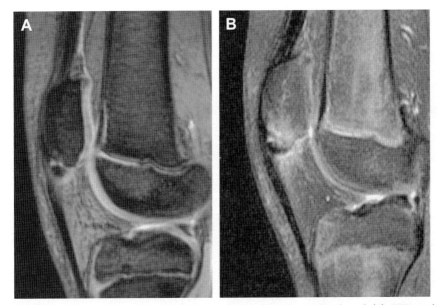

Fig. 31. Sinding-Larsen–Johansson syndrome. (*A*) Gradient echo T2-weighted and (*B*) STIR sagittal images showing fragmentation of the inferior pole of the patella with minor edema within the adjacent tendon and bone.

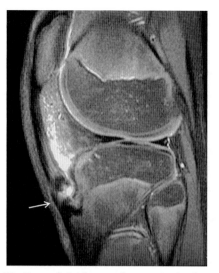

Fig. 32. Osgood Schlatter disease. Sagittal PD FS image showing fragmentation of the tibial tubercle (*arrow*), widening of the adjacent patellar tendon, and a deep infrapatellar bursal effusion.

into adulthood. The diagnosis can be made on clinical grounds and imaging is rarely required. The radiograph will demonstrate a prominent fragmented tibial tubercle. The imaging features on ultrasound and MR imaging are those of distal patellar tendinosis and fragmentation of the immature tibial tubercle, often accompanied by fluid within the deep infrapatellar bursa (**Fig. 32**).

Clinically significant pathology in the quadriceps tendon is unusual. In the asymptomatic population mature bone formation at the tendon insertion is a common finding on radiographs, as is minor high signal within the distal quadriceps tendon on MR imaging. Patients with symptomatic insertional tendinosis will usually show hypervascularity on ultrasound (**Fig. 33**). Quadriceps tendinosis has been shown to be a particular problem in beach volleyball players.[33]

High signal deep to the distal portion of the tendon within the quadriceps fat pad is also a common MR imaging finding of unknown cause. Although this is primarily an incidental finding, there may be an association with anterior knee pain when there is mass effect with indentation of the suprapatellar pouch (**Fig. 34**).[34]

Tumors

The patella is a rare site for bony tumors. Nearly one-half of the lesions are nonneoplastic and two-thirds of neoplasms are benign, the most common lesions being chondroblastoma and giant cell tumor. Aneurysmal bone cyst, Infection, gout, and brown tumors are the commonest nonneoplastic conditions. Most lesions may be identified on a radiograph but MR imaging and CT are usually performed to identify more specific features and demonstrate the extent of the lesion (**Fig. 35**).[35]

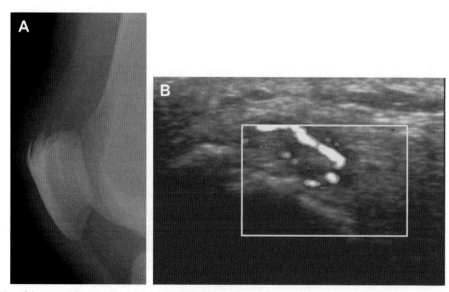

Fig. 33. Quadriceps enthesopathy. (*A*) Lateral radiograph shows mature bone formation at the quadriceps tendon insertion. (*B*) Doppler ultrasound shows marked hypervascularity within the tendon.

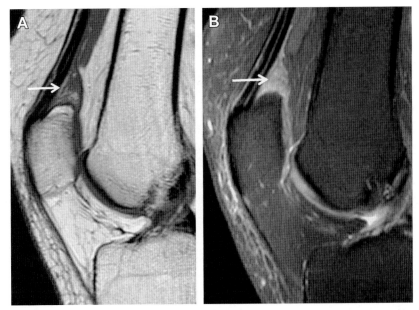

Fig. 34. Quadriceps fat pad edema. (*A*) T1-weighted and (*B*) PD FS sagittal images showing edemalike signal in the quadriceps fat pad with some minor mass effect (*arrows*).

In summary, imaging plays a useful role in the management of patients with symptoms related to the extensor mechanism. MR imaging is an excellent technique for assessing the morphology of the extensor mechanism and for identifying a variety of pathologies. Dynamic imaging of the patellofemoral joint may be helpful in selected cases. Ultrasound is most often used to investigate symptoms related to the tendons or for the assessment of a soft tissue mass. The radiograph has a limited role in the assessment of chronic conditions but is still widely used in the setting of acute trauma.

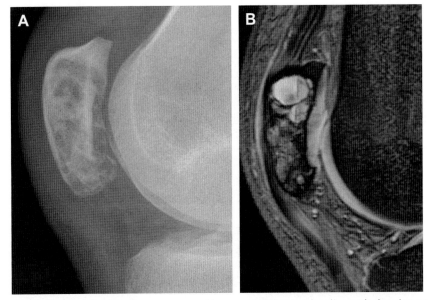

Fig. 35. Chondroblastoma with secondary aneurysmal bone cyst. (*A*) Lateral radiograph showing a well-defined lytic lesion within the patella. (*B*) Sagittal T2-weighted gradient echo image showing solid chondroblastoma involving the inferior portion of the patella, with a cystic component superiorly containing fluid-fluid level representing a secondary aneurysmal bone cyst.

REFERENCES

1. Dirim B, Haghighi P, Trudell D, et al. Medial patellofemoral ligament: cadaveric investigation of anatomy with MRI, MR arthrography, and histologic correlation. Am J Roentgenol 2008;191(2):490–8.

2. Sheehan FT, Derasari A, Fine KM, et al. Q-angle and J-sign: indicative of maltracking subgroups in patellofemoral pain. Clin Orthop Relat Res 2010;468(1):266–75.

3. Draper CE, Besier TF, Fredericson M, et al. Differences in patellofemoral kinematics between weight-bearing and non-weight-bearing conditions in patients with patellofemoral pain. J Orthop Res 2011;29(3):312–7.

4. O'Donnell P, Johnstone C, Watson M, et al. Evaluation of patellar tracking in symptomatic and asymptomatic individuals by magnetic resonance imaging. Skeletal Radiol 2005;34(3):130–5.

5. Borrero CG, Maxwell N, Kavanagh E. MRI findings of prepatellar Morel-Lavallee effusions. Skeletal Radiol 2008;37(5):451–5.

6. Gao GX, Mahadev A, Lee EH. Sleeve fracture of the patella in children. J Orthop Surg (Hong Kong) 2008;16(1):43–6.

7. Dupuis CS, Westra SJ, Makris J, et al. Injuries and conditions of the extensor mechanism of the pediatric knee. Radiographics 2009;29(3):877–86.

8. Haas JP, Collins MS, Stuart MJ. The "sliver sign": a specific radiographic sign of acute lateral patellar dislocation. Skeletal Radiol 2012;41(5):595–601.

9. Pope TL Jr. MR imaging of patellar dislocation and relocation. Semin Ultrasound CT MR 2001;22(4):371–82.

10. Spritzer CE, Courneya DL, Burk DL Jr, et al. Medial retinacular complex injury in acute patellar dislocation: MR findings and surgical implications. Am J Roentgenol 1997;168(1):117–22.

11. Recht MP, Goodwin DW, Winalski CS, et al. MRI of articular cartilage: revisiting current status and future directions. Am J Roentgenol 2005;185(4):899–914.

12. Kendell SD, Helms CA, Rampton JW, et al. MRI appearance of chondral delamination injuries of the knee. Am J Roentgenol 2005;184(5):1486–9.

13. Matokovic D, Matijasevic B, Petric P, et al. A case report of spontaneous concurrent bilateral rupture of the quadriceps tendons in a patient with chronic renal failure. Ther Apher Dial 2010;14(1):104–7.

14. Vahasarja V. Prevalence of chronic knee pain in children and adolescents in northern Finland. Acta Paediatr 1995;84(7):803–5.

15. Collado H, Fredericson M. Patellofemoral pain syndrome. Clin Sports Med 2010;29(3):379–98.

16. Miller TT, Staron RB, Feldman F. Patellar height on sagittal MR imaging of the knee. Am J Roentgenol 1996;167(2):339–41.

17. Dejour H, Walch G, Nove-Josserand L, et al. Factors of patellar instability: an anatomic radiographic study. Knee Surg Sports Traumatol Arthrosc 1994;2(1):19–26.

18. Monk AP, Doll HA, Gibbons CL, et al. The pathoanatomy of patellofemoral subluxation. J Bone Joint Surg Br 2011;93(10):1341–7.

19. Pfirrmann CW, Zanetti M, Romero J, et al. Femoral trochlear dysplasia: MR findings. Radiology 2000;216(3):858–64.

20. Carrillon Y, Abidi H, Dejour D, et al. Patellar instability: assessment on MR images by measuring the lateral trochlear inclination-initial experience. Radiology 2000;216(2):582–5.

21. Anbarasu A, Loughran CF. Saw tooth patellofemoral arthritis. Clin Radiol 2000;55(10):767–9.

22. Kornaat PR, Bloem JL, Ceulemans RY, et al. Osteoarthritis of the knee: association between clinical features and MR imaging findings. Radiology 2006;239(3):811–7.

23. Peters TA, McLean ID. Osteochondritis dissecans of the patellofemoral joint. Am J Sports Med 2000;28(1):63–7.

24. Kavanagh EC, Zoga A, Omar I, et al. MRI findings in bipartite patella. Skeletal Radiol 2007;36(3):209–14.

25. Dupont JY. Synovial plicae of the knee. Controversies and review. Clin Sports Med 1997;16(1):87–122.

26. Jee WH, Choe BY, Kim JM, et al. The plica syndrome: diagnostic value of MRI with arthroscopic correlation. J Comput Assist Tomogr 1998;22(5):814–8.

27. Weckstrom M, Niva MH, Lamminen A, et al. Arthroscopic resection of medial plica of the knee in young adults. Knee 2010;17(2):103–7.

28. Boles CA, Butler J, Lee JA, et al. Magnetic resonance characteristics of medial plica of the knee: correlation with arthroscopic resection. J Comput Assist Tomogr 2004;28(3):397–401.

29. Filardo G, Kon E, Della Villa S, et al. Use of platelet-rich plasma for the treatment of refractory jumper's knee. Int Orthop 2010;34(6):909–15.

30. James SL, Ali K, Pocock C, et al. Ultrasound guided dry needling and autologous blood injection for patellar tendinosis. Br J Sports Med 2007;41(8):518–21 [discussion: 522].

31. Campagna R, Pessis E, Biau DJ, et al. Is Superolateral Hoffa fat pad edema a consequence of impingement between lateral femoral condyle and patellar ligament? Radiology 2012;263(2):469–74.

32. Jibri Z, Martin D, Mansour R, et al. The association of infrapatellar fat pad oedema with patellar maltracking: a case-control study. Skeletal Radiol 2012;41(8):925–31.

33. Pfirrmann CW, Jost B, Pirkl C, et al. Quadriceps tendinosis and patellar tendinosis in professional beach

volleyball players: sonographic findings in correlation with clinical symptoms. Eur Radiol 2008;18(8): 1703–9.

34. Roth C, Jacobson J, Jamadar D, et al. Quadriceps fat pad signal intensity and enlargement on MRI:

prevalence and associated findings. Am J Roentgenol 2004;182(6):1383–7.

35. Singh J, James SL, Kroon HM, et al. Tumour and tumour-like lesions of the patella–a multicentre experience. Eur Radiol 2009;19(3):701–12.

Posterolateral and Posteromedial Corner Injuries of the Knee

Daniel Geiger, MD[a], Eric Chang, MD[b], Mini Pathria, MD[c],
Christine B. Chung, MD[c],*

KEYWORDS

- Knee • Posterolateral • Posteromedial • Corner • Injuries

KEY POINTS

- Posterolateral and posteromedial corners of the knee are complex anatomic regions; detailed knowledge of anatomic structures and relationships is necessary for appropriate assessment at imaging.
- Association between untreated posterolateral and posteromedial corner injuries of the knee and failure of central support structure reconstruction has been established. Accurate diagnosis and characterization of these injuries will improve clinical and surgical outcome.
- Posterolateral and posteromedial corner injuries of the knee may be difficult to diagnose clinically. Classic magnetic resonance imaging patterns allow noninvasive diagnosis that can guide management.

INTRODUCTION

The posterolateral (PLC) and posteromedial (PMC) corners of the knee are anatomic units composed of a complex arrangement of structures. As referenced in their names, they extend both posteriorly[1] and along the lateral and medial aspects of the knee, respectively (**Fig. 1**). As the posterior extension of the lateral and medial supporting structures, they act in conjunction with the central supporting ligaments (anterior and posterior cruciate ligaments) to provide static (capsular and noncapsular ligaments) and dynamic (musculotendinous units and their aponeuroses) articular stability.[2,3] The delineation of fine anatomic detail in these regions and identification of delicate structures are particularly challenging at imaging because of composite anatomy, orientation, and small size of their components. Pathology might be overlooked or misdiagnosed without clear knowledge of the regional morphology, biomechanics, and specific patterns of injury. Moreover, PLC and PMC injuries uncommonly occur in an isolated fashion, more often associated with concomitant injuries that may dominate the clinical picture. Untreated PLC injuries can lead to chronic posterolateral instability[4,5] and PMC deficiencies may cause persistent valgus instability[6]; both conditions lead to poor outcome of anterior cruciate ligament (ACL) and posterior cruciate ligament (PCL) reconstruction. It is therefore imperative, in a postinjury or preoperative setting, to provide the referring physician with an accurate description (when possible) of the PLC and PMC

Disclosure: The authors declare that they have no conflict of interest.
[a] Department of Radiological, Oncological and Pathological Sciences, Sapienza University of Rome, Viale Regina Elena 324, Rome 00161, Italy; [b] VA Healthcare San Diego, 3350 La Jolla Village Drive, La Jolla, CA 92161, USA; [c] Department of Radiology, University of California-San Diego, 408 Dickinson Street, San Diego, CA 92103–8226, USA
* Corresponding author.
E-mail address: cbchung@ucsd.edu

Radiol Clin N Am 51 (2013) 413–432
http://dx.doi.org/10.1016/j.rcl.2012.10.004
0033-8389/13/$ – see front matter Published by Elsevier Inc.

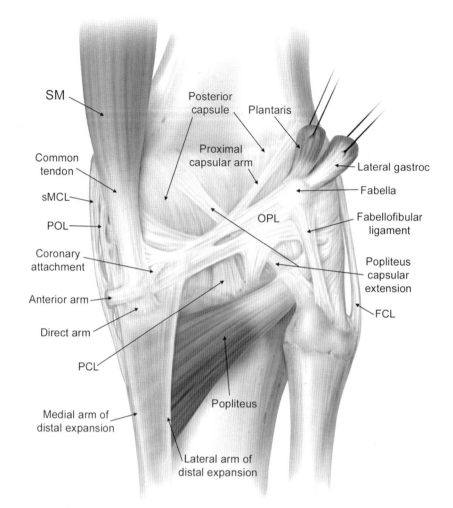

Fig. 1. Posterior aspect of the knee after removal of medial and lateral gastrocnemius muscles and neurovascular structures. SM, semimembranosus muscle; sMCL, superficial medial collateral ligament; FCL, fibular (lateral) collateral ligament; lateral gastroc, lateral gastrocnemius; OPL, oblique popliteal ligament; PCL, posterior cruciate ligament; POL, posterior oblique ligament. (*From* LaPrade RF, Morgan PM, Wentorf FA, et al. The anatomy of the posterior aspect of the knee. An anatomic study. J Bone Joint Surg Am 2007;89(4):758–64; with permission.)

structures. The characterization of structural alteration at imaging will allow a reference for clinical evaluation that can guide surgical approach and interrogation, facilitating optimal treatment, and thereby improving patient outcome. Magnetic resonance imaging (MRI) currently is the gold standard imaging strategy in the evaluation of the soft tissues; therefore, the authors focus mainly on this technique. Ultrasound scan has been established as a complementary technique.[7] Plain films and computed tomography play a role in the evaluation of osseous lesions (bony avulsions, cortical stress changes related to chronic injury). This article discusses the anatomy, basic biomechanics, and common injuries of the PLC and PMC complexes,

presenting the reader with a systematic approach for their evaluation.

POSTEROLATERAL CORNER OF THE KNEE
Anatomy, Biomechanics, and Mechanism of Injuries to the PLC

Seebacher and colleagues[8] in 1982 introduced a three-layered approach in the anatomic description of the lateral supporting structures of the knee, using a similar three-layer concept previously assumed in their description of the medial side supporting structures (**Fig. 2**).[9] In Seebacher's original description of the lateral supporting structures, the *superficial layer (I)* consists of the iliotibial tract

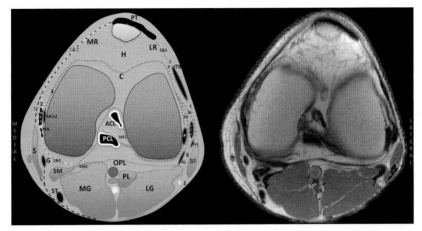

Fig. 2. Axial diagram (*left*) shows layers and anatomic components at the level of the joint line with a corresponding axial T2-weighted MRI (*right*). 1 = first layer, 2 = second layer, 3 = third layer, 3s = third layer (superficial lamina), 3d = third layer (deep lamina), AL, arcuate ligament; BF, biceps femoris and its tendon; C, capsule and H, Hoffa's fat pad; FFL, fabellofibular ligament; G, gracilis muscle tendon; g, lateral inferior genicular artery; ITB, iliotibial band; LCL, lateral collateral ligament; LG, lateral gastrocnemius muscle; LR, lateral retinaculum; MCL, medial collateral ligament; MCLd, deep medial collateral ligament; MFL, meniscofemoral ligament (Humphrey's); MG, medial gastrocnemius muscle; MR, medial retinaculum; OPL, oblique popliteal ligament; P, popliteus muscle tendon; PL, plantaris muscle; POL, posterior oblique ligament; PT, patellar tendon; S, sartorius muscle and its tendon; SM, semimembranosus muscle tendon; SMC, semimembranosus tendon (capsular arm); ST, semitendinosus muscle tendon.

and its expansion anteriorly and the biceps femoris tendon (BFT) and its expansion posteriorly. The peroneal nerve lies deep to it, posterior to the BFT. The *middle layer (II)* is incomplete and consists of the lateral patellar retinaculum anteriorly and the 2 patellofemoral ligaments posteriorly. The proximal patellofemoral ligament joins the lateral intermuscular septum, the distal patellofemoral ligament attaches to the fabella (when present) or at the femoral insertion of the posterolateral joint capsule or lateral head of the gastrocnemius. Included in the middle layer is the patellomeniscal ligament, which travels from the patella to the lateral meniscus, reaching inferiorly the lateral tibial tubercle of Gerdy, running deep to the iliotibial tract. The *deepest layer (III)* is composed of the lateral extent of the joint capsule and is attached to the edges of the tibia and femur. Posterior to the overlying iliotibial tract, the capsule divides into 2 laminae (superficial and deep). The superficial lamina travels superficial to the lateral collateral ligament and ends posteriorly at the fabellofibular ligament. The deeper lamina travels deep to the lateral collateral ligament, passes along and attaches to the edge of the lateral meniscus, giving rise to the coronary ligament and ultimately reaching the arcuate ligament. The deep and superficial laminae of the posterolateral capsule are always separated from each other with the lateral inferior genicular artery, considered an anatomic landmark, between them (see **Fig. 2**). Further cadaveric,[10]

MRI[11–18] and ultrasound scan[7,19] evaluations of specific PLC anatomy followed Seebacher's original work to delineate the imaging counterpart of his anatomic description. Because of the increasing interest in the anatomy and biomechanics of the PLC corner of the knee in the orthopedic literature, the need for standardization and a systematic approach to the nomenclature of the lateral complex structures and PLC has been addressed.[20,21] For a systematic approach to these structures we consider the superficial layer (first layer) comprising the lateral fascia, iliotibial band and biceps femoris tendon. The middle layer (second layer) comprises the patellar retinaculum, and patellofemoral and patellomeniscal ligaments. The deep layer (third layer) consists of the *lateral collateral ligament* (fibular collateral ligament), the *lateral coronary ligament* (lateral meniscotibial ligament), the *arcuate ligament*, the *popliteus tendon-muscle unit*, the *popliteofibular ligament*, the *fabellofibular ligament*, and the lateral joint capsule with its attachment to the lateral meniscus edge. The deep layer is the most anatomically variable of the 3 layers and the one constituting the posterolateral corner of the knee complex.[20] We briefly describe the components of the third inner layer and their anatomic relations.

The lateral collateral ligament (fibular collateral ligament), is an extracapsular structure, has a tubular shape, and measures approximately 3–4 mm in diameter and 7 cm in length. It originates from the lateral femoral condyle, arising from a small depression posterior to the lateral femoral epicondyle and 2 cm proximal to the joint line. It courses distally and posteriorly to attach to the posterior portion of the lateral aspect of the fibular head (see **Fig. 1**).

The lateral coronary ligament (or meniscotibial portion of the midthird lateral capsular ligament or lateral meniscotibial ligament) attaches the lateral meniscus to the lateral tibial plateau and functions as a meniscal stabilizer. The lateral coronary ligament is composed of short confluent ligamentous bands attached to the peripheral portion of the meniscal body and to the lateral tibia several millimeters inferior to the articular surface, occasionally resulting in a small synovial recess.[22,23]

The arcuate ligament has an inverted Y shape. The 2 superior arms consist of a lateral limb (upright), coursing upward along the joint capsule and extending to the lateral femoral condyle, and a medial limb (arcuate), crossing over the popliteal tendon, attaching to the posterior capsule, and merging with the oblique popliteal ligament. The lower limb attaches to the fibular head.[24] The arcuate ligament lies deep to the lateral inferior genicular artery, and its presence is variable, ranging from 24% to 80% in previous studies.[8,25,26]

The popliteus muscle originates from the lateral aspect of the lateral femoral condyle, attaches to the posterior horn of the lateral meniscus via the popliteomeniscal fascicles (anteroinferior, posterosuperior, posteroinferior) and to the apex of the fibula via the popliteofibular fascicles, extending distally to the posteromedial aspect of the tibial shaft (see **Fig. 1**). The popliteus muscle is always present, whereas the posteroinferior popliteomeniscal fascicle may be absent.[26,27]

The popliteofibular ligament originates at the level of the musculotendinous junction of the popliteus muscle and courses distally and laterally to insert on the fibular styloid. The popliteofibular ligament is a wide tendinous band, approximately the same width or wider than the popliteus tendon,[28–31] and is reportedly present in between 94% and 98% of the population.[25,26] The proximal myotendinous portion of the popliteus muscle and the popliteofibular ligament originating from it form an inverted Y-shaped structure. Therefore, the 3 arms of the inverted Y are the superior portion of the popliteus myotendinous unit, the popliteofibular ligament, and the inferior portion of the popliteus myotendinous unit distal to the origin of the popliteofibular ligament.

The fabellofibular ligament is the distal edge of the capsular arm of the short head of the biceps femoris muscle, and, as such, is present in all knees. Usually, it is a delicate structure but is more robust in appearance when the bony fabella is present but less consistent and more subtle in nature when a cartilaginous fabellar analog is present. We would like to reinforce the concept addressed from LaPrade[21] regarding the presence of at least a fabellar cartilaginous analog in every knee. When the fabella is present, the fabellofibular ligament arises from the lateral margin of the fabella, and, when absent, it originates from the posterior aspect of the supracondylar process of the femur.[32] Extending from the fabella or the fabellar analog, the fabellofibular ligament extends toward the fibula, parallel to the lateral collateral ligament, and inserts distally on the lateral aspect of the tip of the fibular head styloid process, posterior to the fibular insertion of the biceps femoris tendon (see **Fig. 1**). Previous studies addressed the variable presence of the fabellofibular ligament, ranging from 51%–87%.[8,26]

Biomechanically the PLC structures resist varus and external rotation forces. With regard to varus forces the lateral collateral ligament is considered the major stabilizer, with a minor contribution from the posterior cruciate ligament and the posterolateral capsule; a minor secondary contribution is made from the anterior cruciate ligament. In relation to external rotation forces, the lateral collateral ligament, popliteofibular ligament, fabellofibular ligament, capsular attachment of the short head of the biceps femoris muscle, and the popliteus tendon play a fundamental role in resisting stress. A role of the PLC in resisting posterior translation of the tibia has been addressed, establishing the popliteomeniscal fascicles as stabilizers of the posterior horn of the lateral meniscus. Isolated injuries of the PLC tend to be rare and commonly occur in conjunction with cruciate ligament lesions. The association of lateral collateral ligament and deep PLC structure injuries increases varus angulation and tibial external rotation, also causing anteroposterior instability of the knee. Deep PLC lesions (preserved lateral collateral ligament), in conjunction with anterior cruciate ligament deficiency, increase anterior translation of the tibia without causing external rotation of the tibia or varus angulation of the joint. When deep PLC structures fail and lateral collateral ligament and anterior cruciate ligament injuries are present, anterior and varus instability with external rotation of the tibia occur. Deep PLC structure deficiency, with lateral collateral ligament and posterior cruciate ligament injury, cause posterior translation, varus angulation, and external rotation of the tibia.[33–42] Posterolateral corner injuries are frequently associated with acute posterior cruciate ligament tears and have been reported in 62% of patients.[43] Therefore, when a posterior cruciate ligament injury is observed, particular attention should be paid to the PLC area. Injuries of the PLC are less common than injuries of the PMC, but because this anatomic area is subject to a greater stress during motion than the medial side, they tend to be more disabling.[13] PLC injuries most commonly occur via a direct blow to the anteromedial aspect of the proximal tibia in the fully extended knee, with the force directed in a posterolateral direction, but can also occur from a hyperextension injury with external rotation.[41,44] Anterior rotatory dislocations (varus stress and hyperextension) and posterior rotatory dislocations (varus stress, posteriorly directed blow to proximal tibia and flexion), are also common mechanisms of injury,[20,45] the latter known as a "dashboard injury." An undetected PLC injury can lead to chronic instability and failure of efforts to reconstruct the central supporting structures because of deficiency of PLC in resisting biomechanical stress.[34,46–49] Testing of the PLC resistance to stress involves varus and external rotation stress tests at different degrees of flexion.[35] The posterolateral rotation test (dial test) is one commonly used for posterolateral instability, assessing increasing external rotation of the tibia in relation to the femur at 30° of knee flexion.

INJURIES TO THE PLC COMPLEX
Soft-tissues Injuries of the PLC

Lateral collateral ligament (fibular collateral ligament)
Alterations to the lateral collateral ligament are a common feature of PLC injuries. In vitro studies addressed the role of the lateral collateral ligament (LCL) as a restraint to PLC instability and varus angulation in static testing. Nielsen and colleagues[50] noted an increase in varus joint opening with marked posterolateral rotatory instability when an LCL lesion is associated with a posterolateral capsule transection rather than an LCL injury alone. Grood and coworkers[51] addressed the increase of varus angulation at partial knee flexion when a PCL injury is combined with an LCL injury. Gollehon and colleagues[52] showed the principal role of the LCL and PLC deep ligament complex in preventing varus and external rotation of the tibia and the increase of varus rotation and posterior translation in combined injuries of the LCL, PCL, and deep lateral complex. However, LaPrade and Terry[33] evaluated 71 patients presenting with a PLC knee injury and signs of instability but at surgery found an injured LCL in only 23% of the knees. Based on this finding, they suggest that an LCL injury should not be the sole determining factor when diagnosing PLC injuries. Lateral collateral ligament

injuries consist of structural alterations that include thickening, tears, soft-tissue avulsions from the femoral attachment, and soft-tissue avulsions (with or without a bony component) from the fibular head. LCL injuries are best visualized in the axial and coronal plane at MRI examination (**Fig. 3**).[5,13,53]

Popliteus muscle and its tendon
Injuries to the popliteus muscle can be intra-articular (at the femoral insertion or at the level of the popliteal hiatus) or extra-articular (muscular or myotendinous portion) in nature, the latter being more frequent. An avulsion at the femoral attachment may appear as an irregular contour of its tendon at the level of the popliteal hiatus with surrounding edema. Partial tears of the myotendinous junction present with increased T2 signal at the level of the muscle-tendon junction on fat suppressed, fluid-sensitive sequences at MRI examination. Complete tendon tears may present as an interruption of the muscle belly appearing as a masslike lesion with surrounding edema.[13] Enlargement of the muscle belly or disruption of muscle fibers may be apparent. Only 8% of all popliteus injuries occur in an isolated fashion,[54] with isolated cases of muscle or tendon lesions

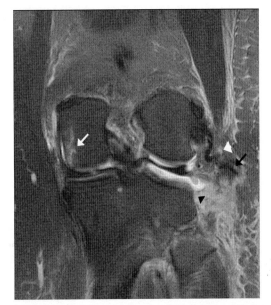

Fig. 3. Coronal proton density (PD) image with fat saturation (FS) of the knee in a patient after reduction of a knee dislocation shows a displaced arcuate fracture fragment (*black arrow*). Additionally, there is disruption of the midportion of the LCL (*white arrowhead*), avulsion of the lateral meniscotibial ligament (soft tissue Segond injury, *black arrowhead*), and a bone contusion at the peripheral aspect of the medial femoral condyle (*white arrow*).

reported in skiers,[55] football,[55–57] soccer,[58,59] rugby,[60] and polo players.[61] Lesions of the popliteus muscle are usually combined with injuries to other knee structures.[13] Brown and colleagues,[54] in their MRI analysis of popliteus injuries (n = 24), reported combined injuries in 92% of cases, with involvement of its muscular portion in 96% of patients. Associated injuries included ACL (17%) or PCL (29%) tears, combined medial (46%) or lateral (25%) meniscal injuries, and medial (8%) or lateral (4%) collateral ligament lesions. Bone bruises or fractures were reported in 33% of patients. Popliteus muscle injuries are best evaluated on the axial and coronal planes (**Fig. 4**), and diagnosis of abnormalities on MR imaging plays a fundamental role in the diagnosis of an injury to the popliteus muscle because of the difficulty in assessing this structure at arthroscopy.[53,62]

Popliteofibular ligament

Visualization and assessment of the popliteofibular ligament can be challenging on MRI. Standard imaging planes (coronal, sagittal, and axial) may depict the structure, but visualization is not always optimal because of its oblique orientation and the delicate nature of the structure; coronal and sagittal planes are in our practice the most useful planes for assessment (**Fig. 5**). Some advocate the use of a coronal oblique plane, oriented parallel to the direction of the popliteus tendon, with one study showing visualization of the popliteofibular tendon improving from 8% to 53% of the knees.[63] Another study compared coronal oblique fat-saturated T2 with isotropic three-dimensional water excitation double-echo steady state (WE-DESS) sequences. The latter sequence improved the identification of the popliteofibular ligament from 71% to 91% of cases.[64]

Injuries to the popliteofibular ligament consist of ligamentous disruption, avulsion from the fibular insertion, partial tearing, and intrasubstance degeneration in the form of signal alteration within the tendon.[53] Surgical reconstruction of a disrupted popliteofibular ligament has been found to be beneficial in patients with posterolateral external rotatory instability of the knee.[65]

Arcuate ligament

The variable presence and subtlety of the arcuate ligament makes assessment difficult[24,66] and makes recognizing injuries of the arcuate ligament complex a challenging proposition. The anatomy of the arcuate ligament is debated[39] and can be considered a thickening of the posterolateral capsule. On sagittal images, the arcuate ligament is best identified on images on which the popliteus tendon and fibular tip are both visualized. The straight limb of the arcuate can be found superficial to the popliteus tendon as a delicate linear low-signal structure attaching to the fibular tip (**Fig. 6**). Dedicated imaging of the PLC in the coronal oblique plane may significantly improve visualization of the arcuate ligament, with an increase from 10% to 46% reported by Yu and colleagues[63] compared with standard coronal imaging.

Increased signal at the level of the posterolateral capsule on fat-saturated fluid-sensitive images should raise concern for capsular disruption and the possibility of associated injury or tear of the arcuate ligament (**Fig. 7**).[53] Injury to the posterolateral capsule has been suggested as one reason why PLC injuries can occasionally present without a significant knee joint effusion.[67] Baker and coworkers[68] operated on 13 patients with acute PCL injuries and posterolateral instability of the knee, identifying tears of the arcuate ligament complex in all 13. Their results suggest that surgical repair of the arcuate ligament complex improves patient outcome in PCL injuries with posterolateral instability,[68] emphasizing the importance of evaluating this structure on preoperative imaging.

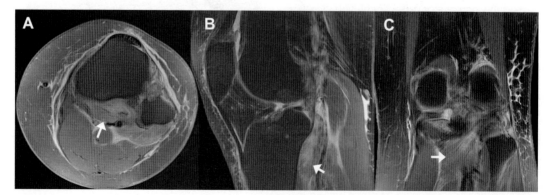

Fig. 4. Axial (*A*), sagittal (*B*), and coronal (*C*) PD FS images show a strain (grade II lesion) at the level of the myotendinous junction of popliteus (*white arrows*) and extensive circumferential soft tissue edema.

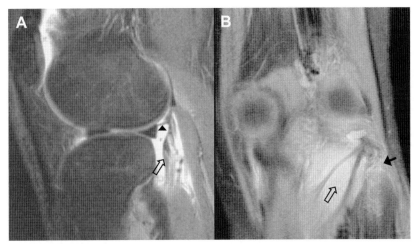

Fig. 5. Sagittal (*A*) and coronal (*B*) T2 FS images show diffuse edema at the level of the PLC and surrounding the myotendinous junction of popliteus compatible with a high-grade strain (*open arrows*). A partial tear of the popliteofibular ligament is present (*black arrow*). The posterosuperior popliteomeniscal fascicle is intact (*black arrowhead*).

Fabellofibular ligament

The fabellofibular ligament is best visualized on MRI in the coronal plane and is located posteriorly to the lateral collateral ligament and at the far posterior tip of the fibular styloid.[12] Yu and colleagues[63] compared visualization of the fabellofibular ligament in the coronal oblique plane with the standard coronal plane imaging and reported an increase in visualization from 34% to 48% on coronal oblique images. The fabellofibular ligament was seen in only 4% in the sagittal plane. Injuries of the fabellofibular ligament include degeneration, tearing and avulsion from the fibular tip (see **Fig. 7**). Avulsion of the fabellofibular ligament can be associated with an avulsive injury of the direct arm of the short head of the biceps femoris tendon.[5,14,53] The inferior lateral genicular artery is a branch of the popliteal artery, which can be used as an anatomic landmark in evaluating the fabellofibular ligament, as it passes around the posterior joint capsule laterally, running anterior to the fabellofibular ligament and posterior to the popliteofibular ligament.[39]

Soft tissue Segond injury (lateral meniscotibial capsular injury)

The soft tissue Segond injury is a soft-tissue avulsion injury described by LaPrade and colleagues,[12]

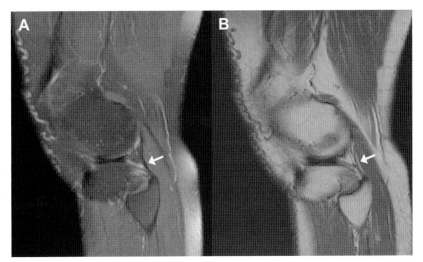

Fig. 6. Sagittal proton density images with (*A*) and without fat saturation (*B*) show an intact arcuate ligament (lateral limb) (*arrows*).

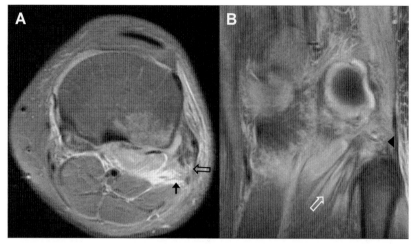

Fig. 7. Axial (*A*) and coronal (*B*) PD FS images show edema in the expected location of the arcuate (*black arrow*) and fabellofibular (*open black arrow and black arrowhead*) ligaments, without clearly identified ligaments suggesting injury of these structures. There is also high T2 signal within the muscle belly and around the myotendinous junction of the popliteus compatible with a grade II strain (*open white arrow*).

consisting of disruption of the conjoined tibial attachment of the anterior arm of the short head of the biceps femoris muscle and the meniscotibial portion of the midthird lateral capsular ligament, with associated proximal retraction or thickening (see **Fig. 3**; **Fig. 8**).

Myotendinous injuries of the lateral head of gastrocnemius

The proximal myotendinous portion of the lateral gastrocnemius muscle is commonly not included in the classic list of the specific anatomic structures composing the PLC.[8] However, different factors determine its participation in knee stability provided by the posterolateral corner structures. Based on several anatomic relationships, it is clear

that this structure serves as an important secondary dynamic stabilizer of the PLC. This is supported by its involvement in accommodating the fabella (or its cartilaginous equivalent) with its attachment to the fabellofibular ligament. Furthermore, the lateral gastrocnemius reinforces the meniscofemoral capsule and is firmly attached to the lateral femoral condyle at the level of the supracondylar process. Clinically, the stabilizing role of the lateral gastrocnemius is recognized in PLC reconstruction, including advancement procedures.[4,69]

Injuries to the gastrocnemius muscle usually involve the distal myotendinous junction of the medial gastrocnemius (tennis leg).[70] Although primary injuries of the lateral gastrocnemius are rare, the lateral gastrocnemius should be evaluated

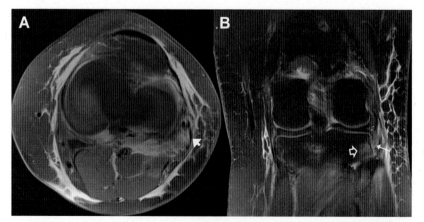

Fig. 8. Axial (*A*) and coronal (*B*) PD FS images show a distal biceps femoris tendon injury (*short white arrow*) and an avulsion of the lateral meniscotibial ligament (*white arrow*) with subjacent bone marrow edema (*open white arrow*), falling in the spectrum of a soft tissue Segond injury.

carefully in cases of posterolateral corner injury because of the secondary stabilizing role of this structure. The lateral gastrocnemius is usually best seen on sagittal images.[12,15,53]

Osseous Alterations Associated with PLC Injuries

Arcuate fracture

This injury is an avulsion fracture at the level of the fibular head (**Fig. 9**). If a pattern of diffuse fibular head edema is present at MRI examination, the injury usually involves the distal lateral collateral ligament insertion and the distal insertion of the biceps femoris tendon to the fibula (LCL and BFT distally form the conjoint tendon). When edema is localized at the medial aspect of the fibular head, the arcuate ligament or popliteofibular insertions are usually involved. Plain films (arcuate sign) and computed tomography (CT) show the bony avulsion at the fibular tip; MRI has a role in depicting ligamentous injuries.[15,71,72] The authors advocate the presence of fibular edema at the level of the fibular head on MRI as a diagnostic clue. In their MRI evaluation of 19 knees presenting with an arcuate sign at conventional radiographic examination, Juhng and colleagues,[71] reported a tear of the posterolateral capsule in 67% of the cases and an injury to the cruciate ligaments in 89% (16 knees) of the cases: 9 knees with a combined ACL and PCL injury, 4 knees with isolated ACL, and 3 knees with isolated PCL injuries. A bone bruise or fracture was present in all cases, with 50% showing an anteromedial femoral condyle bone bruise and 28% showing the same feature at the anteromedial tibia. A meniscal tear was present on the medial or lateral side in 28% and 22% of the cases, respectively. An injury of

the popliteus muscle was evident in 33% of the cases, and all patients had a joint effusion. Huang and coworkers,[72] in their MRI evaluation of 13 knees presenting with an arcuate sign on plain film, found that in 85% of the patients the avulsed bony fragment from the fibula originated either from the attachment of the popliteofibular ligament or the attachment of the popliteofibular, arcuate, and fabellofibular ligaments at the posterosuperior aspect of the fibular styloid process. All patients presented with both PCL and medial collateral ligament (MCL) injury, but no ACL injuries were reported. A popliteus tendon tear was present only in one case, and 77% of the cases had an injury to the arcuate ligament complex, although integrity of the arcuate, popliteofibular, and fabellofibular ligaments could not be fully assessed. The medial meniscus was injured in 38% of the knees and the lateral meniscus in 46%, with arthroscopic confirmation. Bone marrow edema was present in 38% of the patients (anterior lateral tibial plateau, medial tibial plateau, lateral femoral condyle, medial femoral condyle, patella, posterior tibial plateau and fibular head).[72]

Segond fracture

First described in 1879 by Dr Segond,[73] this injury is classically described as a bony avulsion at the tibial attachment of the midthird lateral capsular ligament (**Fig. 10**).[10,12,14,74,75] The midthird lateral capsular ligament is a thickening of the lateral joint capsule that attaches to the lateral femoral condyle and lateral tibia with capsular attachments to the lateral meniscus. It is the lateral equivalent of the deep medial collateral ligament.[21] Its tibial attachment is just posterior to Gerdy's tubercle.[14] The avulsion may also involve the anterior arm of the short head of the biceps

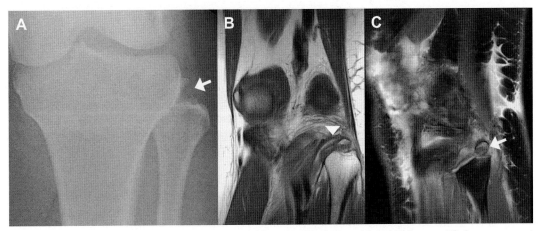

Fig. 9. Frontal radiograph (*A*) coronal PD weighted (*B*) and sagittal T2-weighted FS images (*C*) show an arcuate avulsion fracture (*white arrows*) displaced toward the popliteofibular ligament (*white arrowhead*).

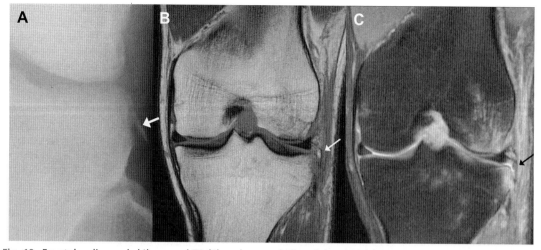

Fig. 10. Frontal radiograph (*A*) coronal T1 (*B*) and coronal T2-weighted FS (*C*) images show a displaced Segond fracture (*white and black arrows*) with surrounding soft tissue and marrow edema.

femoris that joins the midthird lateral capsular ligament at the tibial insertion. Different studies found its association with ACL injuries, meniscal tears, and damage to the PLC structures. Dietz and colleagues,[76] in a study on 20 knees, reported a concomitant ACL injury (confirmed at arthroscopy or physical examination) in 75% of the cases, whereas Goldman and colleagues,[77] in their study on 9 knees, reported an associated ACL injury in 100% of their patients with arthrographic and surgical confirmation. Campos and colleagues[78] suggested the involvement of the iliotibial band and the anterior oblique band of the lateral collateral ligament as important factors in the pathogenesis of the Segond fracture. In their patient population (n = 17) they reported an association with ACL injuries (94%), bone

contusions (82%), meniscal tears (53%), PLC injuries (35%), MCL tears (35%), and popliteus tendon injuries (23%).

Anteromedial femoral bone bruise

The presence of a bone bruise in the anterior aspect of the medial femoral condyle on MRI has been associated with PLC knee injuries in the literature (**Fig. 11**). Ross and colleagues[67] reported a bone contusion in the anterior aspect of the medial femoral condyle in 100% of the knees presenting with a complete lateral complex injury (grade III), although their study was small, only containing 6 patients. Varus force and knee hyperextension are commonly involved, both considered common mechanisms of PLC injuries. Therefore, if an anteromedial femoral condylar bone bruise is present

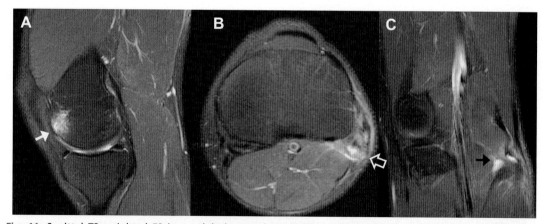

Fig. 11. Sagittal T2-weighted FS image (*A*) shows edema in the anteromedial aspect of the medial femoral condyle (*white arrow*). Axial (*B*) and coronal (*C*) PD FS images from the same patient show edema in the posterolateral corner with high-grade tear of the LCL at the fibular attachment (*open white arrow*), and a high-grade injury of the plantaris muscle (*black arrow*).

Components of the *Posterolateral Corner Complex*	Suggested Imaging Planes for MR Visualization
Lateral collateral ligament	Axial and coronal
Lateral coronary ligament	Coronal
Arcuate ligament	Sagittal
Popliteus myotendinous unit	Axial
Popliteofibular ligament	Coronal, *coronal oblique*[a] and sagittal
Fabellofibular ligament	Coronal and *coronal oblique*[a]
Lateral joint capsule	Axial and coronal
[a] Dedicated imaging plane usually not included in routine MRI protocols.	

on MRI, it is a diagnostic clue that requires a careful evaluation of the PLC complex.

Avulsion of Gerdy's tubercle

The iliotibial band inserts into Gerdy's tubercle on the lateral tibia, and its avulsion can be seen in conjunction with PLC injuries. Isolated injuries of the iliotibial band are infrequent. Ross and colleagues,[67] reported an avulsed iliotibial band in 50% of the knees (6 knees) presenting with a PLC complex injury. Hayes and colleagues[79] developed a mechanism-based classification of complex knee injuries (100 cases) based on patterns of bone marrow edema and ligament injuries seen on MRI and recognized 10 patterns, with injuries based on pure varus force accounting for just 1% (medial tibia and femoral condyle "coup-contrecoup" impactions with ITB and LCL injuries).

This mechanism is rarely seen because varus positioning is normally associated with an internally rotated flexed knee,[79] and additional structures beyond the iliotibial band are usually involved, with concomitant ACL lesions commonly present.[13,80] In their evaluation of avulsion fractures of the lateral femoral condyle in children, Sferopoulos and colleagues[81] reported 2 cases of avulsive fracture of the Gerdy's tubercle. Both of these were sport-related injuries from a direct blow to the medial aspect of the knee while playing football. MRI (**Fig. 12**), CT, and plain radiographs are all able to demonstrate this injury.[81]

Fracture of tibial plateau rim (anterior aspect of the medial plateau)

Fractures of the peripheral anterior margin of the medial tibial plateau have been associated with PLC injuries, and their presence is a useful indicator to raise awareness of a potential PLC injury. Bennett and colleagues[82] evaluated 16 patients with clinically suspected posterolateral corner injuries using MRI and found a tibial plateau fracture in 35%; of these, 83% were at the level of the anterior rim of the medial tibial plateau.

POSTEROMEDIAL CORNER OF THE KNEE
Anatomy, Biomechanics, and Mechanism of Injuries to the PMC

In 1979, Warren and Marshall[9] introduced the concept of a three-layer approach in the evaluation of the medial supporting structures of the knee, dividing those structures in a *superficial layer (I)*, *intermediate layer (II)*, and *capsule proper (III)* (see **Fig. 2**). In their original description, the superficial layer consists of fascial extensions, made by the deep (crural) fascia that invests the sartorius muscle. Posteriorly, it consists of a thin fascial sheet overlying the 2 heads of the gastrocnemius and the popliteal fossa structures. Serving as a support structure to muscle bellies and neurovascular structures in the popliteal region, it may be reinforced by fascial fibers originating from the sartorius, vastus medialis, and fascia at the level of the popliteal fossa. Anteriorly, layer I connects

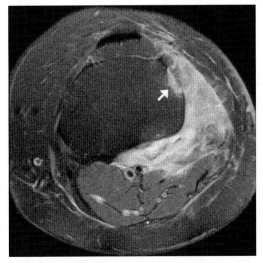

Fig. 12. Axial T2 FS image shows bone marrow edema localized at the level of Gerdy's tubercle (*white arrow*) consistent with an avulsive injury, with extensive edema around the PLC and lateral aspect of the knee.

to layer II to form the medial patellar retinaculum. A fatty tissue layer lies between the superficial layer and the structures deep to it. Anteriorly and distally, the superficial layer joins the tibial periosteum at the level of the sartorius muscle insertion. The gracilis and semitendinosus muscles can be identified more distally as distinct structures with layer I lying superficial and layer II deep to them. The intermediate layer consists of the fibers of the MCL, also called the superficial medial collateral ligament or tibial collateral ligament. At the level of the posteromedial aspect of the knee, the intermediate layer (II) joins the capsule proper (III) and the tendon sheath of the semimembranosus muscle, forming the posteromedial corner pouch surrounding the medial femoral condyle (see **Fig. 2**).[9,83–85] The capsule proper, the deepest of the 3 layers, attaches to the medial meniscus and to the articular margins. Anatomic descriptions of the medial side of the knee describe the MCL as having an anterior vertical component and a posterior oblique component (see **Fig. 1**).[86] The vertical anterior portion measures 1.5 cm in width and 10–11 cm in length, attaching proximally to the medial femoral epicondyle about 5 cm above the joint line, and attaching distally to the medial aspect of the tibial metadiaphysis around 6–7 cm below the joint line. Its distal attachment lies deep to the semitendinosus and gracilis tendons.[83,85,87,88] The intermediate layer (II) and the deeper capsule proper (III) unite posteriorly with the anterior margin of the superficial MCL and the PMC of the knee. The posterior portion of the MCL originates at the proximal attachment of the medial collateral ligament and extends distally in a posterior oblique fashion (at 25° with respect to the anterior vertical portion) to reach the posteromedial aspect of the knee, forming an envelope about the semimembranosus tendon.[88] The posterior oblique portion of the MCL gained its own discrete anatomic consideration in an article from Hughston and Eilers[89] describing the posterior oblique ligament (POL), introducing the concept of the posteromedial corner. To be more specific, the POL has its proximal origin at the adductor tubercle of the medial femoral condyle while the MCL proper (anterior portion) originates around 1 cm anterior and distal to it. The POL also attaches to the medial meniscus at the posteromedial corner of the knee while the superficial MCL does not. The POL comprises 3 arms: the central or tibial arm, attaching to the medial meniscus; the superior or capsular arm, attaching to the posterior joint capsule and proximal portion of the oblique popliteal ligament; and a distal arm, attaching both to the sheath of the semimembranosus tendon and distally to the tibial insertion of the semimembranosus.[89] The MCL

includes a deep thickened component called the deep medial collateral ligament (or deep medial capsular ligament), divided into a meniscofemoral component proximally and a meniscotibial component distally. A bursa separates the deep and superficial fibers of the MCL.

The anatomic structures that comprise the PMC of the knee and participate in its function as a restraint to anteromedial rotary instability (AMRI) are the *distal semimembranosus myotendinous complex*, the *POL*, the *medial portion of the oblique popliteal ligament* (OPL), the *meniscotibial ligament* (distal portion of the deep MCL), and the *posterior horn of the medial meniscus*.[90,91]

The distal semimembranosus myotendinous complex consists of 5 distal insertional arms dividing at the level of the joint line: the direct (principal), capsular, anterior (tibial or reflected), inferior (popliteal) arms, and the OPL expansion.[92] The direct arm travels anteriorly and inserts just below the joint line at the tibial tubercle on the posterior aspect of the medial tibial condyle passing beneath the anterior arm. The anterior arm extends anteriorly, under the posterior oblique ligament to attach to the medial aspect of the proximal tibia just beneath the medial collateral ligament. The inferior arm travels more distally than the direct and anterior arms, passing beneath the POL and the MCL to attach just above the tibial attachment of the MCL. The capsular arm has a deep location and coalesces with the capsular portion of the oblique popliteal ligament. A sixth arm, inserting at the posterior third of the lateral meniscus, has been described in 43% of cases by Kim and colleagues.[93]

The OPL is a lateral extension of the semimembranosus tendon that surrounds the posteromedial joint capsule, extending in a superolateral oblique direction as the largest structure in the posterior knee. The OPL is therefore a component of both the PMC and PLC of the knee and contributes to the posterior joint stabilizers, forming part of the popliteal fossa (see **Fig. 1**; **Fig. 13**). LaPrade and colleagues[1] elegantly showed its anatomic relationships, describing it as a broad fascial band crossing the posterior aspect of the knee in an oblique direction. Medially, the OPL arises from the confluence of the lateral expansion of semimembranosus distally and the capsular arm of the POL proximally. Laterally, the OPL attaches to an osseous or cartilaginous fabella, to the meniscofemoral portion of the posterolateral joint capsule and the plantaris muscle. There is also a fibrous attachment to the lateral aspect of the PCL facet.

Flandry and Perry[94] have described the biomechanics of the medial supporting structures of

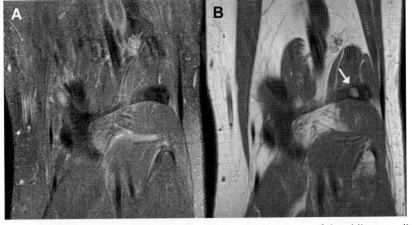

Fig. 13. Coronal FS PD (*A*) and non FS PD (*B*) images show the normal anatomy of the oblique popliteal ligament. Note its attachment to the fabella at the posterolateral aspect of the knee (*arrow*).

the knee with emphasis to the posteromedial corner. With its 5 arms attaching to bone, capsule, medial meniscus, ligaments, and tendon sheaths, the semimembranosus muscle acts as the main dynamic stabilizer of the PMC. If a structure of the PMC fails, the semimembranosus muscle activates itself, eventually developing intrinsic muscle spasm and articular instability. When the semimembranosus muscle contracts, flexion and internal rotation occur, increasing tension in the adjacent ligaments and contributing to joint stability. The semimembranosus also produces traction on the posterior horn of the medial meniscus, reducing the incidence of meniscal injuries caused by compression of the medial femoral condyle. The semimembranosus muscle causes tension on the oblique popliteal ligament and therefore participates in lateral capsular stability. The natural tendency of the POL is to be lax when the knee is flexed and tight when the knee extends. The above mechanism is therefore extremely important, because most knee injuries occur during knee flexion.[40,41] With respect to patterns of injury, patients with symptomatic AMRI almost always have involvement of the POL (99%), with the injury to the semimembranosus (70%) and peripheral meniscal detachment (30%) occurring less frequently.[90] When a grade III MCL injury is present, in conjunction with an anterior cruciate ligament (ACL) injury and medial meniscal tear, a specific pattern of injury has been described, the so-called *O'Donoghue's unhappy triad*.[95] The latter pattern of injury may be associated with PMC injuries. There is a strong association between PMC and ACL injuries,[90] and if those lesions do not occur together, usually an intact PMC compensates for the ACL deficiency to maintain stability. Combined PCL and MCL

injuries are uncommon, and likewise a combination of PCL and lateral support structure injury is rare. Combined ACL-PCL injuries with medial supporting structure involvement occur with equal or greater frequency than on the contralateral side.[6,96–99] Usually an isolated MCL injury is treated conservatively, but the presence of a simultaneous posteromedial corner injury may require surgical intervention because of the potential for AMRI. An accurate evaluation of the PMC at imaging is imperative to guide the clinical and surgical management.

INJURIES TO THE PMC
Soft-tissue Injuries of the PMC

Semimembranosus insertion injuries
Injuries to the distal semimembranosus insertion occur in up to 70% of posteromedial corner injuries[90] and include avulsion fracture at its tibial attachment, partial or complete tendon tears, and tendinosis (**Figs. 14** and **15**). Chan and colleagues[100] reviewed the radiographs and MRI studies of 10 patients with posteromedial tibial plateau injuries, including 5 fractures of the posteromedial tibial plateau and 5 distal semimembranosus insertional injuries, and found an ACL tear in 100% of patients.

Avulsion fractures usually occur at the insertion of the direct arm and may appear as a bone bruise with a fracture line on MRI examination. Partial tears and strains are common and usually involve the capsular arm. At MRI, partial tears and strains manifest as altered signal within an otherwise intact tendon. Complete tears of the semimembranosus, although uncommon, present as a discontinuity of the tendon itself, and are best seen on axial and sagittal images. Tendinosis caused by

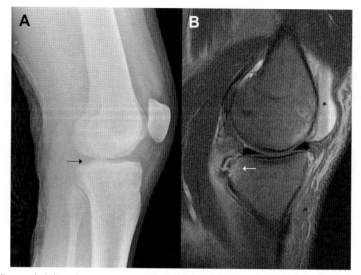

Fig. 14. Lateral radiograph (*A*) and sagittal T2-weighted MR with fat saturation (*B*) show an insertional avulsion injury of the distal semimembranosus tendon, involving both the capsular and direct arms. Note the small bony avulsed fragment (*black arrow*) and resulting bone marrow edema (*white arrow*). A lipohemarthrosis is also evident as a sequela of knee trauma (*asterisk*).

chronic stress is seen as thickening of the tendon insertion. If the capsular arm of the semimembranosus tendon is involved, signal alteration with eventual thickening may be seen at the level of the posterior medial capsular region, contiguous with the POL, and better seen on axial images.[91] The presence of fluid distending the joint capsule may facilitate evaluation of these deep structures. If fluid is absent, the capsular arm appears as a flat structure on the posterior aspect of the medial tibial plateau, indistinguishable from the nearby direct arm, in continuity anteriorly with the anterior arm and posteriorly with the OPL. The anterior arm is better seen on peripheral medial sagittal images, curving anteriorly with an almost horizontal course,

and on coronal images as a round hypointense structure adjacent to the medial tibia, passing under the MCL. The direct arm is usually not visible on MRI. The inferior arm may be seen anteriorly as a low signal intensity structure that extends below the joint line.[92]

Posterior oblique ligament (POL) injuries

As previously mentioned, POL injuries have been found in 99% of surgically treated patients presenting with medial-sided knee injuries and AMRI.[90] Wijdicks and colleagues[101] in their biomechanic cadaveric study on 24 knees, directly evaluated the changes in tensile forces of the POL in an injury state and its relation to the MCL. They applied

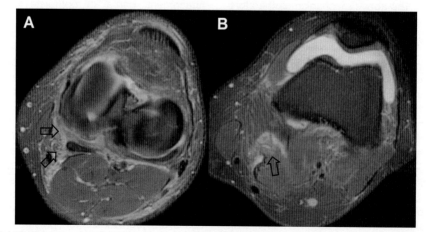

Fig. 15. Axial T2 FS images (*A, B*) show prominent edema within the myotendinous junction of the distal semimembranosus (*black open arrows*) consistent with a strain.

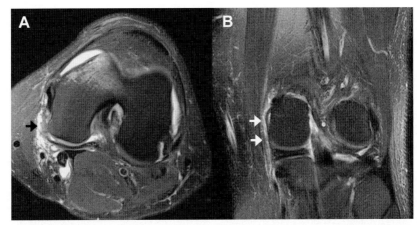

Fig. 16. Axial PD FS image (*A*) shows an irregular POL with surrounding edema consistent with disruption (*black arrow*). Coronal PD FS image (*B*) from a different patient shows an acute on chronic POL injury characterized by thickening of the ligament proximally and partial thickness tearing at femoral attachment with surrounding edema (*white arrows*).

a valgus and external rotation moment to the knee after sectioning the MCL (superficial and deep) and found a significant load increase to the POL compared with a knee with an intact MCL condition. This finding reinforces the concept that in cases of reconstruction or surgical repair, all injured medial knee structures should be restored to reproduce the force relationships between them. Petersen and colleagues,[102] in another kinematic cadaveric study on 10 knees, addressed the importance of the POL as a restraint to posterior tibial translation in PCL-deficient knees, therefore emphasizing the need to specifically evaluate it in cases of combined injuries to PMC structures and the PCL. House and colleagues,[91] recommended

applying the same grading system used for medial collateral ligament injuries to POL injuries (grade I, microscopic tear; grade II, partial tear; grade III, complete tear). POL injuries comprise sprains, partial tears, and complete tears, and are best visualized on axial and coronal planes (**Fig. 16**).

Medial meniscocapsular lesions

The posterior third of the medial meniscus contributes to the dynamic stabilizing function of the PMC because of its intimate anatomic relations with the deep structures, which act as a restraint to posterior translation of the medial femoral condyle on the tibia. Its firm attachment to the tibia is important and guaranteed in part by the meniscotibial portion

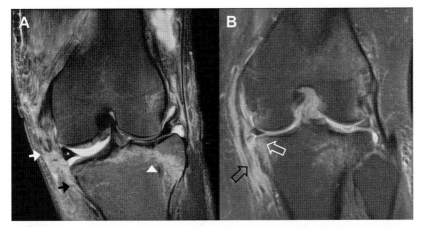

Fig. 17. Coronal PD FS image (*A*) shows disruption of the MCL at the distal midportion (*white arrow*) with associated injury of the meniscotibial fibers of the deep MCL (*black arrow*) and a floating medial meniscus (*asterisk*). An osteochondral impaction fracture of the lateral tibial plateau is also present (*white arrowhead*). Coronal PD FS image (*B*) from a different patient shows a meniscotibial avulsion fracture (Reverse Segond fracture) (*open white arrow*) and a disrupted MCL distally (*open black arrow*).

Components of the *Posteromedial Corner Complex*	Suggested Imaging Planes for MRI Visualization
Distal semimembranosus myotendinous complex	Sagittal and axial
POL	Axial
OPL	Axial and sagittal
Meniscotibial ligament	Coronal
Posterior horn of medial meniscus	Sagittal

of the deep MCL. Meniscal instability may put the PMC under stress, therefore making it more prone to injury.[91] MRI can detect injuries to both the meniscotibial and meniscofemoral portions of the deep MCL, which can be seen as disruption, thickening, or bony avulsion. When a bony avulsion is appreciated at the level of the meniscotibial ligament insertion, the specific lesion is called a *reverse Segond fracture* (**Fig. 17**), which is associated with posterior cruciate ligament rupture.[66,103]

Injuries to the oblique popliteal ligament (OPL)

The OPL is the largest structure along the posterior aspect of the knee[1] (see **Figs. 1** and **13**), and its anatomic contribution to the PMC complex has been established. Morgan and colleagues[104] did an in vitro cadaveric study on 20 knees and defined the role of the OPL as the primary ligamentous restraint to knee hyperextension, describing its participation in genu recurvatum (knee hyperextension) development. The OPL should therefore be carefully assessed on MRI when evaluating the posteromedial corner of the knee.[1,104] On axial and sagittal planes, the OPL appears as a thin deep structure of low signal intensity, indistinguishable in most cases from the posterior capsule, but continuous with the semimembranosus tendon.[92] Injuries to the OPL may manifest as irregularity of this fascialike structure, with encircling edema in the deep posteromedial aspect of the knee. On axial imaging, this finding is appreciable on fluid-sensitive sequences at the level of the joint line.

SUMMARY

The posterolateral and posteromedial corners of the knee represent challenging anatomic regions in musculoskeletal imaging. Plain films and CT are helpful in the assessment of osseous involvement. However, MRI is the imaging modality of choice because of its intrinsic ability to evaluate soft tissue structures, although ultrasound scan can be used as a complementary technique. High field strength MRI is becoming the standard in high-end musculoskeletal imaging services and will lead to future technologic advances that will enhance the visualization of even the most delicate anatomic components. The ability of the

musculoskeletal radiologist to see more, demands a deeper understanding of complex anatomy and specific injury patterns, particularly in those anatomic areas in which anatomy does not follow classical imaging planes and is confined in a narrow space. The posterolateral and posteromedial corner of the knee fall into this category. The underestimation and misinterpretation of reporting injuries in these specific areas can result in a poor patient outcome. For example, chronic posterolateral instability for untreated PLC injuries[4,5] and valgus instability for PMC deficiencies[6] can cause reconstruction of the central supporting structures to fail long term. Therefore, a full appreciation of PMC and PLC structures is of primary importance in the MRI evaluation of the knee to generate a relevant, pertinent, and exhaustive report that will guide the clinical or surgical management of these patients and improve patient outcome.

REFERENCES

1. LaPrade RF, Morgan PM, Wentorf FA, et al. The anatomy of the posterior aspect of the knee. An anatomic study. J Bone Joint Surg Am 2007; 89(4):758–64.
2. Hughston JC, Andrews JR, Cross MJ, et al. Classification of knee ligament instabilities. Part I. The medial compartment and cruciate ligaments. J Bone Joint Surg Am 1976;58(2):159–72.
3. Hughston JC, Andrews JR, Cross MJ, et al. Classification of knee ligament instabilities. Part II. The lateral compartment. J Bone Joint Surg Am 1976; 58(2):173–9.
4. Hughston JC, Jacobson KE. Chronic posterolateral rotatory instability of the knee. J Bone Joint Surg Am 1985;67(3):351–9.
5. Pacholke DA, Helms CA. MRI of the posterolateral corner injury: a concise review. J Magn Reson Imaging 2007;26(2):250–5.
6. Tibor LM, Marchant MH Jr, Taylor DC, et al. Management of medial-sided knee injuries, part 2: posteromedial corner. Am J Sports Med 2011; 39(6):1332–40.
7. Barker RP, Lee JC, Healy JC. Normal sonographic anatomy of the posterolateral corner of the knee. AJR Am J Roentgenol 2009;192(1):73–9.

8. Seebacher JR, Inglis AE, Marshall JL, et al. The structure of the posterolateral aspect of the knee. J Bone Joint Surg Am 1982;64(4):536–41.

9. Warren LF, Marshall JL. The supporting structures and layers on the medial side of the knee: an anatomical analysis. J Bone Joint Surg Am 1979; 61(1):56–62.

10. Terry GC, LaPrade RF. The posterolateral aspect of the knee. Anatomy and surgical approach. Am J Sports Med 1996;24(6):732–9.

11. Veltri DM, Warren RF. Anatomy, biomechanics, and physical findings in posterolateral knee instability. Clin Sports Med 1994;13(3):599–614.

12. LaPrade RF, Gilbert TJ, Bollom TS, et al. The magnetic resonance imaging appearance of individual structures of the posterolateral knee. A prospective study of normal knees and knees with surgically verified grade III injuries. Am J Sports Med 2000;28(2):191–9.

13. Recondo JA, Salvador E, Villanua JA, et al. Lateral stabilizing structures of the knee: functional anatomy and injuries assessed with MR imaging. Radiographics 2000;20(Spec No):S91–102.

14. Haims AH, Medvecky MJ, Pavlovich R Jr, et al. MR imaging of the anatomy of and injuries to the lateral and posterolateral aspects of the knee. AJR Am J Roentgenol 2003;180(3):647–53.

15. Harish S, O'Donnell P, Connell D, et al. Imaging of the posterolateral corner of the knee. Clin Radiol 2006;61(6):457–66.

16. Malone WJ, Koulouris G. MRI of the posterolateral corner of the knee: normal appearance and patterns of injury. Semin Musculoskelet Radiol 2006;10(3):220–8.

17. Bolog N, Hodler J. MR imaging of the posterolateral corner of the knee. Skeletal Radiol 2007; 36(8):715–28.

18. De Maeseneer M, Shahabpour M, Vanderdood K, et al. Posterolateral supporting structures of the knee: findings on anatomic dissection, anatomic slices and MR images. Eur Radiol 2001;11(11): 2170–7.

19. Sekiya JK, Swaringen JC, Wojtys EM, et al. Diagnostic ultrasound evaluation of posterolateral corner knee injuries. Arthroscopy 2010;26(4):494–9.

20. Davies H, Unwin A, Aichroth P. The posterolateral corner of the knee. Anatomy, biomechanics and management of injuries. Injury 2004;35(1):68–75.

21. LaPrade RF. Posterolateral knee injuries: anatomy, evaluation and treatment. New York: Thieme; 2006.

22. El-Khoury GY, Usta HY, Berger RA. Meniscotibial (coronary) ligament tears. Skeletal Radiol 1984; 11(3):191–6.

23. Bikkina RS, Tujo CA, Schraner AB, et al. The "floating" meniscus: MRI in knee trauma and implications for surgery. AJR Am J Roentgenol 2005; 184(1):200–4.

24. Munshi M, Pretterklieber ML, Kwak S, et al. MR imaging, MR arthrography, and specimen correlation of the posterolateral corner of the knee: an anatomic study. AJR Am J Roentgenol 2003; 180(4):1095–101.

25. Sudasna S, Harnsiriwattanagit K. The ligamentous structures of the posterolateral aspect of the knee. Bull Hosp Jt Dis Orthop Inst 1990;50(1): 35–40.

26. Watanabe Y, Moriya H, Takahashi K, et al. Functional anatomy of the posterolateral structures of the knee. Arthroscopy 1993;9(1):57–62.

27. Peduto AJ, Nguyen A, Trudell DJ, et al. Popliteomeniscal fascicles: anatomic considerations using MR arthrography in cadavers. AJR Am J Roentgenol 2008;190(2):442–8.

28. Maynard MJ, Deng X, Wickiewicz TL, et al. The popliteofibular ligament. Rediscovery of a key element in posterolateral stability. Am J Sports Med 1996;24(3):311–6.

29. Shahane SA, Ibbotson C, Strachan R, et al. The popliteofibular ligament. An anatomical study of the posterolateral corner of the knee. J Bone Joint Surg Br 1999;81(4):636–42.

30. Wadia FD, Pimple M, Gajjar SM, et al. An anatomic study of the popliteofibular ligament. Int Orthop 2003;27(3):172–4.

31. McCarthy M, Camarda L, Wijdicks CA, et al. Anatomic posterolateral knee reconstructions require a popliteofibular ligament reconstruction through a tibial tunnel. Am J Sports Med 2010; 38(8):1674–81.

32. Diamantopoulos A, Tokis A, Tzurbakis M, et al. The posterolateral corner of the knee: evaluation under microsurgical dissection. Arthroscopy 2005;21(7): 826–33.

33. LaPrade RF, Terry GC. Injuries to the posterolateral aspect of the knee. Association of anatomic injury patterns with clinical instability. Am J Sports Med 1997;25(4):433–8.

34. LaPrade RF, Resig S, Wentorf F, et al. The effects of grade III posterolateral knee complex injuries on anterior cruciate ligament graft force. A biomechanical analysis. Am J Sports Med 1999;27(4): 469–75.

35. Covey DC. Injuries of the posterolateral corner of the knee. J Bone Joint Surg Am 2001;83-A(1): 106–18.

36. Fanelli GC, Larson RV. Practical management of posterolateral instability of the knee. Arthroscopy 2002;18(2 Suppl 1):1–8.

37. LaPrade RF, Bollom TS, Wentorf FA, et al. Mechanical properties of the posterolateral structures of the knee. Am J Sports Med 2005;33(9):1386–91.

38. Stannard JP, Brown SL, Farris RC, et al. The posterolateral corner of the knee: repair versus reconstruction. Am J Sports Med 2005;33(6):881–8.

39. Moorman CT 3rd, LaPrade RF. Anatomy and biomechanics of the posterolateral corner of the knee. J Knee Surg 2005;18(2):137–45.

40. Resnick D, Kang HS, Petterklieber ML. Internal derangements of joints. 2nd edition. Philadelphia: Saunders Elsevier; 2007.

41. DeLee JC, Drez JD, Miller MD. Orthopaedic sports medicine: principles and practice. 3rd edition. Philadelphia: Saunders Elsevier; 2009.

42. Malone WJ, Verde F, Weiss D, et al. MR imaging of knee instability. Magn Reson Imaging Clin N Am 2009;17(4):697–724, vi–vii.

43. Fanelli GC, Edson CJ. Posterior cruciate ligament injuries in trauma patients: part II. Arthroscopy 1995;11(5):526–9.

44. Baker CL Jr, Norwood LA, Hughston JC. Acute posterolateral rotatory instability of the knee. J Bone Joint Surg Am 1983;65(5):614–8.

45. Fanelli GC, Orcutt DR, Edson CJ. The multiple-ligament injured knee: evaluation, treatment, and results. Arthroscopy 2005;21(4):471–86.

46. O'Brien SJ, Warren RF, Pavlov H, et al. Reconstruction of the chronically insufficient anterior cruciate ligament with the central third of the patellar ligament. J Bone Joint Surg Am 1991;73(2):278–86.

47. Chen FS, Rokito AS, Pitman MI. Acute and chronic posterolateral rotatory instability of the knee. J Am Acad Orthop Surg 2000;8(2):97–110.

48. Harner CD, Vogrin TM, Hoher J, et al. Biomechanical analysis of a posterior cruciate ligament reconstruction. Deficiency of the posterolateral structures as a cause of graft failure. Am J Sports Med 2000; 28(1):32–9.

49. Freeman RT, Duri ZA, Dowd GS. Combined chronic posterior cruciate and posterolateral corner ligamentous injuries: a comparison of posterior cruciate ligament reconstruction with and without reconstruction of the posterolateral corner. Knee 2002;9(4):309–12.

50. Nielsen S, Rasmussen O, Ovesen J, et al. Rotatory instability of cadaver knees after transection of collateral ligaments and capsule. Arch Orthop Trauma Surg 1984;103(3):165–9.

51. Grood ES, Stowers SF, Noyes FR. Limits of movement in the human knee. Effect of sectioning the posterior cruciate ligament and posterolateral structures. J Bone Joint Surg Am 1988;70(1):88–97.

52. Gollehon DL, Torzilli PA, Warren RF. The role of the posterolateral and cruciate ligaments in the stability of the human knee. A biomechanical study. J Bone Joint Surg Am 1987;69(2):233–42.

53. Vinson EN, Major NM, Helms CA. The posterolateral corner of the knee. AJR Am J Roentgenol 2008;190(2):449–58.

54. Brown TR, Quinn SF, Wensel JP, et al. Diagnosis of popliteus injuries with MR imaging. Skeletal Radiol 1995;24(7):511–4.

55. Gruel JB. Isolated avulsion of the popliteus tendon. Arthroscopy 1990;6(2):94–5.

56. Burstein DB, Fischer DA. Isolated rupture of the popliteus tendon in a professional athlete. Arthroscopy 1990;6(3):238–41.

57. Geissler WB, Corso SR, Caspari RB. Isolated rupture of the popliteus with posterior tibial nerve palsy. J Bone Joint Surg Br 1992;74(6):811–3.

58. Guha AR, Gorgees KA, Walker DI. Popliteus tendon rupture: a case report and review of the literature. Br J Sports Med 2003;37(4):358–60.

59. Conroy J, King D, Gibbon A. Isolated rupture of the popliteus tendon in a professional soccer player. Knee 2004;11(1):67–9.

60. Quinlan JF, Webb S, McDonald K, et al. Isolated popliteus rupture at the musculo-tendinous junction. J Knee Surg 2011;24(2):137–40.

61. Winge S, Phadke P. Isolated popliteus muscle rupture in polo players. Knee Surg Sports Traumatol Arthrosc 1996;4(2):89–91.

62. Bencardino JT, Rosenberg ZS, Brown RR, et al. Traumatic musculotendinous injuries of the knee: diagnosis with MR imaging. Radiographics 2000; 20(Spec No):S103–20.

63. Yu JS, Salonen DC, Hodler J, et al. Posterolateral aspect of the knee: improved MR imaging with a coronal oblique technique. Radiology 1996; 198(1):199–204.

64. Rajeswaran G, Lee JC, Healy JC. MRI of the popliteofibular ligament: isotropic 3D WE-DESS versus coronal oblique fat-suppressed T2W MRI. Skeletal Radiol 2007;36(12):1141–6.

65. Zhang H, Feng H, Hong L, et al. Popliteofibular ligament reconstruction for posterolateral external rotation instability of the knee. Knee Surg Sports Traumatol Arthrosc 2009;17(9):1070–7.

66. De Maeseneer M, Shahabpour M, Vanderdood K, et al. Medial meniscocapsular separation: MR imaging criteria and diagnostic pitfalls. Eur J Radiol 2002;41(3):242–52.

67. Ross G, Chapman AW, Newberg AR, et al. Magnetic resonance imaging for the evaluation of acute posterolateral complex injuries of the knee. Am J Sports Med 1997;25(4):444–8.

68. Baker CL Jr, Norwood LA, Hughston JC. Acute combined posterior cruciate and posterolateral instability of the knee. Am J Sports Med 1984; 12(3):204–8.

69. LaPrade RF, Ly TV, Wentorf FA, et al. The posterolateral attachments of the knee: a qualitative and quantitative morphologic analysis of the fibular collateral ligament, popliteus tendon, popliteofibular ligament, and lateral gastrocnemius tendon. Am J Sports Med 2003;31(6): 854–60.

70. Delgado GJ, Chung CB, Lektrakul N, et al. Tennis leg: clinical US study of 141 patients and anatomic

investigation of four cadavers with MR imaging and US. Radiology 2002;224(1):112–9.

71. Juhng SK, Lee JK, Choi SS, et al. MR evaluation of the "arcuate" sign of posterolateral knee instability. AJR Am J Roentgenol 2002;178(3):583–8.

72. Huang GS, Yu JS, Munshi M, et al. Avulsion fracture of the head of the fibula (the "arcuate" sign): MR imaging findings predictive of injuries to the posterolateral ligaments and posterior cruciate ligament. AJR Am J Roentgenol 2003;180(2):381–7.

73. Segond P. Recherches cliniques et expérimentales sur les épanchements sanguins du genou par entorse. 1879.

74. Woods GW, Stanley RF, Tullos HS. Lateral capsular sign: x-ray clue to a significant knee instability. Am J Sports Med 1979;7(1):27–33.

75. Weber WN, Neumann CH, Barakos JA, et al. Lateral tibial rim (Segond) fractures: MR imaging characteristics. Radiology 1991;180(3):731–4.

76. Dietz GW, Wilcox DM, Montgomery JB. Segond tibial condyle fracture: lateral capsular ligament avulsion. Radiology 1986;159(2):467–9.

77. Goldman AB, Pavlov H, Rubenstein D. The Segond fracture of the proximal tibia: a small avulsion that reflects major ligamentous damage. AJR Am J Roentgenol 1988;151(6):1163–7.

78. Campos JC, Chung CB, Lektrakul N, et al. Pathogenesis of the Segond fracture: anatomic and MR imaging evidence of an iliotibial tract or anterior oblique band avulsion. Radiology 2001;219(2):381–6.

79. Hayes CW, Brigido MK, Jamadar DA, et al. Mechanism-based pattern approach to classification of complex injuries of the knee depicted at MR imaging. Radiographics 2000;20(Spec No):S121–34.

80. Gottsegen CJ, Eyer BA, White EA, et al. Avulsion fractures of the knee: imaging findings and clinical significance. Radiographics 2008;28(6):1755–70.

81. Sferopoulos NK, Rafailidis D, Traios S, et al. Avulsion fractures of the lateral tibial condyle in children. Injury 2006;37(1):57–60.

82. Bennett DL, George MJ, El-Khoury GY, et al. Anterior rim tibial plateau fractures and posterolateral corner knee injury. Emerg Radiol 2003;10(2):76–83.

83. Daniel DM, Pedowitz RA, O'Connorr JJ, et al. Daniel's Knee Injuries: Ligament and Cartilage Structure, Function, Injury, and Repair. 2nd ed. Philadelphia: Lippincott Williams & Wilkin; 2003.

84. Ruiz ME, Erickson SJ. Medial and lateral supporting structures of the knee. Normal MR imaging anatomy and pathologic findings. Magn Reson Imaging Clin N Am 1994;2(3):381–99.

85. Loredo R, Hodler J, Pedowitz R, et al. Posteromedial corner of the knee: MR imaging with gross anatomic correlation. Skeletal Radiol 1999;28(6):305–11.

86. LaPrade RF, Engebretsen AH, Ly TV, et al. The anatomy of the medial part of the knee. J Bone Joint Surg Am 2007;89(9):2000–10.

87. Indelicato P. Injury to the medial capsuloligamentous complex. In: Feagin JA, editor. The crucial ligaments: diagnosis and treatment of ligamentous injuries about the knee. New York: Churchill Livingstone; 1994. p. 197–206.

88. Irizarry JM, Recht MP. MR imaging of the knee ligaments and the postoperative knee. Radiol Clin North Am 1997;35(1):45–76.

89. Hughston JC, Eilers AF. The role of the posterior oblique ligament in repairs of acute medial (collateral) ligament tears of the knee. J Bone Joint Surg Am 1973;55(5):923–40.

90. Sims WF, Jacobson KE. The posteromedial corner of the knee: medial-sided injury patterns revisited. Am J Sports Med 2004;32(2):337–45.

91. House CV, Connell DA, Saifuddin A. Posteromedial corner injuries of the knee. Clin Radiol 2007;62(6): 539–46.

92. Beltran J, Matityahu A, Hwang K, et al. The distal semimembranosus complex: normal MR anatomy, variants, biomechanics and pathology. Skeletal Radiol 2003;32(8):435–45.

93. Kim YC, Yoo WK, Chung IH, et al. Tendinous insertion of semimembranosus muscle into the lateral meniscus. Surg Radiol Anat 1997;19(6):365–9.

94. Flandry F, Perry CC. The anatomy and biomechanics of the posteromedial aspect of the knee. In: Fanelli GC, editor. Posterior cruciate ligament injuries. Heidelberg (Germany): Springer; 2000;47.

95. O'Donoghue DH. The unhappy triad: etiology, diagnosis and treatment. Am J Orthop 1964;6: 242–7 PASSIM.

96. Shelbourne KD, Carr DR. Combined anterior and posterior cruciate and medial collateral ligament injury: nonsurgical and delayed surgical treatment. Instr Course Lect 2003;52:413–8.

97. Harner CD, Waltrip RL, Bennett CH, et al. Surgical management of knee dislocations. J Bone Joint Surg Am 2004;86(2):262–73.

98. Kaeding CC, Pedroza AD, Parker RD, et al. Intra-articular findings in the reconstructed multiligament-injured knee. Arthroscopy 2005;21(4):424–30.

99. Halinen J, Lindahl J, Hirvensalo E, et al. Operative and nonoperative treatments of medial collateral ligament rupture with early anterior cruciate ligament reconstruction: a prospective randomized study. Am J Sports Med 2006;34(7):1134–40.

100. Chan KK, Resnick D, Goodwin D, et al. Posteromedial tibial plateau injury including avulsion fracture of the semimembranous tendon insertion site: ancillary sign of anterior cruciate ligament tear at MR imaging. Radiology 1999;211(3):754–8.

101. Wijdicks CA, Griffith CJ, LaPrade RF, et al. Medial knee injury: part 2, load sharing between the posterior oblique ligament and superficial medial collateral ligament. Am J Sports Med 2009;37(9): 1771–6.

102. Petersen W, Loerch S, Schanz S, et al. The role of the posterior oblique ligament in controlling posterior tibial translation in the posterior cruciate ligament-deficient knee. Am J Sports Med 2008;36(3):495–501.

103. Escobedo EM, Mills WJ, Hunter JC. The "reverse Segond" fracture: association with a tear of the posterior cruciate ligament and medial meniscus. AJR Am J Roentgenol 2002;178(4):979–83.

104. Morgan PM, LaPrade RF, Wentorf FA, et al. The role of the oblique popliteal ligament and other structures in preventing knee hyperextension. Am J Sports Med 2010;38(3):550–7.

Imaging of Cysts and Bursae About the Knee

Lynne S. Steinbach, MD[a],*, Kathryn J. Stevens, MD[b]

KEYWORDS

- Bursa • Ganglion cyst • Knee • Imaging • MRI • Cyst mimics

KEY POINTS

- Bursae are fluid-filled synovial lined masses, commonly found around the knee, but most do not communicate with the joint. Repetitive friction, communicating joint fluid, and synovial processes can all cause bursal distention. It is important to be familiar with the expected anatomic locations of bursae and not to confuse them with other pathologic abnormalities.
- Cysts and ganglia are fluid-filled or mucin-filled collections that are not lined with synovium. These cysts or ganglia may be an incidental finding, but can be secondary to underlying internal derangement, such as a meniscal tear or mucoid degeneration of the anterior cruciate ligament.
- Other synovial, vascular, hemorrhagic, and neoplastic lesions can mimic cysts around the knee joint. It is important to use the underlying criteria outlined in the article to distinguish them from each other.

Learning objectives

- Review bursal anatomy around the knee
- Identify imaging features of bursal fluid collections
- Differentiate between bursal fluid and other fluid collections and ganglia occurring around the knee
- Recognize imaging pitfalls and lesions mimicking cysts

INTRODUCTION

Cystic lesions around joints are a common clinical problem and are frequently seen on routine imaging examinations. Histologically, there are two types of cysts: ganglia and synovial cysts (bursae). Ganglia are benign cystic masses lined by a dense fibrous connective tissue capsule that contains internal viscous material. Synovial cysts or bursae are lined by synovial cells and also contain viscous fluid. Both ganglia and bursae have variable communication with the adjacent joint. Bursae are located between surfaces where there is friction and movement, often between different tissues (ie, tendon and bone). Both ganglia and synovial cysts may undergo hemorrhage. Because symptoms and therapy for para-articular cysts do not depend on the histologic composition of the cyst wall, their differentiation may be more of an academic interest than clinical importance. Sometimes ganglia can undergo the process of synovialization, which also makes the distinction less than perfect. However, bursae are seen in predictable locations, which make it easier to distinguish between these two fluid-filled structures with imaging.

The clinical presentation of a para-articular cyst depends on its location, size, mass effect, and relationship to surrounding structures. Para-articular cysts are often asymptomatic and may be

Funding Sources: None.
Conflict of Interest: None.
[a] University of California San Francisco, 505 Parnassus, Suite M392, San Francisco, CA 94143-0628, USA;
[b] Department of Radiology, Stanford University Medical Center, 300 Pasteur Drive, Grant Building Room S-062A, Stanford, CA 94305-5105, USA
* Corresponding author.
E-mail address: lynne.steinbach@ucsf.edu

Radiol Clin N Am 51 (2013) 433–454
http://dx.doi.org/10.1016/j.rcl.2012.10.005

incidentally seen on clinical inspection or imaging examinations.[1] Occasionally, they may cause pain, swelling, nerve compression, erosion, or joint impairment. In rare cases, the clinical presentation of a para-articular cyst may be misleading. For example, rupture of a popliteal cyst may present with sudden onset of pain and swelling in the upper calf, simulating thrombophlebitis.

Para-articular cysts frequently are associated with abnormalities in adjacent joints. For example, parameniscal cysts are always associated with meniscal tears; popliteal cysts are highly associated with internal derangement of the knee, and paralabral cysts of the shoulder and hip are often combined with labral tears.

Asymptomatic para-articular cysts are often treated with observation alone. The treatment of symptomatic cysts depends on the underlying cause. Infectious bursitis usually is treated with antibiotics; noninfectious bursitis usually is treated with steroid injection and immobilization, and cysts that impair joint function may require aspiration or resection. If a cyst is associated with underlying joint disease (eg, parameniscal cyst), it is important to address the underlying joint abnormality to prevent a recurrence of the cyst.

IMAGING

The goal of imaging cysts around joints is to confirm the cystic nature of the lesion, to determine the relationship of the cyst to the joint and to the surrounding structures, and to evaluate the joint for associated disorders. The imaging modalities that may be used to achieve these goals include radiography, arthrography, ultrasound, computed tomography (CT), and magnetic resonance (MR) imaging. Radiographs are usually of limited value for assessing soft tissue abnormalities. They may demonstrate soft tissue swelling, effusion, signs of associated degenerative joint disease, bone erosion, calcification, or calcified loose bodies in a communicating cyst. Arthrography can be helpful in demonstrating the communication of a cyst with the joint cavity. However, cysts may fail to fill when the communication is very narrow or when the cyst is filled with highly viscous fluid. Arthrography offers little information about noncommunicating cysts.

Ultrasound is well suited to screen for suspected cysts. It can be used to demonstrate the location and extent of cysts and can differentiate cysts from noncystic masses. However, ultrasound may not be able to demonstrate subtle sites of joint communication and has limited ability to evaluate for associated intra-articular abnormalities. Furthermore, cysts containing debris or

hyperplastic synovium may simulate solid mass lesions on ultrasound.

CT is an excellent tool in assessing abnormalities of calcified tissues because of its high spatial resolution. However, its value for assessing soft tissue lesions is limited by its low soft tissue contrast. Para-articular cysts are of lower attenuation than muscle and of higher attenuation than fat, and lack of enhancement or rim enhancement will be seen following intravenous contrast administration.

MR imaging is superior to all other imaging modalities for investigating soft tissue abnormalities, particularly for demonstrating the location and extent of the lesion. MRI offers superior soft tissue contrast and multiplanar imaging capabilities and is noninvasive. It demonstrates the exact location and extent of the lesion, its relationship to the joint and surrounding structures, and with the aid of intravenous contrast, can show lack of enhancement, suggesting the cystic nature of the lesion. In addition, MR imaging is very accurate for depicting associated joint disorders, such as meniscal tears, ligamentous abnormalities, and degenerative or inflammatory changes.

In most cases the diagnosis of a cyst is readily established on imaging examinations. However, there are some pitfalls. Atypical cyst content due to debris or hemorrhage may alter the imaging appearance of cysts. Furthermore, chronic inflammation may cause marked thickening of the synovial membrane and, therefore, may simulate a solid soft tissue mass. Necrotic or mucinous neoplasms may also simulate a cyst, although there is usually some solid component that differentiates these more serious masses from the benign cystic lesions.

POSTERIOR KNEE
Popliteal Cysts

Popliteal or Baker's cysts are the most common synovial cysts in the body and arise from the gastrocnemio-semimembranosus bursa, located posterior to the upper portion of the medial femoral condyle, between the medial head of the gastrocnemius muscle and the semimembranosus tendon. The gastrocnemio-semimembranosus bursa is composed of 2 parts, the semimembranosus bursa and the gastrocnemius bursa, which may be partially separated by a central septum.[2] Because of the anatomy of the gastrocnemio-semimembranosus bursa, the typical location of a popliteal cyst is along the medial side of the popliteal fossa; however, popliteal cysts can extend medially, laterally, or superiorly and may be superficial or deep to the semimembranosus and gastrocnemius muscles.[3,4]

Estimation of the incidence of popliteal cysts varies from 5%, based on a series of MR examinations,[5,6] to 32% from a series of arthrograms.[6,7] In a recent series, popliteal cysts were seen in approximately 20% of 102 asymptomatic knees imaged with MR.[1] The maximum diameter of the asymptomatic popliteal cyst was 30 mm in that study. The relatively high incidence of popliteal cysts reported in older arthrographic studies may be caused by distention of communicating but otherwise normal bursae and may not reflect the true incidence of distended popliteal bursae.[5] The incidence of popliteal cysts increases with age. In children they are rare, unless there is underlying arthritic disease.[8] Popliteal cysts usually communicate with the knee joint in adults, and there is a strong association of popliteal cysts with other abnormalities of the knee joint, such as chronic effusion, meniscal tears (particularly tears of the posterior horn of the medial meniscus), tears of the cruciate and collateral ligaments, osteoarthritis, and inflammatory disease.[5–7]

Popliteal cysts typically present clinically as a painless mass along the medial side of the popliteal fossa or the calf. However, large cysts can impair full extension or flexion of the knee. If pain is present, the pain may be caused by the underlying abnormality in the knee joint and not by the cyst itself. Rupture of a popliteal cyst occasionally can produce sudden onset of severe pain in the calf and clinically may resemble thrombophlebitis (pseudothrombophlebitis).[9] Occasionally rupture of a Baker's cyst can also result in compartment syndrome.[10,11]

Arthrography is accurate in demonstrating cysts that communicate with the joint and can also demonstrate underlying abnormalities of the knee joint.[7,12] Arthrography is of limited value for demonstrating those bursae that do not communicate with the joint.

Ultrasound is an excellent modality for screening of a suspected popliteal cyst. Ultrasound is able to demonstrate the location and extent of the cyst and can differentiate popliteal cysts from other mass lesions in the popliteal fossa, such as aneurysms of the popliteal artery and soft tissue tumors.[13] It can also demonstrate the presence of deep venous thrombosis, which may mimic or accompany a popliteal cyst. However, its ability to demonstrate the underlying abnormality of the knee joint is limited. On ultrasound examinations, a popliteal cyst presents as an anechoic mass along the medial side of the popliteal fossa, with smooth borders and occasional septations (Fig. 1). Internal echoes indicate debris, hemorrhage, or infection. Ill-defined fluid spaces between or within the calf muscles may be seen if the popliteal cyst has ruptured. However, sonographic diagnosis of a ruptured popliteal cyst may be difficult.[13]

CT is able to define the location and the extent of a popliteal cyst. The bursa presents as a well-defined homogenous mass with attenuation values similar to that of water (Fig. 2). The adjacent soft tissue planes are typically preserved unless there is rupture.[12] After intravenous contrast administration, enhancement of the cyst wall may be observed.

On MR imaging, popliteal cysts present as well-defined fluid collections at the medial side of the popliteal fossa, which may show septations (Fig. 3).[3,5] In cases of hemorrhage, the signal intensity characteristics on T1-weighted and T2-weighted MR images are altered by blood breakdown products. MR is able to demonstrate intra-articular bodies or debris within the bursa.[3] In cases of ruptured popliteal cysts, MR imaging demonstrates marked edema in the subcutaneous fat and fluid tracking along the fascial planes (Fig. 4)[9] and may suggest the diagnosis of a ruptured popliteal cyst when sonography is negative. Large cysts can also dissect into the thigh or calf musculature[14] and usually retain their smooth contour in comparison to a ruptured cyst (Fig. 5). MR imaging also can demonstrate hemosiderin deposition in the synovial membrane of the gastrocnemio-semimembranosus bursa in cases of pigmented villonodular synovitis.[15,16]

Popliteus Bursa

The popliteus bursa develops at the distal aspect of the tendon sheath of the popliteus muscle (Fig. 6) and can also communicate with the tibiofibular joint.[17] Rupture of the popliteus bursa often simulates inflammation or a muscle strain.[17]

ANTERIOR KNEE
Suprapatellar Bursa

The suprapatellar bursa develops proximal to the knee joint capsule as a separate synovial space between the rectus femoris tendon and the femur. From the third fetal month, the septum between the bursa and the knee joint usually involutes, leading to a single joint space.[18] Communication of the suprapatellar bursa with the knee joint is found in approximately 84% of adults.[19] In most of these cases, a transverse residuum of the septum is present, forming the suprapatellar plica. In the remaining 16%, the bursa is completely separated from the joint by an intact septum.[19] Fluid accumulation in a noncommunicating bursa can clinically mimic a soft tissue tumor above the knee joint.[20] In these cases, focal fluid collections

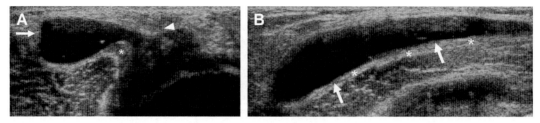

Fig. 1. Transverse (*A*) and longitudinal (*B*) ultrasound images through the popliteal fossa demonstrating an anechoic fluid collection (*arrows*) arising between the semimembranosus tendon (*arrowhead*) and medial gastrocnemius (*asterisks*).

are seen anterior to the distal femoral diaphysis on MR imaging or CT[3,20,21] and may contain bodies (**Fig. 7**). Synovial chondromatosis of the suprapatellar bursa is most often secondary to osteoarthritis of the knee, with the bodies passing through a small portal in a thickened suprapatellar plica, but rarely can be seen as a primary process in an imperforate septum.[22] When bursitis is chronic, a suprapatellar mass with signal intensity similar to skeletal muscle surrounded by fluid may be seen on MR images. In such a case, pigmented villonodular synovitis, synovial hemangioma, or synovial sarcoma should be considered differential diagnoses.[23]

Prepatellar and Infrapatellar Bursae

The prepatellar bursa is usually located anterior to the patella (**Fig. 8**), but can extend lateral or medial to the patella. Cadaveric studies have determined that the prepatellar bursa is a bilaminar or trilaminar structure,[24] although in practice only a single cavity is usually demonstrated on imaging studies. The superficial infrapatellar bursa lies superficial to the tibial tubercle, and the deep infrapatellar bursa

lies between the posterior aspect of the distal patellar tendon and the anterior tibia (see **Fig. 8**). None of these bursae communicate with the knee joint.

Inflammation of the superficial bursae can occur as a result of overuse and may be caused by occupational kneeling or crawling, and, therefore, has been referred to as the carpet-layer's, housemaid's, or clergyman's knee. Septic prepatellar bursitis is usually caused by *Staphylococcus aureus* and can occur as a result of penetrating trauma or may occur secondarily in cases of chronic bursitis.[25] Prepatellar bursitis may also be a manifestation of gout.[26,27]

Prepatellar or superficial infrapatellar bursitis manifests as focal swelling, inflammation, and pain anterior to the patella and anterior to the tibial tubercle, respectively. In carpet-layer's knee, an anechoic fluid collection can be observed in either the prepatellar or the superficial infrapatellar bursa on ultrasound examinations.[28] In addition, hypoechoic thickening of the subcutaneous fat may be present. On MR imaging, prepatellar bursitis presents as a fluid collection anterior to the patella and anterior to the superior part of the patellar tendon

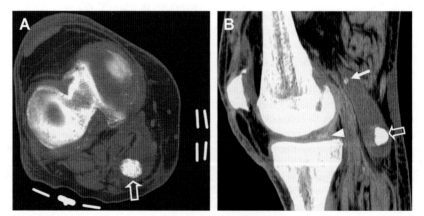

Fig. 2. Axial CT (*A*) and sagittal (*B*) reformat demonstrating a large Baker's cyst containing a loose body (*open arrow*). A smaller loose body is seen superiorly (*arrow*). Incidental chondrocalcinosis is seen in the posterior horn of the medial meniscus (*arrowhead*).

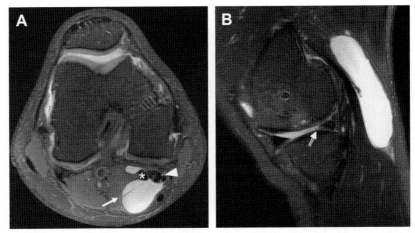

Fig. 3. Axial (*A*) and sagittal (*B*) proton density (PD) fat-saturated (FS) images through the popliteal fossa demonstrate a popliteal cyst arising between the semimembranosus tendon (*arrowhead*) and medial gastrocnemius tendon (*asterisks*). The cyst contains a single thin septation (*arrow*). The patient has a postsurgical change of his posterior horn of the medial meniscus (*double line arrow*), with developing osteoarthritis.

(**Fig. 9**). The signal intensity of the lesion is occasionally heterogeneous because of inflammation or hemorrhage,[3] and the surrounding subcutaneous fat may additionally show heterogeneous signal intensity. In superficial infrapatellar bursitis, focal fluid and inflammatory change is seen in the subcutaneous tissues anterior to the tibial tubercle (**Fig. 10**).

A small fluid-filled deep infrapatellar bursa is seen in a large number (41%) of asymptomatic knees.[1] The diameter of the asymptomatic bursa is usually 14 mm or less. Deep infrapatellar bursitis is characterized by more substantial bursal distention. This bursal distention results from overuse of the knee extensor mechanism and is mainly seen in jumpers and runners. Clinically, deep infrapatellar bursitis presents as anterior knee pain and

simulates patellar tendinitis. On MR images, a fluid collection is seen between the distal part of the patellar tendon and the tibia (**Fig. 11**), and occasionally fluid levels may be seen within the bursa in cases of hemorrhagic bursitis (**Fig. 12**). Similar changes can also be seen in Osgood-Schlatter disease. On T2-weighted images, small amounts of fluid at this location are occasionally seen in asymptomatic individuals and are believed to be incidental findings without clinical significance.[1]

Degloving Injury (Morel-Lavallee Lesion)

The Morel-Lavallee lesion, first described in 1853 by French physician Maurice Morel-Lavallee, is a closed degloving injury that produces a fluid-filled mass at the interface of the subcutaneous

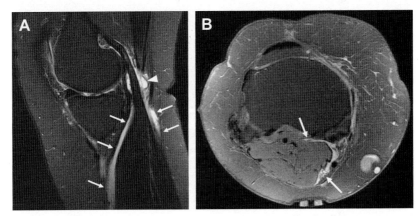

Fig. 4. Sagittal (*A*) and axial (*B*) PD FS images in a patient with acute calf pain demonstrates a small amount of loculated fluid in the expected location of a popliteal cyst (*arrowhead*), with ill-defined fluid tracking distally around the medial gastrocnemius muscle (*arrows*), compatible with a ruptured Baker's cyst.

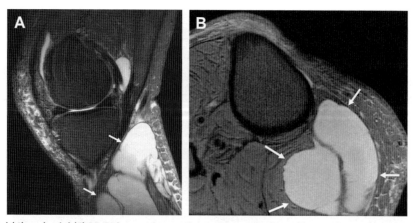

Fig. 5. Sagittal (*A*) and axial (*B*) PD FS images in a patient with a palpable calf mass show a large loculated Baker's cyst dissecting distally into the medial gastrocnemius muscle (*arrows*). The walls of the cyst remain smoothly marginated.

tissue with the fascia. It classically overlies the lateral hip and pelvis and lower back, but can also be seen in the area anterior to the knee, simulating prepatellar bursitis.[29–35]

Prepatellar degloving injuries classically result from a shear injury during contact sports, such as wrestling or football. There is often a blunt tangential force that separates the hypodermis from the underlying fascia. However, in some cases there may be no recollection of a prior traumatic event. The region of injury fills in with blood, lymph, and necrotic fat, creating a fluid collection that is surrounded by granulation tissue. The granulation tissue can organize into a fibrotic pseudocapsule, preventing resorption of fluid. The mass can grow quickly or slowly over the next several months or years and can also be a source for bacterial infection.

Because the material filling in the mass is complex, the mass may have a variable appearance on MR imaging, depending on the age and amount of fat, blood, and lymph tissue contained within. Blood clot and debris may be seen in the acute stage when the collection would have fluid-like signal characteristics on MR imaging. As the hematoma becomes organized, the deoxyhemoglobin converts to methemoglobin, producing increased signal intensity on both T1-weighted and T2-weighted images. The methemoglobin often forms in the periphery and then fills in the center of the lesion. The capsule may contain low signal intensity hemosiderin at this stage.

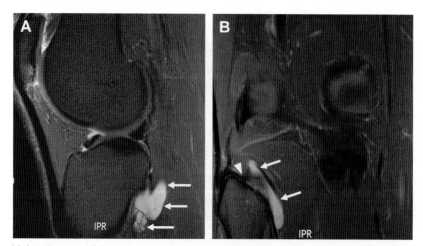

Fig. 6. Sagittal (*A*) and coronal (*B*) T2 FS images in a patient with distended popliteus bursa demonstrating a focal fluid collection lateral to the myotendinous junction of popliteus (*arrows*), in close proximity to the superior tibiofibular joint (*arrowhead*).

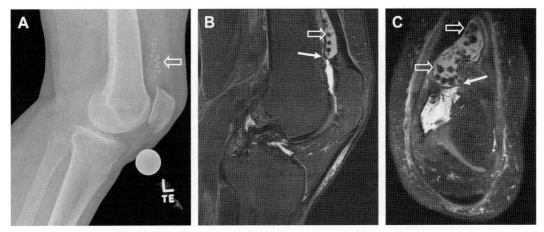

Fig. 7. (A) Lateral radiograph of the knee in a 57-year-old woman demonstrating multiple loose bodies (*open arrow*) in the region of the suprapatellar bursa, compatible with synovial chondromatosis. (B) Sagittal PD FS and (C) coronal T2 FS images demonstrating a thick suprapatellar plica (*arrow*), with multiple loose bodies and more complex fluid in the suprapatellar bursa (*open arrows*).

The blood products may eventually resorb and form a seroma, which can have a range of signal intensities. Fluid-fluid levels and internal septations may also be seen in the mass (**Fig. 13**). The presence of fatty globules within the mass is very specific but not always seen. With time, the pseudocapsule, composed of hemosiderin and fibrous components, develops into a low signal intensity rim around the collection and may show mild enhancement, along with the contents of the lesion, simulating a malignant soft tissue tumor.

Ultrasound is also useful for evaluating Morel-Lavallee lesions and enables aspiration of the collection at the same visit. Depending on the stage of the hematoma, the presentation of the mass may range from anechoic to hyperechoic. Fatty globules present as hyperechoic nodules.

It is helpful to distinguish the Morel-Lavallee lesion from a distended prepatellar bursa because treatment would be different. Most masses related to degloving do not change in size because of the presence of the fibrous pseudocapsule, whereas the dimensions of a prepatellar bursa may wax and wane depending on the pressures placed in that region or the activity of a synovial process.

Although history and clinical examination are the mainstays for the diagnosis of this injury, various features can aid in the distinction of a degloving injury from a bursa or soft tissue tumor. A history of trauma is helpful, but not always present. On imaging, there is often an acute angle at the margin related to peeling back of the subcutaneous fat from the fascia (see **Fig. 13**). The location in the subcutaneous fat is unlikely for a tumor. The degloving injury often extends beyond the confines of a prepatellar bursa, covering a larger region in both the medial-lateral and the craniocaudal dimensions and sometimes extending to the mid thigh.[29] A prepatellar bursa does not usually extend beyond the mid coronal plane medially or laterally, or to the mid thigh. Unlike the prepatellar bursa, a degloving mass does not have a synovial lining and the wall of the collection is often low signal intensity because of the presence of hemosiderin and/or fibrosis. Fatty globules within the mass are also somewhat specific.

Unlike prepatellar bursitis, degloving injuries do not respond significantly to steroid injections because they do not have a synovial lining. The

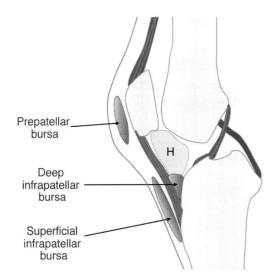

Fig. 8. Sagittal diagram demonstrating the location of the prepatellar and infrapatellar bursae of the anterior knee. H, Hoffa's fat pad.

Prepatellar bursa

Deep infrapatellar bursa

Superficial infrapatellar bursa

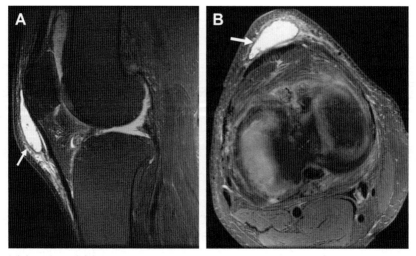

Fig. 9. Sagittal (*A*) and axial (*B*) PD FS images in a patient with moderate prepatellar bursitis demonstrating a well-defined fluid collection anterior to the patella and superior patellar tendon (*arrow*), with mild surrounding inflammatory change.

degloving injury is often treated conservatively with rest and compression.[36] However, aspiration, suction drainage, vasopneumatic cryotherapy, sclerodesis, or resection may be necessary if the lesion is larger or unresponsive to conservative treatment.[31]

MEDIAL KNEE

A variety of bursal spaces exist in close proximity around the posteromedial knee, and knowledge of anatomy in this region is critical to identify the different bursal spaces correctly (**Fig. 14**). Medial bursitis is common and fluid is often seen in more than one bursal space.

Pes Anserine Bursa

The pes anserine bursa is located on the medial aspect of the knee between the conjoined distal tendons of the sartorius, gracilis, and semitendinosus muscles (pes anserinus) and the tibial insertion of the medial collateral ligament (tibial condyle). Acute pes anserine bursitis can occur in athletes as an overuse injury, particularly in long-distance runners.[37] Chronic distention of the bursa with fluid is also frequently seen in obese patients and those with degenerative or inflammatory joint disease.[38,39] Clinically, pes anserine bursitis presents as focal swelling and tenderness inferior to the anteromedial portion of the proximal tibia.[3,40]

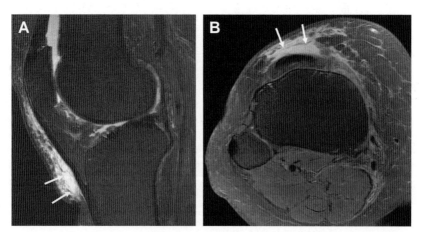

Fig. 10. Sagittal (*A*) and axial (*B*) PD FS images in a patient with anterior knee pain demonstrates an ill-defined fluid collection (*arrows*) in the subcutaneous tissues anterior to the distal patellar tendon with adjacent edema, compatible with superficial infrapatellar bursitis.

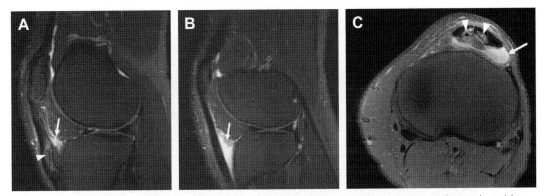

Fig. 11. Sagittal (*A, B*) and axial (*C*) PD FS images in a patient with severe distal patellar tendinopathy, with associated dystrophic ossification (*arrowheads*), bony spurring of the tibial tuberosity, and deep infrapatellar bursitis (*arrows*).

However, patients can also present with more vague medial knee pain, mimicking a medial meniscal tear or medial collateral ligament injury. Fluid distention of the bursa also occurs in asymptomatic individuals.[40]

On CT, fluid distention of the pes anserine bursa presents as a well-delineated low-attenuation cystic structure that lies immediately beneath the pes anserinus.[40] On MR imaging, acute pes anserine bursitis demonstrates as a cyst-like fluid collection adjacent to the medial tibial condyle (**Fig. 15**).[38,41] Chronic bursitis sometimes presents as a solid mass with intermediate signal intensity on proton density weighted MR images and heterogeneous areas of high signal intensity on T2-weighted MR images.[23] The MR appearance of chronic bursitis is less specific than that of acute

bursitis, and the differential diagnosis includes pigmented villonodular bursitis, giant cell tumor of the tendon sheath, synovial hemangioma, and synovial sarcoma.[23,42,43]

Semimembranosus-Tibial Collateral Ligament Bursa

The semimembranosus-tibial collateral ligament (SM-TCL) bursa is consistently present, as shown in a study of 50 cadaver knees,[44] and is located posterior and superior to the pes anserine bursa. The bursa drapes over to the semimembranosus tendon and has the shape of an inverted "U." The superficial part of the bursa lies between the semimembranosus tendon and the medial collateral ligament, and the deep part lies between the

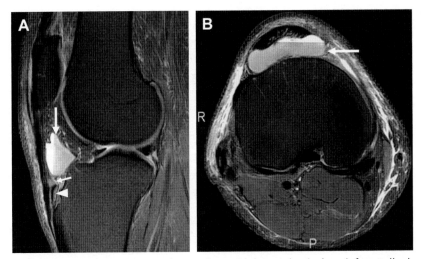

Fig. 12. Sagittal (*A*) and axial (*B*) PD FS images in a patient with hemorrhagic deep infrapatellar bursitis demonstrate a layering fluid level (*arrows*). There is tendinopathy and undersurface tearing of the distal patellar tendon (*small arrow*) and a small ossicle adjacent to the tibial tubercle (*arrowhead*). (*Courtesy of* Phillip Tirman.)

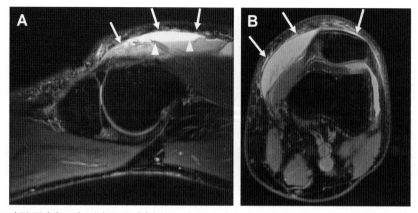

Fig. 13. Sagittal T2 FS (*A*) and axial PD FS (*B*) images in a soccer player 2 days after sustaining a fall on the field. A large complex fluid collection is seen within the prepatellar soft tissues, extending over the medial thigh (*arrows*) compatible with a Morel-Lavallee lesion. A layering fluid level is seen on the horizontally oriented sagittal image (*arrowheads*).

semimembranosus tendon and the medial tibial condyle, thereby decreasing frictional forces on the tendon as it passes between these structures. Inflammation of the SM-TCL bursa results in focal pain over the posteromedial aspect of the knee at the level of the joint line and may clinically simulate a meniscal abnormality or other internal derangement.

On MR imaging, inflammation of the SM-TCL bursa presents as a longitudinal fluid collection along the semimembranosus tendon close to the medial joint line (**Fig. 16**). On sagittal images, the fluid collection typically drapes over the tendon. On coronal images, the bursa has a semilunar configuration, surrounding the tendon at its superior, medial, and inferior aspect. Fluid distention of the SM-TCL bursa can coexist with fluid accumulation in the pes anserine bursa and in the MCL bursa (**Fig. 17**).[38]

Medial Collateral Ligament Bursa

The medial collateral ligament (MCL) bursa, also known as the tibial collateral ligament bursa, is found in approximately 90% of all patients and is located between the deep and superficial fibers of the medial collateral ligament in the central third of the medial knee (**Fig. 18**).[45] The MCL bursa allows the MCL to glide over the bony surfaces of the tibia and femur when the knee is flexed. The MCL bursa can fill with fluid in patients with osteoarthritis, patients with inflammatory arthropathies, such as gout or genu vara, or following trauma.[45] MCL bursitis can cause localized pain over the medial joint line, which clinically may mimic a meniscal tear.

On MR images, the bursa is only seen when it is distended with fluid.[45,46] Fluid collections in the MCL bursa are well defined and vertically oriented, extending along the tibial cortex between the deep

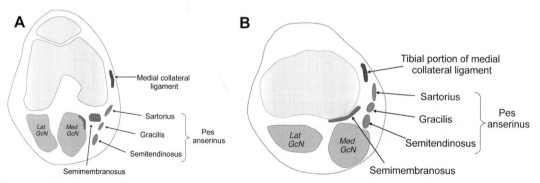

Fig. 14. Axial diagrams of the tendons and ligaments around the posteromedial knee at the level of the distal femur (*A*) and proximal tibia (*B*). Lat GcN, lateral gastrocnemius; Med GcN, medial gastrocnemius.

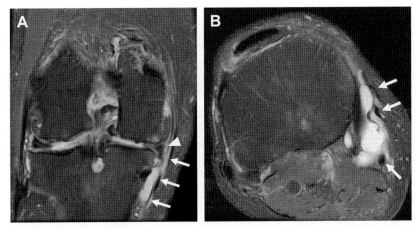

Fig. 15. (*A*) Coronal T2 FS image posterior to the plane of the medial collateral ligament, and (*B*) axial PD FS images of a patient with severe pes anserine bursitis demonstrate a distended, fluid-filled bursa deep to the 3 pes anserine tendons (*arrows*). The medial meniscus is partly extruded (*arrowhead*) and degenerative changes are seen in the medial and lateral compartments of the knee.

and superficial fibers of the MCL, and in most cases along the femur.[45] On axial images the fluid collection often appears bilobed as it protrudes out immediately anterior and posterior to the medial collateral ligament (**Fig. 19**). Differentiation of bursal fluid from a parameniscal cyst can sometimes be difficult, but most tears of the medial meniscus are seen posteromedially, and therefore, most parameniscal cysts will occur posterior to the MCL. High T2 signal in the vicinity of the MCL bursa can also be seen in meniscocapsular separation and peripheral medial meniscal tears, but in these cases the fluid is usually ill-defined and in the perimeniscal soft tissues.[45,46]

LATERAL KNEE
Iliotibial Band Friction Syndrome

Iliotibial band friction syndrome is a common cause of lateral knee pain that is frequently related to intense exercise, as occurs in long-distance runners, football players, and cyclists. It is the sequela of chronic friction between the iliotibial band and the lateral femoral condyle during knee flexion.[47] The localized fluid collections are more likely caused by inflammation of a secondary, or adventitious, bursa rather than a primary bursa.

Iliotibial band friction syndrome manifests on MR imaging as poorly defined high T2 signal intensity, or a circumscribed fluid collection deep to the

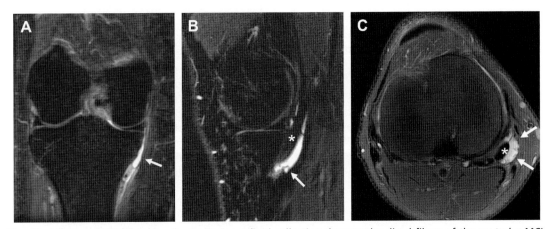

Fig. 16. (*A*) Coronal T2 FS image demonstrates a fluid collection deep to the distal fibers of the posterior MCL (*arrow*). (*B*) Sagittal T2 FS and (*C*) axial PD FS images show a U-shaped fluid collection (*arrows*) draped over the semimembranosus tendon (*asterisk*), compatible with semimembranosus-tibial collateral ligament (SM-TCL) bursitis.

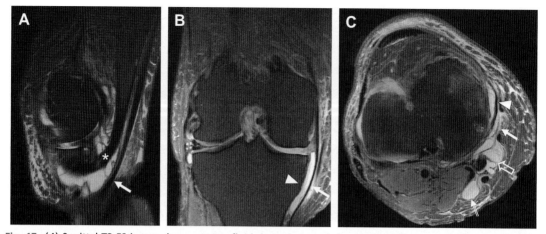

Fig. 17. (*A*) Sagittal T2 FS image demonstrates fluid draped around the semimembranosus tendon (*asterisk*), as well as fluid deep a pes tendon (*arrow*). (*B*) Coronal PD FS demonstrates fluid deep to the tibial portion of the medial collateral ligament (*arrowhead*), as well as deep to a pes tendon (*arrow*). (*C*) Axial PD FS images confirms fluid within the tibial collateral bursa (*arrowhead*), pes anserine bursa (*arrow*), semimembranosus–tibial collateral ligament bursa (*open arrow*), as well as a popliteal cyst (*double line arrow*).

iliotibial band (**Fig. 20**).[48–51] The normal fat signal distal to the vastus lateralis muscle is obliterated on T1-weighted images.

OTHER CYSTIC COLLECTIONS
Parameniscal Cysts

Parameniscal cysts represent encapsulated mass lesions containing synoviallike fluid that are continuous with a meniscus.[52] These cysts are invariably associated with horizontal meniscal tears.[53] Large, clinically apparent cysts are relatively uncommon, whereas small cystic changes in a meniscus are frequently observed microscopically.[52] Two studies performed on symptomatic and asymptomatic knees have shown an incidence of parameniscal cysts in 4% of MR images.[1,54] Parameniscal cysts are formed when synovial fluid is forced through a meniscal tear with accumulation at the meniscocapsular margin.[55] In some series, lateral meniscal cysts have been described as being 3 to 10 times more common than medial meniscal cysts.[56–58] Other studies have shown a higher incidence of medial meniscal cysts, or a more equal occurrence.[54] Medial cysts tend to be larger and more posterior than lateral cysts.

Parameniscal cysts clinically present with pain and swelling. Because of their origin, the swelling is located at the level of the medial or lateral joint line.[3] Diagnosis and treatment of the underlying meniscal tear are important, as parameniscal cysts frequently recur after excision or aspiration, unless the meniscal tear is repaired.

At arthrography, parameniscal cysts typically present as a club-shaped pooling of contrast material at the outer margin of a meniscus. In addition, a serpentine tear in the meniscus can be seen.[59] Ultrasonography shows a partially cystic, frequently septated mass bulging into the para-articular space.[60] The inner border of the cystic mass is closely related to the meniscus. Protrusion of an abnormal meniscus into the cyst may be seen.[52] Occasionally, echogenic areas are seen within the cysts that probably represent debris.[52] Demonstration of the meniscal tear, however, is not possible in most cases,[60] limiting the diagnostic value of ultrasound for meniscal cysts.

On MR images, parameniscal cysts usually present as well-circumscribed, smoothly marginated masses that are adjacent to the meniscus (**Fig. 21**). MR imaging also demonstrates the

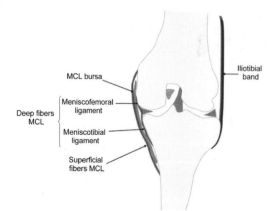

Fig. 18. The location of the MCL bursa, between the deep and superficial fibers of the medial collateral ligament.

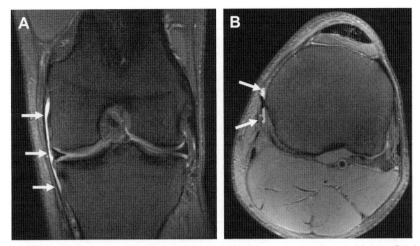

Fig. 19. (A) Coronal T2 FS image shows a thin fluid collection between the deep and superficial fibers of the medial collateral ligament (*arrows*). (B) Axial PD FS image demonstrates a bilobed fluid collection arising deep to the MCL (*arrows*), compatible with mild MCL bursitis.

associated meniscal tear. On T1-weighted MR images, parameniscal cysts are isointense or slightly hypointense to muscle. On T2-weighted MR images, most parameniscal cysts are readily recognized because of their high signal intensity.[58] In contrast to the cyst, parameniscal tears are best visualized on short TE sequences.

Cysts of the Tibiofibular Joint

The proximal tibiofibular joint communicates with the knee joint in approximately 10% of the population.[3] Cysts arising from the proximal tibiofibular joint can cause focal masses, pain, or neuropathy because of compression of the common peroneal

and/or tibial nerves.[3,17,61] Fluid from a tibiofibular joint cyst can extend into the epineurium of the tibial nerve by extruding through a capsular defect, dissecting along the articular branch of the tibial nerve medial to the fibular head and adjacent to the articular branch of the tibial nerve.[62] This dissection can result in denervation of the popliteus muscle. A cyst may also extend laterally around the fibular head, causing either a neural compression or an intraneural ganglion in the peroneal nerve. In some cases this leads to denervation of the tibialis anterior muscle with a resultant foot drop (**Fig. 22**), recently shown to be due to involvement of the tibialis anterior branch of the peroneal nerve.[63] Large proximal tibiofibular joint cysts may erode the

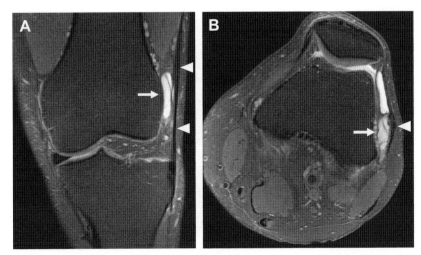

Fig. 20. Coronal (A) and axial (B) PD FS images in a long distance runner with lateral knee pain demonstrate a focal septated fluid collection (*arrow*) between the iliotibial band (*arrowheads*) and lateral femoral condyle, compatible with an adventitial bursa.

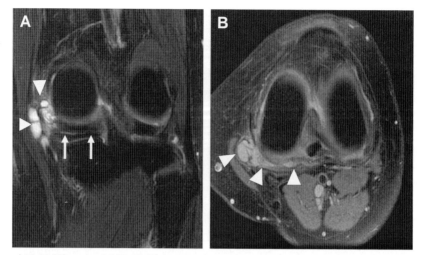

Fig. 21. Coronal T2 FS (*A*) and axial PD FS (*B*) images demonstrating a horizontal cleavage tear of the posterior horn and body of the medial meniscus (*arrows*), with an adjacent multiloculated parameniscal cyst (*arrowheads*).

adjacent bone, simulating a more aggressive lesion.[2] These cysts sometimes communicate with the knee joint during a knee arthrogram and are well seen with ultrasound and MRI.

Ganglia Around the Knee Joint

Ganglia can produce pain and swelling in the knee, but are usually asymptomatic. The cause is unknown but may be related to displacement of synovial tissue during embryogenesis, proliferation of pluripotential mesenchymal cells, migration of synovial fluid into the cyst, and degeneration of connective tissues following trauma. Ganglia can also travel along neurovascular pathways from areas of internal derangement in the joint into the surrounding soft tissues. Ganglia have a predilection for periarticular locations and are mainly seen around the knee joint and around the wrist.[64] They can be attached to a joint capsule or tendon sheath and sometimes have a connection to the synovial cavity. Other possible locations of ganglia are within muscles, ligaments, tendons, or nerves.[58,64–68]

The clinical presentation depends on the location and size of the ganglion. In most cases they are asymptomatic, palpable lesions or they are seen incidentally on imaging examinations. Occasionally, they cause pain and swelling, and rarely, palsy of the peroneal nerve by compression.[65,68]

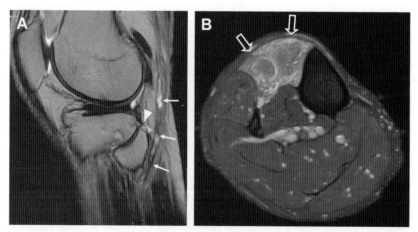

Fig. 22. Sagittal PD (*A*) and axial T2 FS (*B*) images in a 57-year-old man with foot drop. On the sagittal image a thin loculated fluid collection is seen arising from the superior tibiofibular joint (*arrowhead*) and extending into the common peroneal nerve (*arrows*). On the axial images there is acute denervation of the tibialis anterior muscle, manifesting as intramuscular edema (*open arrows*). (*Courtesy of* Ciro Duarte.)

On MR imaging, para-articular ganglia present as well-delineated, rounded, or lobular ("bunch of grapes") lesions (**Fig. 23**). Compared with muscle, they are isointense or slightly hypointense on T1-weighted images and hyperintense on T2-weighted images. The relationship to joint capsules and tendon sheaths is best seen on T2-weighted images. Peripheral, fluid-filled pseudopodia and sharply defined internal septa are very characteristic features of ganglia and, in some cases, these may be seen on MR imaging and not by CT.[64] When located close to the joint line, ganglia resemble parameniscal cysts. In such cases, the absence of a meniscal tear can be used to exclude the possibility of a parameniscal cyst.[58]

Mucoid Degeneration and Ganglia Related to the Cruciate Ligaments

Mucoid degeneration of the cruciate ligaments is characterized by interstitial glycosaminoglycan deposits between the normally aligned collagen bundles, resulting in a thickened ligament with intermediate signal intensity on T1-weighted and diffuse increased T2 signal intensity.[69–72] The synovial lining over the cruciate ligaments may be absent in these cases. Mucoid degeneration is usually seen in middle-aged and elderly patients, but can also occur in young individuals, even under the age of 10 years. Although the cause is uncertain, there are many theories including degeneration, prior trauma, synovial herniation, synovial injury, partial ligament tears, intercondylar notch stenosis, and arthritis. Mucoid degeneration can be mistaken for an anterior cruciate ligament (ACL) tear on MR imaging, but the diffuse nature and thickening of the ACL without a history of acute trauma can aid in the distinction. It is rare that a metastatic lesion might have this appearance.[73]

Mucoid degeneration and mucoid cysts (another term for ganglion associated with cruciate ligaments) are classically thought to represent separate entities; however, some authors have suggested there is a common pathogenesis.[74,75] The authors of this article have seen that cysts can occur within the ligament (**Fig. 24**) or can often dissect out into Hoffa's fat pad, the surrounding bone, and within or outside of the knee joint. In the latter case the authors theorize that they travel along neurovascular pathways, similar to the cysts around the fibula.[62]

Sometimes isolated mucoid cysts are also seen within or around the cruciate ligaments in the absence of mucoid degeneration of the ligament, but these are relatively rare.[76–79] In one study of 1685 consecutive knee MR examinations, there was only a 1% incidence of cruciate ligament ganglion cysts.[76] Generally, the cruciate ligament cysts are located within the intercondylar fossa adjacent to the cruciate ligaments or posterior to the posterior cruciate ligament.[79]

The clinical presentation of mucoid degeneration and mucoid cysts depends on their size and location. Mucoid degeneration may present with pain that simulates a meniscal tear, related to impingement of the enlarged ligament into the lateral compartment of the knee.[72,80] Anterior impingement related to mucoid degeneration of the ACL or a large cyst may present with limited knee extension.[81,82] Other presentations include swelling in the popliteal fossa.[77,81] Less frequent findings are lack of full knee flexion[77] and joint clicking.[83] In most cases, there is no history of antecedent trauma[81] or evidence of joint instability.[81,83,84] Depending on their clinical presentation, conservative treatment is the standard for

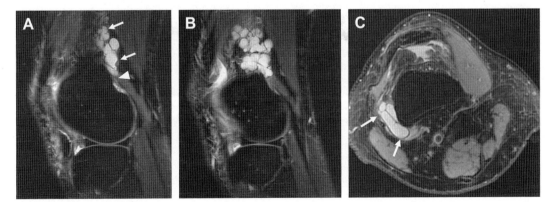

Fig. 23. Sagittal (*A, B*) and axial (*C*) PD FS images of the knee demonstrate a complex, multiloculated cystic lesion (*arrows*) arising adjacent to the lateral gastrocnemius tendon (*arrowhead*) and extending around the posterolateral knee, compatible with a ganglion cyst.

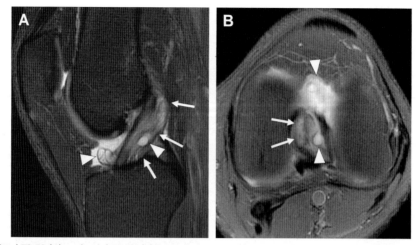

Fig. 24. Sagittal T2 FS (*A*) and axial PD FS (*B*) images demonstrate mucoid degeneration of the ACL, manifesting as a markedly thickened ligament with high T2 signal interspersed between the ACL fibers (*arrows*). There are associated mucoid cysts within the mid portion of the ligament and adjacent to the tibial insertion (*arrowheads*).

mucoid cysts. If there is failure of symptomatic relief, invasive therapy, such as arthroscopic resection[74,81,83,85] or CT-guided puncture,[80,86,87] has been described. Notchplasty can also be performed to keep the ACL from rubbing against the notch or being scraped by osteophytes.[72,82]

On MR imaging, mucoid cysts of the cruciate ligaments present as well as delineated intra-articular masses with signal intensities similar to that of fluid.[77,79] Occasionally there are septations or a peripheral ring of low signal intensity, representing a fibrous capsule.[80] Cysts arising from the posterior cruciate ligament are usually well-defined multilocular lesions. Cysts from the ACL have a rather fusiform configuration because they tend to align along the fibers of the ligament.[79] Although the MR imaging features of intra-articular ganglion cysts are typical, differential diagnosis may include extension from mucoid degeneration of the cruciate ligaments as described earlier, synovial chondromatosis, intra-articularly dissecting parameniscal cysts, synovial hemangiomas, and hematomas.[2] Because of their signal characteristics, intraligamentous cysts have the potential to mimic a tear of a cruciate ligament on MR images. However, most cysts are diagnosed correctly, because they are more focal with a round or oval configuration.

Hoffa's Fat Pad Ganglion

Hoffa's fat pad is an intracapsular, extrasynovial structure in the anterior aspect of the knee that lies below the patella, posterior to the patellar tendon, and anterior to the femorotibial articulation. The fat pad may have a vertical or horizontal

cleft that can fill with fluid.[88] Sometimes a ganglion may be seen in Hoffa's fat pad. Although the cause is not known, speculation includes trauma and transverse ligament degeneration.[89] We have also seen many cases thought to result from extension of ACL mucoid degeneration or ganglia into this structure. In these cases it is important to look at the surrounding structures for abnormalities.

Hoffa's fat pad ganglia are typically rounded fluid signal intensity structures that may be unilocular or multilocular (**Fig. 25**). They should be distinguished from several other entities including the horizontal cleft of the fat pad that is not encapsulated, extension of a parameniscal cyst associated with a meniscal tear, or an ACL ganglion into the fat pad. Other synovial processes that present with a mass can lie in this region, including localized nodular synovitis, synovial osteochondromatosis, and chondroma, but these are usually distinguished from a ganglion by their heterogenous signal intensity.

Lesions that Mimic Cysts Around the Knee Joint

On MR imaging, some entities simulate ganglia or bursae, including synovial chondromatosis, synovial hemangioma, and other vascular and soft tissue masses.

Synovial chondromatosis can demonstrate similar signal intensities on T1-weighted and T2-weighted images to cystic lesions. However, synovial chondromatosis typically demonstrates a lobulated, cauliflower-like appearance and often contains low signal intensity areas indicating

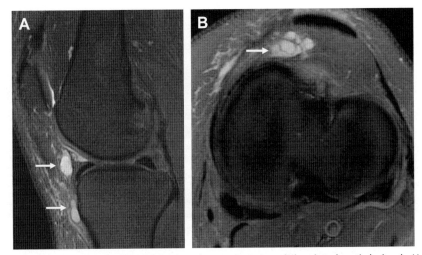

Fig. 25. Sagittal T2 FS (*A*) and axial PD FS (*B*) images demonstrate a multiloculated cystic lesion in Hoffa's fat pad medially, compatible with a ganglion cyst (*arrows*).

calcification or ossification.[90] Enhancement may also be helpful to differentiate uncalcified cartilage from synovial fluid.[91]

Synovial hemangiomas are uncommon, but usually involve the anterior compartment of the knee.[91] They can be differentiated from cysts by their lobulated configuration, ectatic and occasionally branching vessels, and enhancement characteristics after intravenous contrast administration (**Fig. 26**).[2]

Popliteal artery aneurysms lie in the popliteal fossa and frequently form from atherosclerotic disease. They are located in the central posterior aspect of the popliteal fossa, which is not the typical location of a bursa, and rarely have signal characteristics that simulate a ganglion. Popliteal

aneurysms are usually round with heterogenous signal, including areas of high T1 signal intensity and low T2 signal intensity because of blood products. Ultrasound and MR angiography can determine the vascular nature of these masses.[92]

Cystic adventitial disease of the popliteal artery presents with ganglia in the adventitia of the artery that compromise blood flow (**Fig. 27**).[92] Compromised blood flow can result in calf claudication and usually presents in men between the ages of 20 and 50 years. Some of the cysts may communicate with the joint, and it is possible that some of these cysts are created by intra-articular abnormalities, such as mucoid degeneration of the cruciate ligaments that extend along neurovascular pathways outside of the joint.

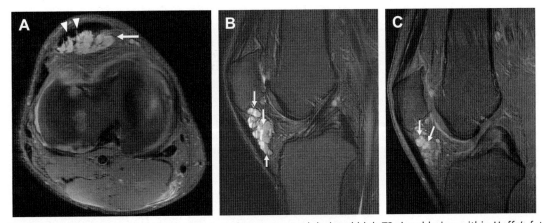

Fig. 26. Axial (*A*) and sagittal (*B*) T2 FS images demonstrate a lobulated high T2 signal lesion within Hoffa's fat pad, with multiple fluid levels (*arrows*), compatible with a hemangioma. The hemangioma shows early infiltration into the patellar tendon (*arrowheads*). (*C*) Sagittal T1 FS after gadolinium demonstrates areas of early enhancement (*arrows*).

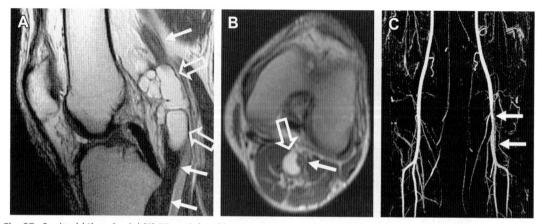

Fig. 27. Sagittal (*A*) and axial (*B*) PD-weighted images demonstrate a multiloculated cystic lesion (*open arrows*) in the popliteal fossa centrally, intimately associated with the popliteal vessels (*arrows*). (*C*) Coronal CT angiogram demonstrates narrowing of the popliteal artery in the region of cystic adventitial disease on the left (*arrows*).

The location in the popliteal artery aids in distinction from a bursa or simple ganglion.

Soft tissue tumors that have predominantly homogeneous increased signal intensity on T2 weighting and lie near or inside of joints can mimic bursae or ganglia. Juxta-articular myxomas are benign, well-circumscribed masses that contain glycosaminoglyan and can simulate a bursa or ganglion on superficial evaluation. Because they are relatively hypovascular, myxomas tend to peripherally enhance on MR imaging, similar to the bursa and ganglion, but may have enhancing intralesional septa (**Fig. 28**).[93] Myxoid sarcomas, nerve sheath tumors, and desmoid tumors are also seen around joints, but usually have a more heterogenous signal and enhancement that helps distinguish them from a bursa or ganglion. Necrotic tumors may simulate a cyst or hematoma. These masses often have a thickened irregular wall, septae, and heterogeneous signal. Occasionally, soft tissue masses, including sarcomas, are homogeneous in signal intensity, but they usually show solid characteristics following contrast administration or on ultrasound (**Fig. 29**). Intra-articular synovial sarcomas are very rare but could potentially mimic intra-articular ganglion cysts. However, contrast-enhancing nodular components in these cases would raise the suspicion of a neoplastic process.

Hematomas can also simulate cysts, but may demonstrate fluid-fluid levels or high signal intensity on T1-weighted images because of methemoglobin. Large focal dilatations of popliteal veins may show signal intensities similar to that of a cyst on MR imaging. However, continuity of the lesion to feeding vessels and demonstration of

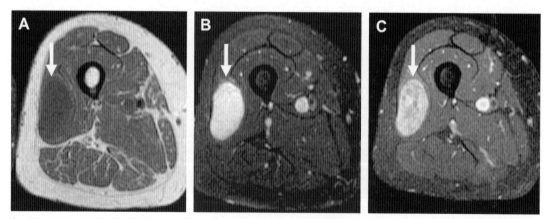

Fig. 28. Axial T1 (*A*), T2 FS (*B*), and (*C*) T1 FS after gadolinium demonstrate a rounded, low T1, high T2 signal intensity lesion in the vastus lateralis muscle (*arrows*) compatible with an intramuscular myxoma. Heterogeneous enhancement is seen after gadolinium.

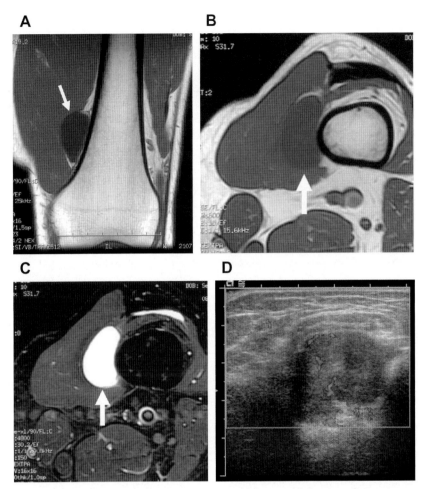

Fig. 29. Coronal (*A*) and axial (*B*) T1-weighted images and axial T2 FS (*C*) images of a young man referred for ultrasound-guided aspiration of a "cyst" in the left lower leg (*arrows*) demonstrate a well-defined, homogeneous low T1/high T2 lesion medially in the thigh, subjacent to the vastus medialis and intermedius. However, on color Doppler ultrasound (*D*), the mass is solid, with internal vascularity, subsequently shown to be a myxoid liposarcoma.

venous flow patterns by Doppler ultrasound enable a diagnosis of popliteal vein varices.[3]

SUMMARY

Cystic lesions around the knee joint are common and are frequently encountered in daily practice. The cysts may communicate directly with the knee joint, may arise from a noncommunicating bursa, or may lie within the surrounding soft tissues. The causes and clinical implications of these cysts differ considerably. Many cysts are encountered incidentally and are treated with observation. Occasionally, cysts may cause pain or impair joint function and, therefore, may require resection or aspiration. Some cysts are secondary to an underlying abnormality of the joint, including internal derangement and meniscal tears. It is important for the radiologist to be familiar with the cause of the cystic structure to

diagnose and treat these lesions and any abnormalities associated with them properly.

REFERENCES

1. Tschirch FT, Schmid MR, Pfirrmann CW, et al. Prevalence and size of meniscal cysts, ganglionic cysts, synovial cysts of the popliteal space, fluid-filled bursae, and other fluid collections in asymptomatic knees on MR imaging. AJR Am J Roentgenol 2003;180:1431–6.
2. Lee KR, Cox GG, Neff JR, et al. Cystic masses of the knee: arthrographic and CT evaluation. AJR Am J Roentgenol 1987;148:329–34.
3. Janzen DL, Peterfy CG, Forbes JR, et al. Cystic lesions around the knee joint: MR imaging findings. AJR Am J Roentgenol 1994;163:155–61.
4. Pavlov H, Steinbach L, Fried SH. A posterior ascending popliteal cyst mimicking thrombophlebitis

following total knee arthroplasty (TKA). Clin Orthop Relat Res 1983;179:204–8.

5. Fielding JR, Franklin PD, Kustan J. Popliteal cysts: a reassessment using magnetic resonance imaging. Skeletal Radiol 1991;20:433–5.

6. Handy JR. Popliteal cysts in adults: a review. Semin Arthritis Rheum 2001;31:108–18.

7. Wolfe RD, Colloff B. Popliteal cysts. An arthrographic study and review of the literature. J Bone Joint Surg Am 1972;54:1057–63.

8. Szer IS, Klein-Gitelman M, DeNardo BA, et al. Ultrasonography in the study of prevalence and clinical evolution of popliteal cysts in children with knee effusions. J Rheumatol 1992;19:458–62.

9. Munk PL, Vellet AD, Levin MF. Leaking Baker's cyst detected by magnetic resonance imaging. Can Assoc Radiol J 1993;44:125–8.

10. Klovning J, Beadle T. Compartment syndrome secondary to spontaneous rupture of a Baker's cyst. J La State Med Soc 2007;159:43–4.

11. Schimizzi AL, Jamali AA, Herbst KD, et al. Acute compartment syndrome due to ruptured Baker cyst after nonsurgical management of an anterior cruciate ligament tear: a case report. Am J Sports Med 2006;34:657–60.

12. Schwimmer M, Edelstein G, Heiken JP, et al. Synovial cysts of the knee: CT evaluation. Radiology 1985;154:175–7.

13. Pathria MN, Zlatkin M, Sartoris DJ, et al. Ultrasonography of the popliteal fossa and lower extremities. Radiol Clin North Am 1988;26:77–85.

14. Fang CS, McCarthy CL, McNally EG. Intramuscular dissection of Baker's cysts: report on three cases. Skeletal Radiol 2004;33:367–71.

15. Meehan PL, Daftari T. Pigmented villonodular synovitis presenting as a popliteal cyst in a child. A case report. J Bone Joint Surg Am 1994;76:593–5.

16. Steinbach LS, Neumann CH, Stoller DW, et al. MRI of the knee in diffuse pigmented villonodular synovitis. Clin Imaging 1989;13:305–16.

17. Wigley RD. Popliteal cysts: variations on a theme of Baker. Semin Arthritis Rheum 1982;12:1–10.

18. Deutsch AL, Resnick D, Dalinka MK, et al. Synovial plicae of the knee. Radiology 1981;141:627–34.

19. Zidorn T. Classification of the suprapatellar septum considering ontogenetic development. Arthroscopy 1992;8:459–64.

20. Ehlinger M, Moser T, Adam P, et al. Complete suprapatellar plica presenting like a tumor. Orthop Traumatol Surg Res 2009;95:447–50.

21. Yamamoto T, Akisue T, Marui T, et al. Isolated suprapatellar bursitis: computed tomographic and arthroscopic findings. Arthroscopy 2003;19:E10.

22. Boya H, Pinar H, Ozcan O. Synovial osteochondromatosis of the suprapatellar bursa with an imperforate suprapatellar plica. Arthroscopy 2002;18:E17.

23. Zeiss J, Coombs RJ, Booth RL Jr, et al. Chronic bursitis presenting as a mass in the pes anserine bursa: MR diagnosis. J Comput Assist Tomogr 1993;17:137–40.

24. Aguiar RO, Viegas FC, Fernandez RY, et al. The prepatellar bursa: cadaveric investigation of regional anatomy with MRI after sonographically guided bursography. AJR Am J Roentgenol 2007;188:W355–8.

25. Cea-Pereiro JC, Garcia-Meijide J, Mera-Varela A, et al. A comparison between septic bursitis caused by Staphylococcus aureus and those caused by other organisms. Clin Rheumatol 2001;20:10–4.

26. Dawn B, Williams JK, Walker SE. Prepatellar bursitis: a unique presentation of tophaceous gout in an normouricemic patient. J Rheumatol 1997;24:976–8.

27. Yood RA. Gout presenting with recurrent acute prepatellar bursitis before the onset of arthritis. J Rheumatol 1985;12:1204–5.

28. Myllymaki T, Tikkakoski T, Typpo T, et al. Carpetlayer's knee. An ultrasonographic study. Acta Radiol 1993;34:496–9.

29. Borrero CG, Maxwell N, Kavanagh E. MRI findings of prepatellar Morel-Lavallee effusions. Skeletal Radiol 2008;37:451–5.

30. Hak DJ, Olson SA, Matta JM. Diagnosis and management of closed internal degloving injuries associated with pelvic and acetabular fractures: the Morel-Lavallee lesion. J Trauma 1997;42:1046–51.

31. van Gennip S, van Bokhoven SC, van den Eede E. Pain at the knee: the Morel-Lavallee lesion, a case series. Clin J Sport Med 2012;22:163–6.

32. Yahyavi-Firouz-Abadi N, Demertzis JL. Prepatellar Morel-Lavallee effusion. Skeletal Radiol 2012;42:127–8.

33. Ciaschini M, Sundaram M. Radiologic case study. Prepatellar Morel-Lavallee lesion. Orthopedics 2008;31:626, 719–21.

34. Mellado JM, Bencardino JT. Morel-Lavallee lesion: review with emphasis on MR imaging. Magn Reson Imaging Clin N Am 2005;13:775–82.

35. Mellado JM, Perez del Palomar L, Diaz L, et al. A. Long-standing Morel-Lavallee lesions of the trochanteric region and proximal thigh: MRI features in five patients. AJR Am J Roentgenol 2004;182:1289–94.

36. Tejwani SG, Cohen SB, Bradley JP. Management of Morel-Lavallee lesion of the knee: twenty-seven cases in the national football league. Am J Sports Med 2007;35:1162–7.

37. Safran MR, Fu FH. Uncommon causes of knee pain in the athlete. Orthop Clin North Am 1995;26:547–59.

38. Forbes JR, Helms CA, Janzen DL. Acute pes anserine bursitis: MR imaging. Radiology 1995;194:525–7.

39. Grover RP, Rakhra KS. Pes anserine bursitis - an extra-articular manifestation of gout. Bull NYU Hosp Jt Dis 2010;68:46–50.

40. Hall FM, Joffe N. CT imaging of the anserine bursa. AJR Am J Roentgenol 1988;150:1107–8.

41. Rennie WJ, Saifuddin A. Pes anserine bursitis: incidence in symptomatic knees and clinical presentation. Skeletal Radiol 2005;34:395–8.

42. Maheshwari AV, Muro-Cacho CA, Pitcher JD Jr. Pigmented villonodular bursitis/diffuse giant cell tumor of the pes anserine bursa: a report of two cases and review of literature. Knee 2007;14:402–7.

43. Zhao H, Maheshwari AV, Kumar D, et al. Giant cell tumor of the pes anserine bursa (extra-articular pigmented villonodular bursitis): a case report and review of the literature. Case Report Med 2011; 2011:491470.

44. Hennigan SP, Schneck CD, Mesgarzadeh M, et al. The semimembranosus-tibial collateral ligament bursa. Anatomical study and magnetic resonance imaging. J Bone Joint Surg Am 1994;76:1322–7.

45. De Maeseneer M, Shahabpour M, Van Roy F, et al. MR imaging of the medial collateral ligament bursa: findings in patients and anatomic data derived from cadavers. AJR Am J Roentgenol 2001;177:911–7.

46. Lee JK, Yao L. Tibial collateral ligament bursa: MR imaging. Radiology 1991;178:855–7.

47. Fredericson M, Wolf C. Iliotibial band syndrome in runners: innovations in treatment. Sports Med 2005;35:451–9.

48. Ekman EF, Pope T, Martin DF, et al. Magnetic resonance imaging of iliotibial band syndrome. Am J Sports Med 1994;22:851–4.

49. Muhle C, Ahn JM, Yeh L, et al. Iliotibial band friction syndrome: MR imaging findings in 16 patients and MR arthrographic study of six cadaveric knees. Radiology 1999;212:103–10.

50. Murphy BJ, Hechtman KS, Uribe JW, et al. Iliotibial band friction syndrome: MR imaging findings. Radiology 1992;185:569–71.

51. Nishimura G, Yamato M, Tamai K, et al. MR findings in iliotibial band syndrome. Skeletal Radiol 1997;26: 533–7.

52. Coral A, van Holsbeeck M, Adler RS. Imaging of meniscal cyst of the knee in three cases. Skeletal Radiol 1989;18:451–5.

53. Ferrer-Roca O, Vilalta C. Lesions of the meniscus. Part II: horizontal cleavages and lateral cysts. Clin Orthop Relat Res 1980;146:301–7.

54. Campbell SE, Sanders TG, Morrison WB. MR imaging of meniscal cysts: incidence, location, and clinical significance. AJR Am J Roentgenol 2001;177:409–13.

55. Barrie HJ. The pathogenesis and significance of meniscal cysts. J Bone Joint Surg Br 1979;61-B:184–9.

56. Murphey MD, Gross TM, Rosenthal HG, et al. Magnetic resonance imaging of soft tissue and cystic masses about the knee. Top Magn Reson Imaging 1993;5:263–82.

57. Tasker AD, Ostlere SJ. Relative incidence and morphology of lateral and medial meniscal cysts detected by magnetic resonance imaging. Clin Radiol 1995;50:778–81.

58. Burk DL Jr, Dalinka MK, Kanal E, et al. Meniscal and ganglion cysts of the knee: MR evaluation. AJR Am J Roentgenol 1988;150:331–6.

59. Schuldt DR, Wolfe RD. Clinical and arthrographic findings in meniscal cysts. Radiology 1980;134:49–52.

60. Peetrons P, Allaer D, Jeanmart L. Cysts of the semilunar cartilages of the knee: a new approach by ultrasound imaging. A study of six cases and review of the literature. J Ultrasound Med 1990;9:333–7.

61. Spinner RJ, Desy NM, Amrami KK. Sequential tibial and peroneal intraneural ganglia arising from the superior tibiofibular joint. Skeletal Radiol 2008;37: 79–84.

62. Spinner RJ, Mokhtarzadeh A, Schiefer TK, et al. The clinico-anatomic explanation for tibial intraneural ganglion cysts arising from the superior tibiofibular joint. Skeletal Radiol 2007;36:281–92.

63. Hebert-Blouin MN, Amrami KK, Wang H, et al. Tibialis anterior branch involvement in fibular intraneural ganglia. Muscle Nerve 2010;41:524–32.

64. Feldman F, Singson RD, Staron RB. Magnetic resonance imaging of para-articular and ectopic ganglia. Skeletal Radiol 1989;18:353–8.

65. Gambari PI, Giuliani G, Poppi M, et al. Ganglionic cysts of the peroneal nerve at the knee: CT and surgical correlation. J Comput Assist Tomogr 1990; 14:801–3.

66. Malghem J, Vande berg BC, Lebon C, et al. Ganglion cysts of the knee: articular communication revealed by delayed radiography and CT after arthrography. AJR Am J Roentgenol 1998;170:1579–83.

67. Scapinelli R. A synovial ganglion of the popliteus tendon simulating a parameniscal cyst. Two case reports. J Bone Joint Surg Am 1988;70:1085–6.

68. Stener B. Unusual ganglion cysts in the neighbourhood of the knee joint. A report of six cases–three with involvement of the peroneal nerve. Acta Orthop Scand 1969;40:392–401.

69. Kumar A, Bickerstaff DR, Grimwood JS, et al. Mucoid cystic degeneration of the cruciate ligament. J Bone Joint Surg Br 1999;81:304–5.

70. Fernandes JL, Viana SL, Mendonca JL, et al. Mucoid degeneration of the anterior cruciate ligament: magnetic resonance imaging findings of an underdiagnosed entity. Acta Radiol 2008;49:75–9.

71. McIntyre J, Moelleken S, Tirman P. Mucoid degeneration of the anterior cruciate ligament mistaken for ligamentous tears. Skeletal Radiol 2001;30:312–5.

72. Narvekar A, Gajjar S. Mucoid degeneration of the anterior cruciate ligament. Arthroscopy 2004;20: 141–6.

73. Shelly MJ, Dheer S, Kavanagh EC. Metastatic adenocarcinoma of the lung mimicking mucoid degeneration of the anterior cruciate ligament. Ir J Med Sci 2010;179:309–11.

74. Bergin D, Morrison WB, Carrino JA, et al. Anterior cruciate ligament ganglia and mucoid

degeneration: coexistence and clinical correlation. AJR Am J Roentgenol 2004;182:1283–7.

75. Lintz F, Pujol N, Boisrenoult P, et al. Anterior cruciate ligament mucoid degeneration: a review of the literature and management guidelines. Knee Surg Sports Traumatol Arthrosc 2011;19:1326–33.

76. Kim MG, Kim BH, Choi JA, et al. Intra-articular ganglion cysts of the knee: clinical and MR imaging features. Eur Radiol 2001;11:834–40.

77. Garcia A, Hodler J, Vaughn L, et al. Case report 677. Intraarticular ganglion arising from the posterior cruciate-ligament. Skeletal Radiol 1991;20: 373–5.

78. Levine J. A ganglion of the anterior cruciate ligament. Surgery 1948;24:836–40.

79. Recht MP, Applegate G, Kaplan P, et al. The MR appearance of cruciate ganglion cysts: a report of 16 cases. Skeletal Radiol 1994;23:597–600.

80. Nokes SR, Koonce TW, Montanez J. Ganglion cysts of the cruciate ligaments of the knee: recognition on MR images and CT-guided aspiration. AJR Am J Roentgenol 1994;162:1503.

81. Yasuda K, Majima T. Intra-articular ganglion blocking extension of the knee: brief report. J Bone Joint Surg Br 1988;70:837.

82. Kim TH, Lee DH, Lee SH, et al. Arthroscopic treatment of mucoid hypertrophy of the anterior cruciate ligament. Arthroscopy 2008;24:642–9.

83. Chang W, Rose DJ. Ganglion cysts of the anterior cruciate ligament. A case report. Bull Hosp Jt Dis Orthop Inst 1988;48:182–6.

84. Kaempffe F, D'Amato C. An unusual intra-articular ganglion of the knee with interosseous extension. A case report. J Bone Joint Surg Am 1989;71:773–5.

85. Bromley JW, Cohen P. Ganglion of the posterior cruciate ligament: report of a case. J Bone Joint Surg Am 1965;47:1247–9.

86. Antonacci VP, Foster T, Fenlon H, et al. Technical report: CT-guided aspiration of anterior cruciate ligament ganglion cysts. Clin Radiol 1998;53:771–3.

87. Campagnolo DI, Davis BA, Blacksin MF. Computed tomography–guided aspiration of a ganglion cyst of the anterior cruciate ligament: a case report. Arch Phys Med Rehabil 1996;77:732–3.

88. Ozkur A, Adaletli I, Sirikci A, et al. Hoffa's recess in the infrapatellar fat pad of the knee on MR imaging. Surg Radiol Anat 2005;27:61–3.

89. Saddik D, McNally EG, Richardson M. MRI of Hoffa's fat pad. Skeletal Radiol 2004;33:433–44.

90. Kramer J, Recht M, Deely DM, et al. MR appearance of idiopathic synovial osteochondromatosis. J Comput Assist Tomogr 1993;17:772–6.

91. Helpert C, Davies AM, Evans N, et al. Differential diagnosis of tumours and tumour-like lesions of the infrapatellar (Hoffa's) fat pad: pictorial review with an emphasis on MR imaging. Eur Radiol 2004;14:2337–46.

92. Holden A, Merrilees S, Mitchell N, et al. Magnetic resonance imaging of popliteal artery pathologies. Eur J Radiol 2008;67:159–68.

93. Iwasko N, Steinbach LS, Disler D, et al. Imaging findings in Mazabraud's syndrome: seven new cases. Skeletal Radiol 2002;31:81–7.

Imaging Evaluation of Traumatic Ligamentous Injuries of the Ankle and Foot

Anna Nazarenko, MD[a,*], Luis S. Beltran, MD[b],
Jenny T. Bencardino, MD[b]

KEYWORDS

- Ankle • Sprain • Traumatic • Anatomy • Ligament

KEY POINTS

- Ankle sprains can cause a significant financial burden, time lost to injury, and long-term disability.
- Magnetic resonance (MR) imaging is well known to depict normal ankle anatomy, ligamentous injury of the ankle, or associated conditions of ankle sprain.
- Accepted MR imaging findings of acute ligamentous injury, usually within the first 3 weeks, include discontinuity, detachment, irregular contour, thinning, and increased intraligamentous signal on T2-weighted images indicating edema or hemorrhage.

INTRODUCTION

Epidemiology

Ankle injuries are very common in sports worldwide, with many publications in the medical literature devoted to this topic. Ankle trauma accounts for 10% to 30% of all sports injuries, with ankle sprains representing the most common type. A recent international review by Fong and colleagues[1] reported the ankle as the second most common location to be affected in sports injuries, preceded only by the knee. Ankle sprains account for more than 90% of injuries in many sports, including football, hockey, basketball, martial arts, and indoor volleyball.

In the United States, it is estimated that 2 million acute ankle sprains occur each year, averaging $318 to $914 per sprain.[2] Waterman and colleagues[3] reported that almost half of the ankle sprains occurred during athletic activity, most commonly in basketball, football, soccer, and running. The incidence rate of ankle sprains presenting to the emergency department was 2.15 per 1000 person-years, occurring more commonly between 15 to 19 years of age. In comparison, epidemiologic studies in Europe have reported the incidence rates of ankle sprains to be 5 to 7 per 1000 person-years, with the highest incidence in the 10- to 19-year-old age group.[4,5] Although the investigators did not hypothesize as to why the difference in incidence exist,[3–5] it may reflect different availability or popularity of sports in the United States and Europe.

Clinical Considerations

In the acute phase of lateral ankle injury, clinical examination can only accurately diagnose the ligaments involved in 50% of sprains.[6] However, at 5 days after the injury, when the pain and swelling have diminished, the sensitivity and specificity of the physical examination increases to 96% and 84%, respectively.[7] Ankle sprains can cause a significant financial burden, time lost to injury, and long-term disability.[2,8] In a recent review by van Rijn and colleagues,[9] 33% of patients

Disclosures: None.
[a] Department of Radiology, Maimonides Medical Center, 4802 10th Avenue, Brooklyn, NY 11219, USA;
[b] Department of Radiology, NYU Hospital for Joint Diseases, NYU Langone Medical Center, 301 East 17th Street, New York, NY 10003, USA
* Corresponding author.
E-mail address: Anazarenko@maimonidesmed.org

Radiol Clin N Am 51 (2013) 455–478
http://dx.doi.org/10.1016/j.rcl.2012.11.004

had residual symptoms 1 year following an ankle sprain, and ankle resprains ranged from 3% to 34% within 2 weeks to 96 months after the initial injury. Recurrent sprains have been linked to an increase in the risk of posttraumatic ankle arthrosis.[10]

Diagnostic Imaging

Magnetic resonance (MR) imaging, MR arthrography, conventional arthrography, ultrasound, computer tomography (CT) scan, and radiography have all been described in the imaging of ankle sprain.[11] In clinical practice, MR imaging and CT scans are generally not routinely performed in the setting of an acute ankle sprain. MR evaluation is usually reserved for highly competitive athletes and ballet dancers in whom primary ligamentous repair is contemplated and people with chronic ankle instability.[12–15]

MR imaging is able to elegantly depict normal ankle anatomy, ligamentous injuries of the ankle, and pathologic conditions of other structures commonly occurring in conjunction with ankle sprains.[16–18] MR imaging readily demonstrates the complex anatomy of the ankle ligaments.[19] The limitations of MR imaging are cost, time, availability, motion artifact, and low predictive value for the chronic sequelae following acute injury.[14] On MR images, normal ankle ligaments are seen as low-signal-intensity structures connecting nearby bones, usually outlined delimited by surrounding fat signal.[20] Signal heterogeneity, striations, and apparent areas of discontinuity may be noted in normal ligaments, such as the posterior talofibular ligament, posterior tibiotalar component of the deltoid ligament, and anterior inferior tibiofibular ligament.[15,21] This appearance typically results from fat interposed between the ligamentous fascicles.[17]

MR imaging findings of acute ligamentous injury include discontinuity, detachment, contour irregularity, thinning, and increased intraligamentous signal on T2-weighted images (WI) indicating edema or hemorrhage.[16,22] Secondary findings on T2-WI include extravasation of joint fluid or hemorrhage into the adjacent soft tissues, joint effusion, tenosynovial effusion, bone avulsion at the ligamentous insertion, and bone contusion.[18,22–24] In subacute or chronic tears, the edema and hemorrhage have typically reabsorbed, and only direct morphologic changes can be seen. Common findings include signal heterogeneity, waviness, thickening, thinning, elongation, and poor or nonvisualization of the ligament.[19,22] Decreased signal of the surrounding fat on both T1- and T2-WI is often seen because of scarring or synovial proliferation.[19]

Numerous MR protocols have been advocated for optimal visualization of the ligaments, including 3-dimensional (3D) imaging[23] as well as imaging the ankle with the foot in varying degrees of dorsiflexion, plantar flexion, and/or the neutral position.[14,16,25] Routine MR imaging of the ankle is performed in the axial, coronal, and sagittal planes. Generally, axial and coronal imaging with the foot in dorsiflexion and plantar flexion allow visualization of the ligaments in their entirety.[21] The sagittal images are rarely useful for visualizing the ligaments. The ligaments are almost consistently seen on routine orthogonal ankle imaging as long as the foot is mildly plantar flexed and thin slices of 3 mm thickness are obtained. The foot is imaged in the oblique axial plane (ie, parallel to the long axis of the metatarsal bones), the oblique coronal plane (ie, perpendicular to the long axis of the metatarsals), and the oblique sagittal plane (**Box 1**).[15]

Box 1
Routine MR imaging protocol performed in the oblique axial plane, the oblique coronal plane, and the oblique sagittal plane

Routine MR Imaging Protocol

Mild plantar flexion ($\sim$20°) decreases magic angle effect, accentuates the fat plane between the peroneal tendons, and allows better visualization of the calcaneofibular ligament.

An extremity surface coil enhances spatial resolution. A wrist coil or another small dedicated coil is often used to evaluate the forefoot.

T1-weighted (repetition time/echo time = 600/20 ms)

MR images are obtained with a 12- to 16-cm field of view, a 256 $\times$ 192 to 512 acquisition matrix, 1 to 2 signals acquired, and a 3- to 5-mm section thickness, interleaved.

Marrow abnormalities are best evaluated with fat-suppression techniques, such as fat-suppressed proton-density–weighted imaging or short tau inversion recovery (STIR) sequences (1500/20; inversion time = 100–150 ms).

Susceptibility to gradient inhomogeneity makes fat suppression techniques more challenging than STIR techniques in imaging the ankle and foot.

Cartilage abnormalities are best visualized using high-resolution intermediate proton-density or 3D gradient-echo sequences.

Data from Rosenberg ZS, Beltran J, Bencardino JT. From the RSNA Refresher Courses. Radiological Society of North America. MR imaging of the ankle and foot. Radiographics 2000;20:S153–79.

BIOMECHANICS
Functional Anatomy

The ankle joint has 3 articulations (tibiotalar, subtalar, and distal tibiofibular syndesmosis) supported by 3 ligamentous groups (lateral collateral, medial collateral, and syndesmosis).[26] The joints are stabilized by the congruity of the articular surfaces (loaded joint), static ligamentous restraints, and dynamic muscle-tendon units.[27] The lateral collateral ligament complex is subdivided into the anterior talofibular ligament (ATFL), the calcaneofibular ligament (CFL), and the posterior talofibular ligament (PTFL). The medial collateral ligamentous complex, or deltoid ligament complex, has 5 bands: the anterior and posterior tibiotalar, tibiospring, tibiocalcaneal, and tibionavicular ligaments. The tibiofibular syndesmosis is comprised of the interosseous membrane and the anteroinferior tibiofibular ligament (AITFL), posteroinferior tibiofibular ligament (PITFL), interosseous ligament (IOL), and the inferior transverse ligament (ITL).[26]

Triplanar Motion

All 3 joints work as a unit to allow coordinated movement of the rear foot in a triplanar motion (sagittal, frontal, and transverse) (Box 2).[27–30] The coupled motion of the ankle and subtalar joints allow for simultaneous motions in all 3 planes resulting in inversion, eversion, pronation, and supination.[28,31] During non–weight bearing, pronation can be described as dorsiflexion, eversion, and abduction/external rotation, whereas supination is plantar flexion, inversion, and adduction/internal rotation. During weight bearing, pronation can be defined as plantar flexion, eversion, and adduction/internal rotation, whereas supination is dorsiflexion, inversion, and abduction/external rotation.[28] Inversion at the subtalar joint occurs when the medial border of the foot elevates and the lateral border of the foot depresses, ranging from 20° to 30°, whereas eversion is the elevation of the lateral border and depression of the medial border of the foot, ranging from 5° to 15°.[31]

CLINICAL SYNDROMES
High Ankle Sprain

Epidemiology
High ankle or tibiofibular syndesmotic sprains compose approximately 7% of ankle sprains.[32] In athletes, the incidence has been reported as high as 40%.[33] Syndesmotic sprains are common in collision sports, such as American football, skiing, running/jumping, ice hockey, and soccer.[31,33,34]

Box 2
Movements at the level of the tibiotalar joint in a triplanar motion (sagittal, frontal, and transverse)

Trimalar Movements

Sagittal plane: The movements are mainly in the tibiotalar joint and are defined as dorsiflexion (ie, the tip of the dorsum of the foot moves toward the anterior aspect of the tibia) and plantar flexion (ie, the tip of the foot turns downward away from the tibia).[27,29] The range of motion is reported to be 10° to 51° for dorsiflexion and 15° to 56° for plantar flexion.[29,30] The talus is wedge shaped (wider anteriorly) and in dorsiflexion engages between the medial and lateral malleoli. In plantar flexion, the anterior aspect of the talus moves out of the mortise as it internally rotates and supinates, decreasing the stability of the ankle in this position.[31]

Frontal plane: The axis of rotation is about the sagittal plane with little movement (eversion and inversion) in isolation with an intact tibiotalar joint.[27]

Horizontal/transverse plane: The tibiotalar joint moves in internal rotation (the tip of the foot turns medially) and in external rotation (the tip of the foot turns laterally). The vertical axis is through the talus. The isolated degree of rotation is considered to be small.[28,29]

Functional anatomy
The interosseous membrane has an important role in limiting the lateral displacement of the fibula during weight bearing and load sharing with the fibula.[31,35] The distal interosseous (tibiofibular) ligament acts as a spring during dorsiflexion of the ankle joint, allowing for minimal separation of the medial and lateral malleoli.[36]

Clinical considerations and mechanism of injury
The 2 most common causes of syndesmotic injury are excessive external rotation and hyperdorsiflexion. External rotation forces the talus laterally, which pushes the fibula laterally from the mortise.[31] Isolated external rotation usually leads first to the rupture of the anterior aspect of the deltoid ligament or fracture of the medial malleolus. This is followed by the involvement of the AITFL, the superficial PITFL, the ITL, the interosseous membrane, and lastly a spiral fracture to the fibula or Maisonneuve fracture.[37] In football players, the main mechanism is a direct blow to the lateral leg of a downed player or a blow to the lateral knee while the foot is planted in external rotation while the body is rotating in the opposite

direction. In skiing injuries, the foot is fixed in place when the external rotational and forces are applied.[31] The PITFL is usually injured concomitantly with the AITFL.[37]

Diagnostic imaging

On radiography, the talotibial angle is normally 83° ± 4°, the medial clear space is less than 3 mm, and the talar tilt difference is 2 mm.[38] The height of the tibiofibular recess in normal patients is 0.54 ± 0.68 cm (**Fig. 1**). In acute injury, the tibiofibular recess measures 1.2 ± 0.92 cm compared with 1.4 ± 0.57 cm in chronic injury.[39] Isolated AITFL injuries may have no associated swelling, making clinical diagnosis difficult. Vogl and colleagues[40] reported that the sensitivity and specificity of contrast-enhanced T1-weighted MR imaging sequences in detecting disruption of the AITFL was 100% and 83%, respectively.[40] Oae and colleagues[41] compared MR imaging and arthroscopy, using arthroscopy as the gold standard, based on 2 criteria: (1) ligament discontinuity and (2) wavy/curved contour or nonvisualization of the ligament (**Table 1**). The accuracy of ankle arthroscopy has been reported to be 100% in diagnosing syndesmotic disruption compared with 64% by mortise radiography and 48% by anteroposterior (AP) radiography.[38]

MR imaging findings associated with trauma to the syndesmotic ligaments include blurring, lateral fibular subluxation, fibular shortening, tibiofibular diastasis, and fluid-like signal. Interosseous membrane injuries are seen as linear hyperintensity at the level of the distal tibia and fibula on heavily T2-WI, fat-suppressed proton-density–weighted (FS PD) fast spin echo (FSE), or short tau inversion recovery (STIR) images. Low-signal-intensity foci can represent hemosiderin, fibrosis, or calcifications.[26] Brown and colleagues[39] reported that distal tibiofibular syndesmosis sprains are highly associated with ATFL injury (74%), tibiofibular joint incongruity in chronic injury (33%), bone bruise in acute injury (24%), and an osteochondral lesion of the talar dome in both acute and chronic injury (28%).

AITFL/PITFL The AITFL and PITFL are usually seen on 2 or more sequential axial and coronal MR images at the level of the tibial plafond and talar dome. On axial images, they often seem striated and discontinuous. The morphology of the talus and the distal fibula can be used to distinguish the anterior and posterior inferior tibiofibular ligaments from the anterior and posterior talofibular ligaments on axial MR images (T1 and T2 weighted). The talar dome at the level of the tibiofibular ligaments is somewhat square. Additionally, the tibiofibular ligaments insert into the fibula above the malleolar fossa where the cross section of the fibula is round (**Fig. 2**).[19]

The AITFL is trapezoidal and comprised of multiple fiber bands.[16,19,24] It originates from the longitudinal tubercle of the lateral malleolus, courses superomedially, and attaches on the anterolateral tubercle of the tibia.[31] In the horizontal plane, the AITFL makes a 35° angle with the coronal axis of the tibial plafond and a 65° angle with its sagittal axis.[42] The AITFL is 20% intra-articular and makes contact with the lateral ridge of the trochlear surface of the talus in plantar flexion.[26]

The anatomic variations of the AITFL can be classified into 5 categories based on the number of fascicles, presence or absence of separations between the fascicles, attachment of inferior fascicle to the main portion of the ligament, and presence of a separate accessory inferior fascicle.[43] The accessory AITFL ligament, also referred to the distal fascicle or Bassett ligament, is present in 21% to 92% of human ankles in cadaveric and MR imaging studies. This accessory ligament is a triangular horizontal band, which is separated from the other AITFL bands by a triangular fat-filled space. It usually runs inferior and parallel to the AITFL.[36] The PITFL is triangular and has a broad tibial insertion. It originates from the posterior tubercle of the tibia and courses inferolaterally to the posterior lateral malleolus.

Sprain injuries of the AITFL manifest as attenuation, laxity, or discontinuity of the ligament on MR imaging. Other findings include periarticular

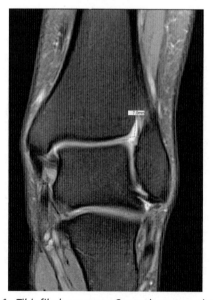

Fig. 1. *Tibiofibular recess.* Coronal proton density with fat saturation showing the height of the tibiofibular recess to be 7.0 mm, which is within normal limits.

Table 1
The sensitivity specificity and accuracy of MR imaging in detecting disruption of the AITFL, using arthroscopy as the gold standard

		Sensitivity (%)	Specificity (%)	Accuracy (%)
AITFL	Criteria 1	100	70	84
	Criteria 1 and 2	100	93	97
PITFL	Criteria 1	100	94	95
	Criteria 1 and 2	100	100	100

Criterion 1, ligament discontinuity; criterion 2, wavy/curved contour or nonvisualization of ligament.
Data from Oae K, Takao M, Naito K, et al. Injury of the tibiofibular syndesmosis: value of MR imaging for diagnosis. Radiology 2003;227(1):155–61.

edema or hemorrhage in the subcutaneous tissues anterior to the torn ligament, which may extend between the torn ends of the ligament in continuity with the tibiofibular recess of the ankle joint. Injuries of the PITFL can also have a similar appearance (**Figs. 3** and **4**).[40] A pitfall of imaging for AITFL tears is its variable appearance; the AITFL can be thick or thin in absence of pathologic conditions. Both the AITFL and PITFL can mimic intra-articular loose bodies on the sagittal plane because of their transverse course. Therefore, it is important to find associated morphologic and signal changes of the ligaments supportive of sprain.[44]

ITL/intermalleolar ligament/IOL The ITL is a strong, thick, deep component of the PITFL. Whether the ITL and distal PITFL form one anatomic unit or are 2 distinct structures is controversial.[31] The ITL can be considered a labrumlike extension of the tibial articular surface with more horizontal orientation as compared with the remainder of the PITFL fibers.[17] It attaches to the osteochondral junction on the posteromedial aspect of the distal fibula.[31] During plantar flexion, the ITL is tightly positioned between the posterior tibial margins and the PTFL.[45] It functions to limit the talus from posterior translation and increases the stability of the joint.[31] This ligament is best visualized on coronal and axial oblique planes parallel to the PITFL.[17,26,46] However, the labrumlike characteristics are best seen on the sagittal plane (**Fig. 5**). On coronal plantar flexion images, the ITL and PTFL ligaments approximate and may overlap.[16]

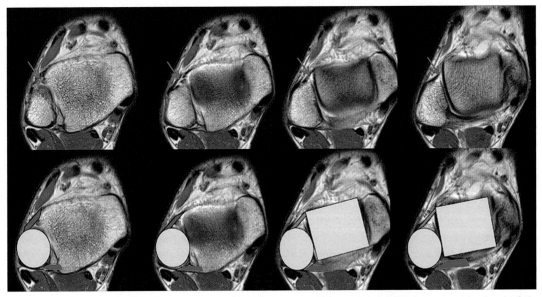

Fig. 2. *Normal tibiofibular ligaments.* Consecutive axial intermediate-weighted MR images at the level of the tibiotalar joint. The syndesmotic ligaments are demonstrated as hypointense bands and include the AITFL (*green arrows*) and the PITFL (*blue arrows*). Geometric figures help localize the levels of visualization of the lateral ankle ligaments. At the level of the AITFL (*green band*) and the PITFL (*blue band*), the talar dome and the fibula are square and ovoid, respectively. Note a broader attachment of the PITFL into the posterolateral talus.

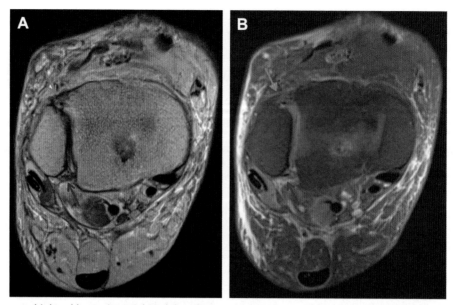

Fig. 3. *Remote high ankle sprain.* Axial PD (*A*) and FS PD (*B*) MR images through the tibial plafond demonstrate an irregular wavy contour and signal heterogeneity of both the AITFL (*green arrow*) and the PITFL (*blue arrow*). The fluid-sensitive sequence helps demonstrate mildly increased signal within both the ligaments. The findings are compatible with a remote partial tear of the AITFL and PITFL.

The intermalleolar ligament (IML), or the posterior IML, is a normal variant of the posterior ankle joint. The reported frequency of the IML is 19% on MR imaging and 56% to 82% on dissected anatomic specimens. On MR imaging the IML may appear as a thick hypointense band or as 2 to 3 parallel strips traversing between the ITL and PTFL. The IML originates within the malleolar fossa, superior to the origin of the PTFL, and courses obliquely to insert into the posteromedial tibial cortex, medial to the site of insertion of the ITL.[46,47] The IOL is the lowest end of the interosseous membrane as it thickens.[31] The IOL is a multi fascicular broad ligament that originates in the fibular notch of the tibia and courses obliquely to attach on the anteroinferior triangular segment of the distal medial fibular shaft above the tibiotalar joint.[17] This ligament may be completely absent.[19]

Lateral Ankle Sprains: Inversion Injuries

Epidemiology

Lateral ankle injuries account for up to 20% of all sports injuries and up to 45% of injuries in basketball.[48] Out of these, the ATFL is injured in 83%, the CFL in 67%, and the PTFL in 34%.[49] Avulsion fractures of the lateral ankle ligaments are not infrequent and can be seen in up to 26% of severe inversion injuries.[50] The CFL has 2.0 to 3.5 times greater maximum load compared with the ATFL,

which likely explains the high prevalence and incidence of ATFL injuries.[51]

Functional anatomy

The lateral ligament complex acts as a static stabilizer of the ankle, limiting excessive inversion-type motion.[52] A recent study by de Asla and colleagues[53] showed that the ATFL elongates during plantar flexion and supination, whereas the CFL increases in length with dorsiflexion and pronation. The 2 ligaments seem to have opposing movements: one shortens whereas the other one elongates. They concluded that under excessive loading conditions, the ATFL may be more susceptible to injury in plantar flexion and supination, whereas the CFL may be more susceptible to injury in dorsiflexion and pronation.

Clinical considerations and mechanism of injury

Patients usually have localized tenderness over the ATFL at 4 to 7 days following injury.[54] The anterior drawer and talar tilt tests are provocative maneuvers used to assess the integrity of the lateral ligaments, specifically the ATFL and the CFL.[55] Residual symptoms after lateral ankle sprain affect 37% of patients at 6 months.[34] Approximately 20% of acute ankle sprains develop functional or mechanical instability, resulting in a diagnosis of chronic ankle instability (CAI).[54] CAI is defined as mechanical and/or functional instability.[27] CAI is associated with a history

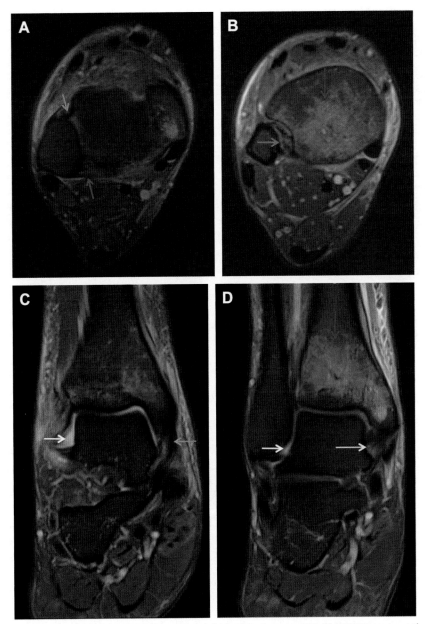

Fig. 4. *Recent high ankle sprain and tibial fracture.* Axial (*A, B*) and coronal (*C, D*) FS PD images at the level of the tibiotalar joint demonstrate a lax wavy contour of the AITFL (*green arrow*), whereas the PITFL appears thickened, discontinuous, and bright (*blue arrow*). Sprain of the oblique/syndesmotic ligament (*red arrow*) and incomplete fracture of the distal tibia outlined by extensive marrow edema (*purple arrow*) are also seen. Concomitant sprain of the superficial tibiospring (*orange arrow*) and deep posterior tibiotalar (*yellow arrow*) components of the deltoid ligament complex are seen. Note a small ankle joint effusion (*white arrow*).

of 2 or more ankle sprains, difficulty walking with uneasiness/apprehension on uneven surfaces, and/or a history of the ankle giving way.[34,54]

Injury to the lateral complex typically occurs during forced plantar flexion and inversion.[26,54] The center of gravity is shifted to the lateral border of the leg causing the ankle to roll inward at a high velocity.[56] In a situation of loading the ball of the foot in landing from a jump or fall a tear along the long course of the ligaments may occur. The mechanism is usually of the twisting type, with both dorsiflexion and internal rotation resulting in a midsubstance rupture of the ATFL, CFL, and the intervening capsule.[26] The predictable pattern of injury involves first the ATFL, followed by the CFL, and then the PTFL.[57]

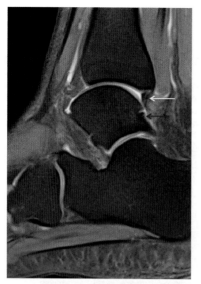

Fig. 5. *Inferior transverse ligament.* PD FS sagittal image of the ankle. The white arrow is pointing to the ITL. This ligament is best visualized on coronal and axial oblique planes parallel to the PITFL. However, the labrumlike characteristics are best seen on the sagittal plane. The blue arrow represents the PTFL.

Diagnostic imaging

Various imaging modalities have been studied in imaging the lateral ankle ligaments (Table 2). The initial inflammatory phase occurring after an ankle sprain lasts 1 to 3 days. In this phase, a hematoma can form between the torn tendon ends. In the reparative phase, occurring 3 to 5 days after the injury, the torn ligament heals through formation of fibroblastic proliferative tissue.[56] It has been reported that if the sprain occurs close to the bony attachment, there is often delayed healing. On MR imaging defects within the substance of the ATFL can be seen within 2 weeks after trauma.[22] During the remodeling phase (15–28 days), the ligament forms collagen fibers that align longitudinally and cross-link.[56] By this time the edema and hemorrhage have usually resolved and the ligament's altered morphology is better visualized. Observed changes include attenuation, thickening, thinning, elongation, or waviness. Periarticular edema is commonly present until up to the seventh week after the injury; however, edema associated with ATFL and CFL injuries usually resolves by the fourth week.[22,64] After 7 weeks, the visualized defect closes, leaving either a thin hypoplastic or thick hyperplastic ligament.[22]

ATFL The ATFL is best imaged on axial T1 or high-resolution PD MR images, appearing as a flat, thin, homogeneous band of low signal intensity arising from the anterior margin of the lateral malleolus and coursing anteromedially downward to attach onto the neck of the talus, just anterior to the fibular articular cartilage (Fig. 6).[16,20,65] At the level of the talofibular ligaments, the talus is oblong and

Table 2
Imaging modalities that can be used in the assessment of lateral ankle sprains

Imaging of the Lateral Ankle Ligaments	
Ultrasound	Ultrasound accuracy is reported as high as 95% and 90% for acute sprains of the ATFL and CFL, respectively. Findings include discontinuity, hypoechogenicity, or lack of visualization.[58,59]
Radiography	Talar tilt test is evaluated on stress AP radiographs and is considered positive if there is a 5° difference compared with the uninjured ankle or a 10° absolute value.[54]
CT scan	3D CT is useful in the evaluation of ATFL lesions, particularly chronic injury. Accuracy in diagnosing ATFL sprain is reported as high as 94%.[60]
Arthrography	Arthrography within 48 hours of acute injury has a sensitivity and specificity of 96% and 71%, respectively.[61]
MR arthrography	MR arthrography may be superior to MR imaging for the assessment of lateral collateral ligament injuries. In a series of 17 patients with chronic ankle instability, MR arthrography was found to be 100% and 82% accurate, whereas conventional MR imaging was only 59% and 63% accurate in detecting ATFL and CFL tears, respectively.[62]
MR imaging	MR imaging has a reported sensitivity and specificity of 83% and 77% when compared with arthrography for the detection of CFL tears.[63] 3D FISP imaging has a reported accuracy of 94% for detecting ATFL and CFL tears. Compared with operative findings, the sensitivity and specificity for diagnosing rupture of the ATFL and the CFL was 100% and 50% and 92% and 100%, respectively.[23]

Abbreviation: FISP, Fast imaging with steady-state precession.

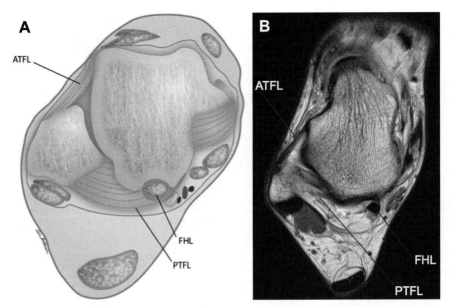

Fig. 6. *Normal talofibular ligaments.* (*A*) The normal ATFL, PTFL, and flexor hallucis longus (FHL) tendon with corresponding (*B*) axial PD MR image depicts a taut ATFL measuring 2 to 3 mm in thickness. The PTFL has a striated appearance because of interspersed fat. The PTFL fibers form the roof of the fibro-osseous tunnel along the posterior aspect of the talus in which the FHL tendon traverses the ankle joint (seen best on the schematic).

the sinus tarsi is partially visualized, serving as landmarks in localization. The lower portion of the fibular malleolus has a crescentic configuration, which forms the malleolar fossa (**Fig. 7**).[15] When the foot is positioned in neutral or plantar flexion the orientation of the ATFL is 45° to the coronal plane of the tibia.[26] Studies have shown that the ATFL is 13 to 25 mm in length, 7 to 11 mm in width, and 2 to 3 mm thick.[65,66]

ATFL tears are usually associated with a capsular rupture and extravasation of joint fluid into the anterolateral soft tissues; on fluid-sensitive sequences native joint fluid outlines the ATFL.[15,16,26] On axial T1 or PD MR images the ligament may be indistinct or thickened with associated signal heterogeneity. On FS T2 FSE fluidlike signal intensity is often seen within the torn ATFL fibers.[26] A complete tear of the ATFL can be seen as a fluid-filled defect across the ruptured ligament with retraction of wavy/lax fibers. Intrasubstance tears can be seen as abnormal increased STIR or T2 signal within the ligament, indicating edema or hemorrhage.[67] Chronic tears may manifest either as severe attenuation or as thickening secondary to scarring. In chronic injuries granulation/scar tissue beneath the ATFL in the anterolateral gutter can form a triangular shape. This is often referred to as a *meniscoid* lesion because of its similar morphology to a meniscus in the knee; this tissue can be a cause of impingement in the ankle (**Figs. 8** and **9**).[15]

CFL The CFL is large, strong, and cordlike. It arises from the deep aspect of the inferior tip of the lateral malleolus and courses posteroinferiorly to attach to the lateral aspect of the calcaneus, just about the retro-trochlear eminence. The CFL crosses both the tibiotalar and subtalar joints and is located deep to the peroneal tendons.[16,26,65] It is best seen on axial and coronal images (**Fig. 10**).[15] On axial images the peroneal retinaculum can sometimes be mistaken for the CFL, although the peroneal retinaculum is located superficial to the peroneal tendons.[16] On sequential T1-weighted coronal images the CFL is depicted in cross section as a thin, homogenous low-signal-intensity structure deep to the peroneal tendons.[15,20] The ligament is best depicted on axial images in plantar flexion.[19] The CFL should be clearly identified to avoid confusing it with a loose body or an avulsion fracture of the calcaneus, particularly in the coronal plane.[68] The CFL has an average length of 36 mm, a width of 5 mm, and a thickness of 2 mm.[65]

CFL tears are characterized by indistinctness of the ligament fibers and signal heterogeneity. The ligament is frequently thickened with obliteration of the surrounding fat planes.[15,26] Thickening of the superior peroneal retinaculum and peroneal tenosynovial effusions are also commonly seen with CFL tears because of a communication between the tibiotalar joint and the peroneal tendon sheath.[22]

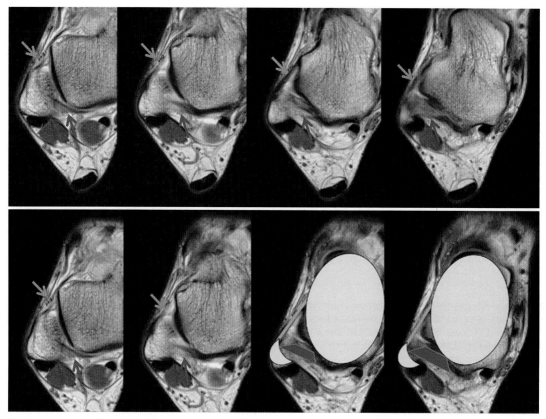

Fig. 7. *Normal talofibular ligaments.* Consecutive PD axial images at the level of the ATFL (*green arrow and band*) and the PTFL (*blue arrow and band*). The normal ATFL and PTFL appear as taught hypointense linear structures. The last 2 images on the bottom row demonstrate that at this level, the talar dome and the fibula are oblong and crescentic in configuration, respectively.

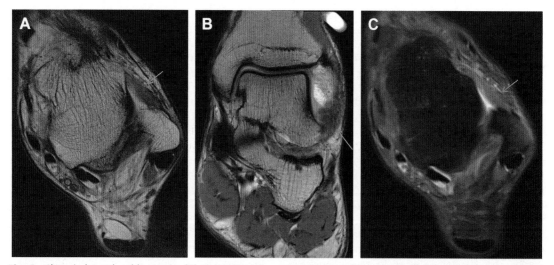

Fig. 8. *Chronic lateral ankle sprain.* (*A*) Axial PD, (*B*) coronal PD, and (*C*) axial FS PD MR images demonstrate a thickened ATFL (*green arrow*) with intermediate signal. Note the deep undersurface of the ATFL has an irregular wavy contour, most likely secondary to scarring and synovitis. These findings are consistent with a chronic inversion sprain.

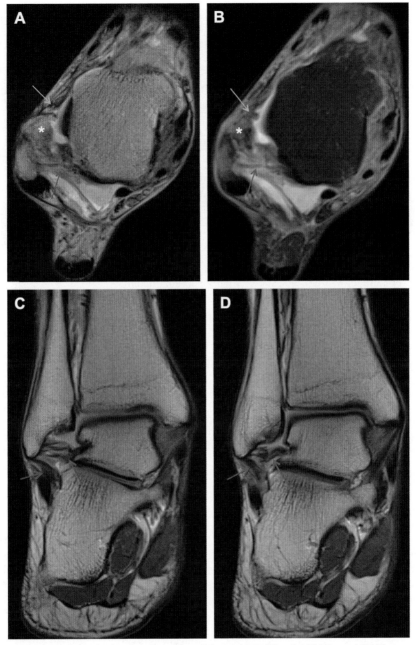

Fig. 9. *Chronic anterior talofibular ligament avulsion.* (*A*) Axial PD, (*B*) axial FS PD, and (*C, D*) sequential coronal PD MR images from posterior to anterior (*left to right*) demonstrate complete disruption of the ATFL (*green arrows*) at its fibular insertion site, associated with a nonhealed fracture of the lateral malleolar tip (*asterisk*). The PTFL (*blue arrow*) shows hyperintense signal and an irregular wavy contour consistent with a partial tear. The CFL (*red arrow*) appear thickened consistent with a healed sprain.

PTFL The PTFL is inhomogeneous, thick, multi fascicular, and considered the strongest and deepest ligament of the lateral collateral complex.[20,26] The PTFL is intracapsular but extra-synovial.[26] On axial and coronal images the PTFL has a fan-shaped configuration, extending infero-medially from the deep aspect of the lateral malleolus to attach on the mid to posterior aspect of the talus.[16,19,20]

The PTFL often shows marked signal heteroge-neity and thickening caused by the presence of fat striations, which should not be misinterpreted as a tear.[19] Sprains involving the PTFL manifest as high T2 signal within the ligament, which has an

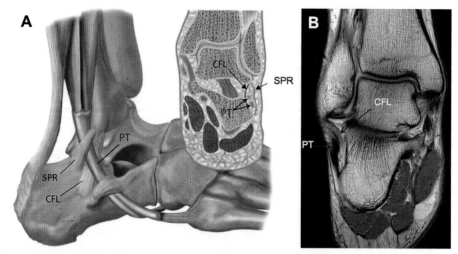

Fig. 10. *Normal CFL.* (*A*) Sagittal illustration, with a coronal inset, showing the CFL deep to the peroneal tendon sheath. (*B*) Coronal PD MR image correlating to the inset in (*A*). The peroneal tendon (PT) is seen superficial to the CFL (illustrated by Salvador Beltran). SPR, superior peroneal retinaculum.

irregular wavy contour (see **Fig. 9**). The PTFL and the posterior IML course transversely behind the tibiotalar joint and frequently are seen as punctuate low-signal-intensity structures posteriorly in the sagittal plane, potentially mimicking intra-articular bodies in the posterior ankle. It is important to carefully track each of these ligaments from their origin to their insertions on orthogonal imaging planes to avoid this pitfall.[44]

Medial Ankle Sprains: Eversion Injury

Epidemiology
Injuries of the deltoid ligament complex accounted for approximately 5% of ankle sprains in a study by Waterman and colleagues.[32] Medial ankle sprains were more commonly seen in men's rugby, gymnastics, and soccer. Male athletes were 3 times more likely to experience medial ankle sprains than female athletes. Up to 10% of deltoid ligament complex sprains are associated with syndesmotic injuries (see **Fig. 4**).[26]

Functional anatomy
The ligamentous complex is triangular/deltoid shaped and can be subdivided into 2 obliquely oriented parallel groups. The more superficial ligaments include the tibionavicular ligament (TNL), tibiospring ligament (TSL), and tibiocalcaneal ligament (TCL), whereas the deeper ligaments include the anterior tibiotalar ligament (aTTL) and posterior tibiotalar ligament (pTTL) (**Fig. 11**).[16] The deep portion of the deltoid ligament is intra-articular and surrounded by synovium.[69] The pTTL is considered the strongest component, followed by the TSL, TNL and TCL.[70] The deltoid ligament

complex stabilizes the ankle against valgus, pronation, and external rotational forces on the talus.[29,69,71,72]

Clinical considerations and mechanism of injury
Medial ankle sprains are usually more painful than their lateral counterpart, and mechanical instability is characteristic.[26] The eversion stress test is considered a reliable clinical examination.[71] Acute injuries are usually clinically apparent with hematoma and tenderness over the medial ankle.[69] Chronic sprains are characterized by chronic insufficiency, pain, medial gutter tenderness, and hindfoot valgus during weight bearing and pronation. Complete tears can sometimes be seen in conjunction with lateral malleolar and bimalleolar fractures.[71]

Acute injury usually occurs with eversion forces resulting in valgus stress and/or internal rotation forces causing pronation stress.[71] Deep ligament tears are more common than superficial tears, and partial tears are more common than full-thickness tears.[26,69] Sprains of the deep components of the deltoid ligament are frequently noted in patients after inversion injuries.[15,19]

Diagnostic imaging
On routine MR imaging positioning the foot in dorsiflexion optimizes visualization of the more posterior components of the deltoid ligament in the coronal plane, such as the TSL and deep TTL.[19] Most ligaments are best seen in the coronal plane. Axial images are reserved for evaluating the tendons and surrounding neurovascular structures, which may be injured in association with deltoid ligament injury.[16] The 3D Fourier transform

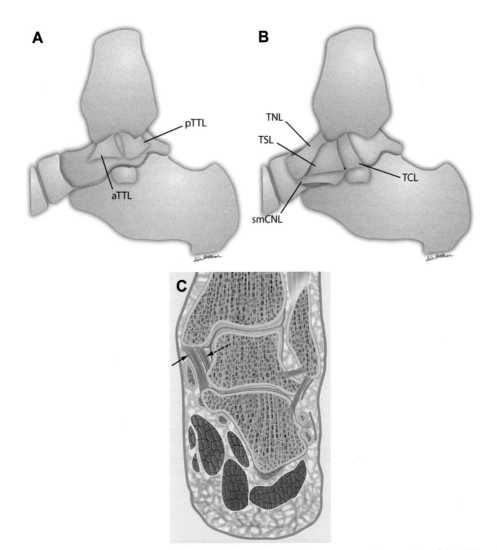

Fig. 11. Deltoid *ligament complex*. (*A*) The deep layer of the deltoid ligament complex consists of the aTTL and the pTTL. (*B*) The superficial layer consists of the TNL, TSL, and TCL. The TSL, which is often the only visible superficial deltoid component, converges with the superomedial calcaneonavicular ligament (smCNL) component of the spring ligament complex at the level of the sustentaculum tali of the calcaneus. (*C*) Coronal illustration (illustrated by Salvador Beltran) showing the superficial (*solid arrow*) and deep (*dashed arrow*) layers of the deltoid ligament complex.

gradient-recalled echo MR images are useful for visualizing the various components along their orthogonal plane.[19] The position of the foot is not critical with this MR sequence. Reformatting images in coronal oblique planes along the expected course of each ligament, obtained from a paramedial sagittal plane, are considered useful to better delineate the ligaments.[70] Ultrasonography has been shown to be a highly accurate diagnostic modality in assessing deltoid ligament injury in the setting of supination external rotation fractures of the ankle.[73]

Superficial The superficial group of ligaments arises from the anterior colliculus of the medial malleolus and fans out anteriorly and posteriorly.[26,70] The TNL is a homogeneous, thin, low-signal band that attaches at the talus and crosses both the ankle and talonavicular joints inferiorly to insert on the medial navicular tuberosity.[16,20] This ligament shares a distal attachment with the posterior tibial tendon (PTT) and superior part of the spring (plantar calcaneonavicular) ligament. The TNL and the aTTL form part of the tibiotalar and talonavicular joints.[16] The TNL is sometimes difficult to discern on routine coronal images because of its oblique forward course and may require oblique coronal planes to be visualized on a single image.[19] The TNL has a mean thickness of 1 to 2 mm.[74]

The full length of the TCL is frequently seen on a single routine coronal image, appearing as a homogeneous band of low signal intensity attached to the posterior sustentaculum tali.[16,20,74] It may be difficult to distinguish the TCL from the TSL because of its close proximity.[74] The TSL courses downward, across the ankle and anterior subtalar joints, to attach to the lateral aspect of the superomedial oblique band of the spring ligament (SL).[69,71,74] Mengiardi and colleagues[74] reported the TSL to be the second largest component of the deltoid ligament with an average thickness of 2 mm (1–4 mm). Both the TSL and the TNL were found to be significantly thicker in men as compared with women. The PTT and its sheath course posteromedial to the deltoid ligament and come in direct contact with the TSL and the pTTL.[16] The PTT serves to maintain the medial arch of the foot, and is often associated with pathologic conditions of the SL and TSL related to medial ankle instability.[69]

Deep The deep components of the deltoid complex are shorter and arise from the intercollicular/malleolar groove.[26,70] The aTTL is thin, multi fascicular, and has a broad insertion more anteriorly on the talar body and neck. This ligament is best seen on coronal images in 50% to 84% of normal asymptomatic ankles.[70,74] The pTTL is a low-signal, thick band with a rectangular shape. It courses posteroinferiorly and broadly attaches to the medial surface of the talus as far posteriorly as the posteromedial talar tubercle.[20,26,70] This ligament is generally regarded as the thickest ligament, ranging in thickness from 6 to 11 mm.[74] It is normal for this ligament to have a heterogeneous appearance and striations caused by interposed fat.[19,70,74]

In high-grade sprains, high T2 signal can be seen on fat-saturated PD or T2-weighted MR images, with associated fluid-filled gaps or complete discontinuity of the ligament.[69] Findings include intermediate signal intensity on T1-WI or PD-weighted images, amorphous hyperintensity on FS PD FSE, indistinct margins and loss of fiber striation in the TTL, or masslike morphology with associated hemorrhage and edema (**Fig. 12**).[26] A potential pitfall is that asymptomatic patients older than 45 years have variable increased T2-weighted signal in the anterior TTL, TNL, and TSL.[74]

Other associated injuries include medial malleolar fractures, distal avulsion fractures, osteochondral lesions of the talus, lateral collateral and syndesmotic ligament injuries, and SL and PTT injuries.[69] More than 60% of posterior TTL injuries are caused by avulsion.[70]

Posttraumatic Sinus Tarsi Syndrome

Epidemiology
Sinus tarsi syndrome (STS) is caused by trauma in 70% of cases.[75,76] Klein and Spreitzer[77] reported that lateral collateral ligament tears were found to be present in about 79% of cases of STS, and lateral collateral ligament injuries had abnormal signal within the region of the sinus tarsi in 39% of cases.

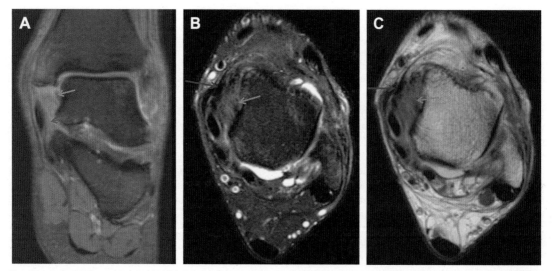

Fig. 12. *Deltoid ligament sprain.* (*A*) Coronal FS PD, (*B*) axial PD FS, and (*C*) axial PD show hyperintense signal of the deep (*green arrow*) and superficial (*blue arrow*) layers of the deltoid ligament complex. There is also loss of the normal striated appearance of the posterior tibiotalar component of the deep deltoid ligament complex (*green arrow*).

Functional anatomy

The sinus tarsi (ST) ligaments, nerves, and vessels play an important role in stabilization and proprioception of the subtalar joint.[67] The ST can be divided into the superficial, intermediate, and deep layers. The superficial layer includes the lateral root of the inferior extensor retinaculum (IER), lateral talocalcaneal (TL) ligament, CFL, posterior TL ligament, and the medial TL ligament. The intermediate layer includes the cervical ligament and intermediate root of the IER. The deep layer contains the interosseous TL ligament and medial root of the IER.[26] The interosseous TL and cervical ligaments are both important in the overall function of the lateral ankle and hindfoot complex. The cervical ligament also acts to limit inversion.[75]

Clinical considerations and mechanism of injury

Patients with STS present with pain exacerbated with weight bearing along the lateral aspect of the foot.[25] Patients usually have subjective sensation of instability of the hindfoot, especially when walking on uneven ground.[75] However, there is usually little objective evidence of instability.[77] STS is usually a chronic condition primarily because acute ST injury is confounded by swelling of the ankle from other ankle sprains.[76]

ST injury commonly develops after an inversion injury.[25,57,77] The IOL is subject to traction and torsional stresses and is taut in supination and relaxed in pronation of the foot. Progressive inversion of the heel without dorsiflexion or extension induces rupture of the ATFL and CFL ligaments, followed by the interosseous TL ligament.[75]

Diagnostic imaging

Before the advent of MR imaging the only techniques for diagnosing STS were arthrography, which showed lack of filling of the anterior recesses of the subtalar joint, or clinically with relief of pain following local anesthetic or steroid injection.[75,77] MR imaging has dramatically improved our ability to demonstrate normal anatomy and pathologic conditions of the ST.[25,67] The ST is a wedge-shaped space in the lateral aspect of the ankle, between the inferior aspect of the talus and the superior aspect of the calcaneus.[25,75] The osseous walls of the ST are irregular and covered by multiple vascular foramina.[25,75]

The TL, or interosseous, ligament is broad and strong and is comprised of a single band medially. The posterior and medial fibers extend from the inferior aspect of the ST laterally to the superior aspect of the deepest portion of the tarsal canal. Laterally, 2 bands are seen separated by fat, vessels, and nerves. The most anterior division of the TL ligament is the cervical ligament, which extends from a small tubercle on the inferior lateral aspect of the neck of the talus onto the dorsal surface of the calcaneus. This ligament can be seen as a low-signal-intensity band, which is better appreciated on sagittal MR images rather than coronal. On T1-weighted MR imaging the TL ligament is seen deep within the tarsal canal as a fanlike structure.[75] The cervical ligament can be seen as a medial structure within the ST extending from the inferior aspect of the talus to the superior aspect of the calcaneus and is best seen on sagittal and coronal planes.[25]

STS can be diagnosed on T1-WI and PD-weighted MR imaging by effacement of the ST fat with or without injury to the ligaments (**Fig. 13, Table 3**).[26] Associated findings include osteoarthritis of the subtalar joint with subchondral cysts, bone marrow edema of the talus or calcaneus at the level of the ligament, PTT tear, and/or contrast enhancement of hypertrophied synovium.[19,57,75,77,78]

Posttraumatic Flat Foot Deformity: SL Complex

Epidemiology

SL injury is usually associated with PTT dysfunction in middle-aged women.[79]

Functional anatomy

The SL complex, or plantar calcaneonavicular ligament, is a hammocklike structure that extends from the sustentaculum tali of the calcaneus to the posteromedial process of the navicular.[80,81] Despite its name the SL is not elastic.[82] The complex consists of 3 ligaments: superomedial (SM), inferior plantar longitudinal (IPL), and medioplantar oblique (MPO) (**Fig. 14**).[80,81,83] The SM component is the most often torn and plays the most impact on the stability of the SL.[80] The SL, along with the anterior and middle facets of the calcaneus and the proximal articular surface of the navicular, compose the acetabulum pedis.[82] This complex supports the talar head and is, thus, critical for static stabilization of the medial longitudinal arch of the foot and for supporting the head of the talus.[80]

Clinical considerations and mechanism of injury

SL dysfunction causes talar plantar flexion and hindfoot valgus, resulting in acquired flatfoot deformity (pes planovalgus) caused by the loss of support of the longitudinal arch of the foot.[80,81] It has been observed that hindfoot deformity is most severe when both the SL and the PTT are injured.[84] Tears of the plantar components of the SL complex as a result of macrotrauma can

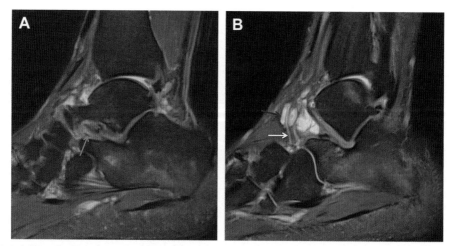

Fig. 13. *STS.* (*A*) Sagittal FS PD image shows diffuse edema of the sinus tarsi fat (*green arrow*). (*B*) Sagittal FS PD image demonstrates a ganglion cyst (*blue arrow*) extending from the sinus tarsi along the roots of the extensor retinaculum (*white arrow*) into the dorsal aspect ankle.

be seen in the young athletic population in association with talar head impaction injuries.[85]

Diagnostic imaging

The sensitivity and specificity of detecting SL rupture or laxity with MR imaging has been reported to be 54% to 77% and 100%, respectively.[86] Rule and colleagues[87] described the SL as a low-signal-intensity band on T2-WI, which overall is best seen in the oblique sagittal and axial planes. However, other studies have noted that the SM band is particularly best viewed in the coronal and axial planes.[81] In between the PTT and the SM band of the SL there is a gliding zone comprised of fibrocartilage, which measures 1 to 3 mm.[69,74] Sometimes it is difficult to differentiate the PTT, the gliding zone, and the SM band of the SL. Findings that may help differentiate these structures include the SM's larger size and vertical

orientation. The SM originates from the superomedial aspect of the sustentaculum tali and travels obliquely, wrapping around the tuberosity of the navicular, to attach in a fanlike fashion to the superomedial navicular bone. The SM band runs immediately deep to the distal PTT. The SM fibers merge with the superficial tibiospring fibers of the deltoid ligament complex, close to their insertion on the sustentaculum tali.[80,83] The average thickness of the SM is 3 mm (2–5 mm).[83]

The MPO and IPL bands of the SL complex are located more inferior than the SM band and are considered weaker than the SM band.[24,87] The MPO band originates from a notch located between the anterior and middle articular facets of the calcaneus, referred to as the coronoid fossa. It fans out to attach to the medial plantar aspect of the navicular bone. This band is generally long and best seen on axial and coronal images.[82,83,88] The IPL ligament is short, thick, and originates from the coronoid fossa of the calcaneus, anterior to the MPO band. It courses obliquely to attach on the inferior beak of the navicular bone and is best seen on sagittal, coronal, or coronal oblique planes. The average thickness of the IPL is 4 mm (2–6 mm).[83]

On MR imaging, findings of sprains of the SL can include heterogeneous or increased signal on fluid-sensitive sequences, thickening, ligament laxity, waviness or a full-thickness gap (**Fig. 15**).[67,80,81] Other findings include PTT tendinopathy, surrounding edema, and impaction injuries of the talar head.[81] A recent study by Desai and colleagues[82] described the SL recess as a fluid-filled space that communicates with the talocalcaneonavicular joint between the MPO and IPL

Table 3
MR imaging findings of STS

I	Diffuse ST infiltration that has low T1 and high T2 signal intensity compatible with inflammation and chronic synovitis
II	Diffuse infiltration of the ST by a low T1 and low T2 signal intensity mass consistent with fibrosis
III	Abnormal fluid collections consistent with synovial cysts

Data from Klein MA, Spreitzer AM. MR imaging of the tarsal sinus and canal: normal anatomy, pathologic findings, and features of the sinus tarsi syndrome. Radiology 1993;186(1):233–40.

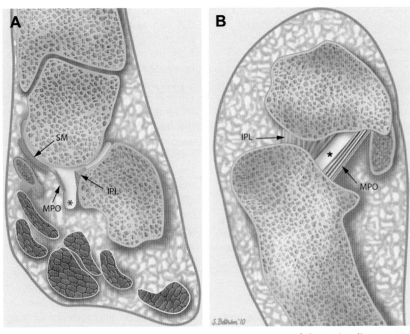

Fig. 14. *SL complex.* (*A*) Coronal illustration shows the three components of the spring ligament complex, which include the SM, MPO, and IPL bands. (*B*) Axial illustration shows the MPO and IPL originating along the plantar aspect of the calcaneus and inserting on the plantar aspect of the navicular. There is a normal synovial lined SL recess (*asterisk*) between the IPL and MPO, which communicates with the talonavicular joint and can become distended with fluid in the presence of a joint effusion.

components of the SL (see **Fig. 14**). The average size of the recess is 0.4 cm (0.2–0.9 cm) × 0.8 cm (0.4–1.5 cm) in transverse and craniocaudal dimensions, respectively. The SL recess is best visualized on axial images when the tibiotalar joint is distended with fluid. It has a teardrop shape on coronal and sagittal images, and is oriented in the antero-medial direction on the axial plane, paralleling the

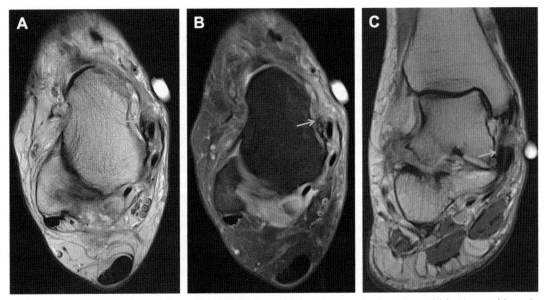

Fig. 15. *Sprain of the SL.* (*A*) Axial PD, (*B*) axial PD FS, and (*C*) coronal PD images show thickening and hyperintense signal in the superomedial band of the spring ligament (*arrow*) with surrounding edema.

SL. The SL recess should not be misinterpreted as a tear of the SL, synovial cyst, or ganglion cyst.[82]

Lisfranc Ligament

Epidemiology

Midfoot sprains are more common in athletes and have been reported to occur in up to 4% of American football.[89] Low-impact injures of the midfoot may result in a Lisfranc ligament sprain. High-impact injures result in Lisfranc fracture subluxation/dislocation, accounting for 0.2% of all fractures and less than 1% of dislocations.[26] The importance of recognizing this injury lies in its poor long-term prognosis when treatment is inadequate, inappropriate, or delayed.[90] Chronic pain, functional loss, and arthrosis are the potential sequelae of delayed or inappropriate treatment.[90,91] The rate of missed diagnosis of Lisfranc injuries is up to 35%.[92]

Functional anatomy

The Lisfranc joint, also known as the tarsometatarsal (TMT) joint, is a complex system comprised of osseous (tarsometatarsal, intertarsal, and intermetatarsal), articular surfaces, and soft tissue components (articular capsules, TMT ligaments, and tendons).[93] The intermetatarsal and TMT ligaments are part of the thick joint capsule, whereas the Lisfranc ligament is a discrete structure, which has been somewhat variably described in the literature as consisting of plantar and dorsal bundles.[94] One classification system described in the literature includes dividing the Lisfranc complex into 3 groups: dorsal, interosseous, and plantar components.[93] In general, the dorsal components are weaker than the plantar components.[90,91,95]

Five metatarsal bases and the distal row of tarsal bones, connected by TMT ligaments, make up the Lisfranc joint. The TMT ligaments are composed of dorsal, interosseous, plantar, intermetatarsal, and intertarsal ligaments. There are 7 dorsal TMT ligaments, which appear as short, flat, homogeneous, low-signal strips that are best seen on sagittal or coronal MR images.[93] The Lisfranc ligament, the first of 3 interosseous TMT ligaments, originates from the lateral cortex of the first/medial cuneiform and connects to the medial cortex of the second metatarsal base plantarly (Fig. 16).[91,93,95,96]

The second plantar TMT ligament (also termed the plantar Lisfranc ligament) originates from the inferolateral surface of the medial cuneiform below the Lisfranc ligament, splitting into 2 bands. The superficial short thin band attaches to the base of second metatarsal and a thicker, longer band courses to attach to the third metatarsal. This ligament is best visualized on the long-axis axial and transverse oblique imaging planes but can also be seen in the short axis coronal plane. The Lisfranc ligament and the plantar Lisfranc ligament both have an oblique anterolateral orientation.[93]

Clinical considerations and mechanism of injury

Patients with Lisfranc injuries present with pain at the TMT joint of the midfoot and cannot bear weight on the affected foot. Popping or snapping, midfoot edema, shortening of the foot, limited forefoot abduction or adduction, and/or plantar ecchymosis may also be seen.[26,95] The functional status can be evaluated by assessing gait, the medial arch, weight bearing on toes, or the pronation-abduction test.[95]

The mechanisms of injury can be divided into direct and indirect trauma. Direct trauma from a blow or a crush injury, such as dropping a weight on the foot, is less common than indirect trauma.[26,67,97] Indirect forces include forced plantar flexion and forefoot abduction.[91] Plantar flexion injuries are more common in the setting of Lisfranc fracture dislocations.[97] In this position, the forefoot acts as an extension of the lower extremity. When the full-body-weight force is applied on the Lisfranc joint, and the TMT can no longer support the tension across the dorsum of the midfoot, the joint gives way.[91,97] Specifically, the weaker dorsal components are the first to give way.[97] This mechanism is similar to a misstep off of a curb, with the forefoot rolled over by the body.[91] The dorsal band maintains plantar flexion and often develops partial tears.[67] Forefoot abduction injuries occur in players with cleats when the foot is planted and rotates to change direction.[91] A similar mechanism is a fall from a horse when the foot is caught in the stirrup.[95,98]

Diagnostic imaging

Lisfranc injuries are associated with fractures in up to 90% of cases, most commonly involving the medial aspect of the second metatarsal base or the distal lateral aspect of the middle cuneiform.[92,99] Myerson described small cortical avulsions as the fleck sign on radiography.[99] CT is considered a good diagnostic tool in detecting fractures not seen on radiography and/or MR imaging, and subtle misalignment not seen on radiographs.[90] MR is more sensitive than CT in identifying the extent of posttraumatic bone marrow edema and the number of bones of the tarsus affected, but is similar to CT in detecting malalignment.[26,67]

MR imaging is superior in demonstrating the ligaments of the midfoot.[90] Hatem and colleagues[100] showed that Lisfranc ligament disruption is demonstrated on MR imaging even in the setting of normal

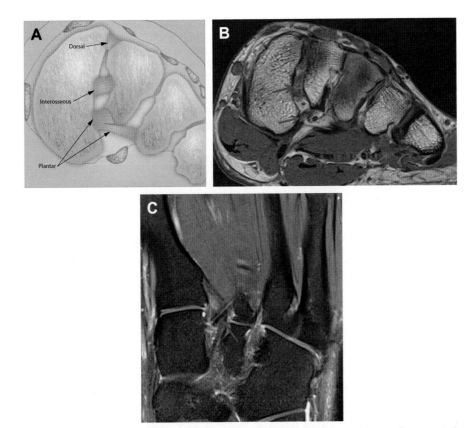

Fig. 16. *Normal Lisfranc ligament* (*A*) with corresponding (*B*) PD MR image in the short-axis coronal plane and (*C*) long-axis axial FS PD MR image showing the Lisfranc ligament complex. The dorsal band (*green arrow*) originates along the dorsolateral aspect of the medial cuneiform and inserts along the dorsomedial aspect of the base of the second metatarsal. The interosseous band (*blue arrow*) originates along the central lateral aspect of the medial cuneiform and inserts along the central medial aspect of the base of the second metatarsal. The plantar band (*red arrow*) originates at the plantar lateral aspect of the medial cuneiform and inserts into the plantar medial aspect of the base of the second and third metatarsals.

weight-bearing radiographs. On radiography, diastasis between the base of the first and second metatarsal greater than 2 mm on weight bearing is suggestive of a Lisfranc ligament tear.[67] Complete tears are seen as displacement of the second metatarsal and medial cuneiform.[67] It has been suggested that non–weight-bearing radiographs miss up to 10% of TMT injuries.[101] Other positive radiographic findings include malalignment of the lateral margins of the first metatarsal and medial cuneiform and the medial margins of the fourth metatarsal and cuboid.[90]

There are 2 types of Lisfranc injuries: homolateral and divergent.[26] Myerson and colleagues[99] described a classification system based on segmental pattern of injury (**Table 4**). On MR imaging the Lisfranc ligament is usually well seen on oblique axial long-axis MR images of the foot. The short-axis oblique coronal and oblique sagittal images are less effective in visualizing the ligament. The ligament is depicted as a homogenous band of

Table 4 Classification of Lisfranc injuries	
Type A	Total incongruity of the TMT joint with homolateral or dorsoplantar displacement of the first to fifth metatarsals
Type B	Partial incongruity with medial dislocation of the first metatarsals and lateral dislocation of the second to the fifth metatarsals
Type C	Divergent, with partial or total displacement of the first metatarsal medially and the lesser metatarsals laterally

Data from Myerson M, Fisher R, Burgess A. Fracture dislocations of the tarsometatarsal joints: end results correlated with pathology and treatment. Foot Ankle 1986;6(5): 225–42.

low signal intensity, which courses obliquely from the medial cuneiform to the base of the second metatarsal (see **Fig. 16**).[19] In a recent study by Castro and colleagues[93] the length, width, and thickness range for the Lisfranc ligament was 7 to 11 mm, 4 to 8 mm, and 5 to 9 mm, respectively.

In a small study of 11 patients with TMT injuries MR imaging afforded detection of Lisfranc ligament tears, which were depicted as either complete absence or fragmentation of the ligament (**Fig. 17**).[102] Commonly associated fractures occur at the base of second or third metatarsals, the medial aspect of the medial and middle cuneiforms,

or the navicular bone. Other findings include fraying or tearing of the Lisfranc ligament with or without synovitis, subchondral bone marrow edema at the TMT joints suggestive of a chip fracture or trabecular fracture, capsular edema and tears, lateral column shortening, disruption of the dorsal arch, arterial injury, and marrow edema in the displaced metatarsals or medial and middle cuneiforms.[26]

TREATMENT IMPLICATIONS

Immediate care of ligament sprains, usually within the first 24 hours, is commonly in the form of RICE

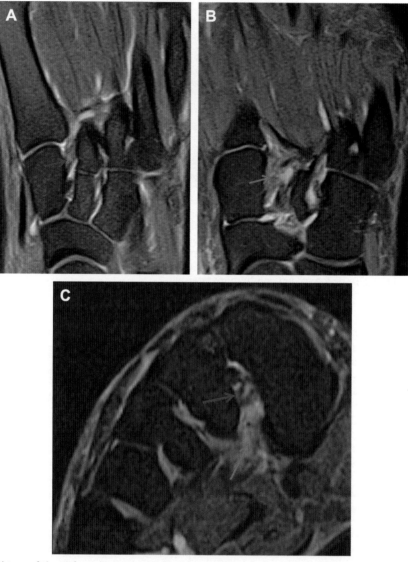

Fig. 17. *Partial tear of the Lisfranc ligament.* (*A, B*) Long-axis axial FS PD and (*C*) short-axis coronal FFS PD images showing hyperintense signal in the interosseous component (*blue arrow*) of the Lisfranc ligament complex with surrounding edema. The plantar component of the Lisfranc ligament (*red arrow*) is discontinuous and replaced by fluidlike signal consistent with a high-grade tear.

(rest, ice, compression, elevation).[11,103] Ice cooling, or cryotherapy, and the use of nonsteroidal antiinflammatory drugs may enhance the healing process and speed up the recovery. Low-grade sprains (grades I–II) are treated conservatively, with a preference for functional rehabilitation over immobilization. Functional rehabilitation includes strengthening exercises and motion restoration.[103] Some reported methods include an air cast, elastic brace, elastic support bandage, training on wobble board, ankle disk training, imagery, and a resistive walking boot. The treatment of a severe sprain (grade III) is controversial in the literature. A suggested approach is to treat with conservative functional measures; if this fails, surgical repair may be performed.[11]

In summary, current MR imaging technology provides exquisite delineation of the ankle ligaments. In particular, clear depiction of the normal anatomy and the typical morphologic changes involving the ligamentous structures of the ankle following sprain injury is widespread in today's MR clinical practice.

REFERENCES

1. Fong DT, Hong YY, Chan LK, et al. A systematic review on ankle injury and ankle sprain in sports. Sports Med 2007;37(1):73–94.
2. Soboroff SH, Pappius EM, Komaroff AL. Benefits, risks, and costs of alternative approaches to the evaluation and treatment of severe ankle sprain. Clin Orthop Relat Res 1984;183:160–8.
3. Waterman BR, Owens BD, Davey S, et al. The epidemiology of ankle sprains in the United States. J Bone Joint Surg Am 2010;92(13):2279–84.
4. Bridgman S, Clement D, Downing A, et al. Population based epidemiology of ankle sprains attending accident and emergency units in the West Midlands of England, and a survey of UK practice for severe ankle sprains. Emerg Med J 2003;20(6): 508–10.
5. Hølmer P, Søndergaard L, Konradsen L, et al. Epidemiology of sprains in the lateral ankle and foot. Foot Ankle Int 1994;15(2):72–4.
6. Raatikainen T, Putkonen M, Puranen J. Arthrography, clinical examination, and stress radiograph in the diagnosis of acute injury to the lateral ligaments of the ankle. Am J Sports Med 1992;20(1):2–6.
7. van Dijk CN, Lim LS, Bossuyt PM, et al. Physical examination is sufficient for the diagnosis of sprained ankles. J Bone Joint Surg Br 1996;78(6): 958–62.
8. Yeung MS, Chan KM, So CH, et al. An epidemiological survey on ankle sprain. Br J Sports Med 1994;28(2):112–6.
9. van Rijn RM, van Os AG, Bernsen RM, et al. What is the clinical course of acute ankle sprains? A systematic literature review. Am J Med 2008; 121(4):324–31.
10. Harrington KD. Degenerative arthritis of the ankle secondary to long-standing lateral ligament instability. J Bone Joint Surg Am 1979;61(3):354–61.
11. Fong DT, Chan YY, Mok KM, et al. Understanding acute ankle ligamentous sprain injury in sports. Sports Med Arthrosc Rehabil Ther Technol 2009; 1(1):14.
12. Hamilton WG. Foot and ankle injuries in dancers. Clin Sports Med 1988;7(1):143–73.
13. Kannus P, Renström P. Treatment for acute tears of the lateral ligaments of the ankle. Operation, cast, or early controlled mobilization. J Bone Joint Surg Am 1991;73(2):305–12.
14. Griffith JF, Brockwell JJ. Diagnosis and imaging of ankle instability. Foot Ankle Clin 2006;11(3):475–96.
15. Rosenberg ZS, Beltran J, Bencardino JT. From the RSNA refresher courses. Radiological Society of North America. MR imaging of the ankle and foot. Radiographics 2000;20:S153–79.
16. Schneck CD, Mesgarzadeh M, Bonakdarpour A, et al. MR imaging of the most commonly injured ankle ligaments. Part I. Normal anatomy. Radiology 1992;184(2):499–506.
17. Boonthathip M, Chen L, Trudell DJ, et al. Tibiofibular syndesmotic ligaments: MR arthrography in cadavers with anatomic correlation. Radiology 2010;254(3):827–36.
18. Labovitz JM, Schweitzer ME. Occult osseous injuries after ankle sprains: incidence, location, pattern, and age. Foot Ankle Int 1998;19(10):661–7.
19. Rosenberg ZS, Beltran J. Magnetic resonance imaging and computed tomography of the ankle and foot. In: Myerson MS, editor. Foot and ankle disorders, vol. 1. Philadelphia: Saunders; 1998. p. 123–56.
20. Muhle C, Frank LR, Rand T, et al. Collateral ligaments of the ankle: high-resolution MR imaging with a local gradient coil and anatomic correlation in cadavers. Radiographics 1999;19(3):673–83.
21. Mesgarzadeh MM, Schneck CD, Tehranzadeh JJ, et al. Magnetic resonance imaging of ankle ligaments. Emphasis on anatomy and injuries to lateral collateral ligaments. Magn Reson Imaging Clin N Am 1994;2(1):39–58.
22. Labovitz JM, Schweitzer ME, Larka UB, et al. Magnetic resonance imaging of ankle ligament injuries correlated with time. J Am Podiatr Med Assoc 1998;88(8):387–93.
23. Verhaven EF, Shahabpour MM, Handelberg FW, et al. The accuracy of three-dimensional magnetic resonance imaging in the diagnosis of ruptures of the lateral ligaments of the ankle. Am J Sports Med 1991;19(6):583–7.

24. Schneck CD, Mesgarzadeh MM, Bonakdarpour AA. MR imaging of the most commonly injured ankle ligaments. Part II. Ligament injuries. Radiology 1992;184(2):507–12.

25. Beltran JJ, Munchow AM, Khabiri HH, et al. Ligaments of the lateral aspect of the ankle and sinus tarsi: an MR imaging study. Radiology 1990;177(2):455–8.

26. Stoller DW, Ferkel RD. The ankle and foot (2 Volume Set). In: Stoller DW, editor. Magnetic resonance imaging in orthopaedics and sports medicine. 3rd edition. Baltimore: Lippincott Williams & Wilkins; 2007. p. 733–1050.

27. Hertel J. Functional anatomy, pathomechanics, and pathophysiology of lateral ankle instability. J Athl Train 2002;37(4):364–75.

28. Rockar P Jr. The subtalar joint: anatomy and joint motion. J Orthop Sports Phys Ther 1995;21(6):361–72.

29. Rasmussen O. Stability of the ankle joint. Analysis of the function and traumatology of the ankle ligaments. Acta Orthop Scand Suppl 1985;211:1–75.

30. Close J. Some applications of the functional anatomy of the ankle joint. J Bone Joint Surg Am 1956;38(4):761–81.

31. Norkus SA, Floyd RT. The anatomy and mechanisms of syndesmotic ankle sprains. J Athl Train 2001;36(1):68–73.

32. Waterman BR, Belmont PJ, Cameron KL, et al. Risk factors for syndesmotic and medial ankle sprain: role of sex, sport, and level of competition. Am J Sports Med 2011;39(5):992–8.

33. Boytim MJ, Fischer DA, Neumann L. Syndesmotic ankle sprains. Am J Sports Med 1991;19(3):294–8.

34. Gerber JP, Williams GN, Scoville CR, et al. Persistent disability associated with ankle sprains: a prospective examination of an athletic population. Foot Ankle Int 1998;19(10):653–60.

35. Skraba JS, Greenwald AS. The role of the interosseous membrane on tibiofibular weight bearing. Foot Ankle 1984;4(6):301–4.

36. Hermans JJ, Beumer A, De Jong TA, et al. Anatomy of the distal tibiofibular syndesmosis in adults: a pictorial essay with a multimodality approach. J Anat 2010;217(6):633–45.

37. Dattani R, Patnaik S, Kantak A, et al. Injuries to the tibiofibular syndesmosis. J Bone Joint Surg Br 2008;90(4):405–10.

38. Takao M, Ochi M, Naito K, et al. Arthroscopic diagnosis of tibiofibular syndesmosis disruption. Arthroscopy 2001;17(8):836–43.

39. Brown KW, Morrison WB, Schweitzer ME, et al. MRI findings associated with distal tibiofibular syndesmosis injury. AJR Am J Roentgenol 2004;182(1):131–6.

40. Vogl TJ, Hochmuth KK, Diebold TT, et al. Magnetic resonance imaging in the diagnosis of acute injured distal tibiofibular syndesmosis. Invest Radiol 1997;32(7):401–9.

41. Oae K, Takao M, Naito K, et al. Injury of the tibiofibular syndesmosis: value of MR imaging for diagnosis. Radiology 2003;227(1):155–61.

42. Ebraheim NA, Taser F, Shafiq Q, et al. Anatomical evaluation and clinical importance of the tibiofibular syndesmosis ligaments. Surg Radiol Anat 2006;28(2):142–9.

43. Ray RG, Kriz BM. Anterior inferior tibiofibular ligament. Variations and relationship to the talus. J Am Podiatr Med Assoc 1991;81(9):479–85.

44. Gyftopoulos S. Normal variants and pitfalls in MR imaging of the ankle and foot. Magn Reson Imaging Clin N Am 2010;18(4):691–705.

45. Muhle C, Frank LR, Rand T, et al. Tibiofibular syndesmosis: high-resolution MRI using a local gradient coil. J Comput Assist Tomogr 1998;22(6):938–44.

46. Rosenberg ZS, Cheung YY, Beltran JJ, et al. Posterior intermalleolar ligament of the ankle: normal anatomy and MR imaging features. AJR Am J Roentgenol 1995;165(2):387–90.

47. Oh CS. Anatomic variations and MRI of the intermalleolar ligament. AJR Am J Roentgenol 2006;186(4):943–7.

48. Sandelin J. Acute sports injuries: a clinical and epidemiological study [dissertation]. Helsinki: University of Helsinki; 1988. p. 1–66.

49. Fallat L, Grimm DJ, Saracco JA. Sprained ankle syndrome: prevalence and analysis of 639 acute injuries. J Foot Ankle Surg 1998;37(4):280–5.

50. Haraguchi N, Toga H, Shiba N, et al. Avulsion fracture of the lateral ankle ligament complex in severe inversion injury. Am J Sports Med 2007;35(7):1144–52.

51. Attarian DE, McCrackin HJ, DeVito DP, et al. Biomechanical characteristics of human ankle ligaments. Foot Ankle 1985;6(2):54–8.

52. Safran MR, Benedetti RS, Bartolozzi AR, et al. Lateral ankle sprains: a comprehensive review: part 1: etiology, pathoanatomy, histopathogenesis, and diagnosis. Med Sci Sports Exerc 1999;31(Suppl 7):S429–37.

53. de Asla RJ, Kozánek M, Wan L, et al. Function of anterior talofibular and calcaneofibular ligaments during in-vivo motion of the ankle joint complex. J Orthop Surg Res 2009;4(1):7.

54. Chan KW, Ding BC, Mroczek KJ. Acute and chronic lateral ankle instability in the athlete. Bull NYU Hosp Jt Dis 2011;69(1):17–26.

55. Bahr RR, Pena FF, Shine JJ, et al. Mechanics of the anterior drawer and talar tilt tests. A cadaveric study of lateral ligament injuries of the ankle. Acta Orthop Scand 1997;68(5):435–41.

56. Dubin JC, Comeau DD, McClelland RI, et al. Lateral and syndesmotic ankle sprain injuries: a narrative literature review. J Chiropr Med 2011;10(3):204–19.

57. Bencardino J, Rosenberg Z. MR imaging in sports injuries of the foot and ankle. Magn Reson Imaging Clin N Am 1999;7(1):131–49.

58. Peetrons PP, Creteur VV, Bacq CC. Sonography of ankle ligaments. J Clin Ultrasound 2004;32(9):491–9.

59. Campbell D, Menz A, Isaacs J. Dynamic ankle ultrasonography. A new imaging technique for acute ankle ligament injuries. Am J Sports Med 1994;22(6):855–8.

60. Nakasa T, Fukuhara K, Adachi N. Evaluation of anterior talofibular ligament lesion using 3-dimensional computed tomography. J Comput Assist Tomogr 2006;30(3):543–7.

61. van Dijk CN, Molenaar AH, Cohen RH, et al. Value of arthrography after supination trauma of the ankle. Skeletal Radiol 1998;27(5):256–61.

62. Chandnani VP, Harper MT, Ficke JR, et al. Chronic ankle instability: evaluation with MR arthrography, MR imaging, and stress radiography. Radiology 1994;192(1):189–94.

63. Oloff LM, Sullivan BT, Heard GS, et al. Magnetic resonance imaging of traumatized ligaments of the ankle. J Am Podiatr Med Assoc 1992;82(1):25–32.

64. Rijke AM, Goitz HT, McCue FC III, et al. Magnetic resonance imaging of injury to the lateral ankle ligaments. Am J Sports Med 1993;21(4):528–34.

65. Dimmick S, Kennedy D, Daunt N. Evaluation of thickness and appearance of anterior talofibular and calcaneofibular ligaments in normal versus abnormal ankles with MRI. J Med Imaging Radiat Oncol 2008;52(6):559–63.

66. Milner CE, Soames RW. Anatomy of the collateral ligaments of the human ankle joint. Foot Ankle Int 1998;19(11):757–60.

67. Cheung Y, Rosenberg ZS. MR imaging of ligamentous abnormalities of the ankle and foot. Magn Reson Imaging Clin N Am 2001;9(3):507–31.

68. Bencardino JT, Rosenberg ZS. Normal variants and pitfalls in MR imaging of the ankle and foot. Magn Reson Imaging Clin N Am 2001;9(3):447–63.

69. Chhabra A, Subhawong TK, Carrino JA. MR imaging of deltoid ligament pathologic findings and associated impingement syndromes. Radiographics 2010;30(3):751–61.

70. Klein M. MR imaging of the ankle: normal and abnormal findings in the medial collateral ligament. AJR Am J Roentgenol 1994;162(2):377–83.

71. Hintermann B, Knupp M, Pagenstert GI. Deltoid ligament injuries: diagnosis and management. Foot Ankle Clin 2006;11(3):625–37.

72. Rasmussen OO, Kromann-Andersen CC, Boe SS. Deltoid ligament. Functional analysis of the medial collateral ligamentous apparatus of the ankle joint. Acta Orthop Scand 1983;54(1):36–44.

73. Henari S, Banks LN, Radiovanovic I, et al. Ultrasonography as a diagnostic tool in assessing deltoid ligament injury in supination external rotation fractures of the ankle. Orthopedics 2011;34(10):e639–43.

74. Mengiardi B, Pfirrmann CW, Vienne P, et al. Medial collateral ligament complex of the ankle: MR appearance in asymptomatic subjects. Radiology 2007;242(3):817–24.

75. Beltran J. Sinus tarsi syndrome. Magn Reson Imaging Clin N Am 1994;2(1):59–65.

76. Breitenseher MJ, Haller JJ, Kukla CC, et al. MRI of the sinus tarsi in acute ankle sprain injuries. J Comput Assist Tomogr 1997;21(2):274–9.

77. Klein MA, Spreitzer AM. MR imaging of the tarsal sinus and canal: normal anatomy, pathologic findings, and features of the sinus tarsi syndrome. Radiology 1993;186(1):233–40.

78. Lowy AA, Schilero JJ, Kanat IO. Sinus tarsi syndrome: a postoperative analysis. J Foot Surg 1985;24(2):108–12.

79. Balen PF, Helms CA. Association of posterior tibial tendon injury with spring ligament injury, sinus tarsi abnormality, and plantar fasciitis on MR imaging. AJR Am J Roentgenol 2001;176(5):1137–43.

80. Toye LR, Helms CA, Hoffman BD, et al. MRI of spring ligament tears. AJR Am J Roentgenol 2005;184(5):1475–80.

81. Ting AY, Morrison WB, Kavanagh EC. MR imaging of midfoot injury. Magn Reson Imaging Clin N Am 2008;16(1):105–15.

82. Desai KR, Beltran LS, Bencardino JT, et al. The spring ligament recess of the talocalcaneonavicular joint: depiction on MR images with cadaveric and histologic correlation. AJR Am J Roentgenol 2011;196(5):1145–50.

83. Mengiardi B, Zanetti M, Schottle PB, et al. Spring ligament complex: MR imaging-anatomic correlation and findings in asymptomatic subjects. Radiology 2005;237(1):242–9.

84. Gazdag AR, Cracchiolo A. Rupture of the posterior tibial tendon. Evaluation of injury of the spring ligament and clinical assessment of tendon transfer and ligament repair. J Bone Joint Surg Am 1997;79(5):675–81.

85. Kavanagh EC, Koulouris G, Gopez A, et al. MRI of rupture of the spring ligament complex with talocuboid impaction. Skeletal Radiol 2007;36(6):555–8.

86. Yao LL, Gentili AA, Cracchiolo AA. MR imaging findings in spring ligament insufficiency. Skeletal Radiol 1999;28(5):245–50.

87. Rule JJ, Yao LL, Seeger LL. Spring ligament of the ankle: normal MR anatomy. AJR Am J Roentgenol 1993;161(6):1241–4.

88. Taniguchi AA, Tanaka YY, Takakura YY, et al. Anatomy of the spring ligament. J Bone Joint Surg Am 2003;85(11):2174–8.

89. Meyer S, Callaghan J, Albright J, et al. Midfoot sprains in collegiate football players. Am J Sports Med 1994;22(3):392–401.

90. Gupta RT, Wadhwa RP, Learch TJ, et al. Lisfranc injury: imaging findings for this important but often-missed diagnosis. Curr Probl Diagn Radiol 2008;37(3):115–26.

91. Hatem SF. Imaging of Lisfranc injury and midfoot sprain. Radiol Clin North Am 2008;46(6):1045–60.

92. Vuori JP, Aro HT. Lisfranc joint injuries: trauma mechanisms and associated injuries. J Trauma 1993; 35(1):40–5.

93. Castro M, Melao L, Canella C, et al. Lisfranc joint ligamentous complex: MRI with anatomic correlation in cadavers. AJR Am J Roentgenol 2010; 195(6):W447–55.

94. MacMahon PJ, Dheer S, Raikin SM, et al. MRI of injuries to the first interosseous cuneometatarsal (Lisfranc) ligament. Skeletal Radiol 2008;38(3):255–60.

95. Mullen JE, O'Malley MJ. Sprains—residual instability of subtalar, Lisfranc joints, and turf toe. Clin Sports Med 2004;23(1):97–121.

96. Kura HH, Luo ZP, Kitaoka HB, et al. Mechanical behavior of the Lisfranc and dorsal cuneometatarsal ligaments: in vitro biomechanical study. J Orthop Trauma 2001;15(2):107–10.

97. Curtis MJ, Myerson MM, Szura BB. Tarsometatarsal joint injuries in the athlete. Am J Sports Med 1993; 21(4):497–502.

98. Mantas J, Burks RT. Lisfranc injuries in the athlete. Clin Sports Med 1994;13(4):719–30.

99. Myerson M, Fisher R, Burgess A. Fracture dislocations of the tarsometatarsal joints: end results correlated with pathology and treatment. Foot Ankle 1986;6(5):225–42.

100. Hatem SF, Davis A, Sundaram M. Your diagnosis? Midfoot sprain: Lisfranc ligament disruption. Orthopedics 2005;28(1):2–7.

101. Arntz CT, Veith RG, Hansen ST. Fractures and fracture-dislocations of the tarsometatarsal joint. J Bone Joint Surg Am 1988;70(2):173–81.

102. Resnick D, Niwayama G. Osteonecrosis: diagnostic techniques, specific situations, and complications. In: Resnick D, Niwayama G, editors. Diagnosis of bone and joint disorders. Philadelphia: W, B. Saunders; 1995. p. 3495–558.

103. Ivins D. Acute ankle sprain: an update. Am Fam Physician 2006;74(10):1714–20.

Ankle Impingement Syndromes

Simon Dimmick, BPTHY, MBBS (Hons), FRANZCR[a,b],
James Linklater, MBBS, FRANZCR[c,*]

KEYWORDS

- Ankle • Ankle impingement • Ankle injuries • Ankle MR imaging

KEY POINTS

- Impingement is a clinical syndrome of end-range joint pain or motion restriction caused by the direct mechanical abutment of bone or soft tissues.
- Imaging can show osseous and soft tissue diseases and anatomic variations that can predispose to impingent syndromes.
- The presence of synovitis, pericapsular edema, and bone marrow edema in association with osseous and soft tissue diseases and anatomic variants that predispose to impingement symptoms are, in the appropriate clinical context, suggestive of a degree of active impingement.
- Common sites of impingement in the ankle include posterior, posteromedial, anteromedial, anterolateral, and less commonly, direct anterior.

INTRODUCTION

Impingement is a clinical syndrome of end-range joint pain or motion restriction caused by the direct mechanical abutment of bone or soft tissues. Impingement syndromes in the ankle are classified according to location and by the type of underlying bony or soft tissue disease. Posttraumatic synovitis, intra-articular fibrous bands/scar tissue, capsular scarring, or developmental and acquired bony spurs or prominences are the most common causes of ankle impingement. Sites of impingement at the ankle include anterolateral, anterior, anteromedial, posteromedial, and posterior. This article reviews the potential sites of impingement around the ankle, relevant anatomy, mechanism and pathogenesis of each impingement syndrome, clinical features, approach to imaging, imaging findings, differential diagnosis, and management.

ANTEROLATERAL IMPINGEMENT
Anatomy of the Anterolateral Gutter

The anterolateral gutter (ALG) or recess of the talocrural (ankle) joint is a triangular space. The boundaries of the ALG are formed by the tibia posteromedially, the fibula laterally, anteriorly by the anterior talofibular ligament (ATFL) and the ankle capsule, inferiorly by the calcaneofibular ligament (CFL) and superiorly by the anterior inferior tibiofibular ligament (AITFL) (Fig. 1). The site of insertion of the inferior fascicle of the AITFL on the lateral malleolus is variable, with resultant variation in the degree of inferior extension into the ALG. The ALG may contain some fluid in normal individuals. During ankle dorsiflexion, the anterolateral border of the talus protrudes into the ALG, displacing any native joint fluid.[1]

Pathogenesis and Mechanism of Anterolateral Impingement

Anterolateral soft tissue impingement most commonly occurs as a complication of a plantar flexion-inversion injury and resultant tear of the ATFL and ALG capsule.[2] An associated hemarthrosis and fibrinous debris within the joint may result in a posttraumatic synovitis in the ALG.[3] The synovitis may impinge on the anterolateral

Disclosure: The authors have nothing to disclose. There is no conflict of interest.
[a] Department of Radiology, Royal North Shore Hospital, Pacific Highway, St Leonards, New South Wales 2065, Australia; [b] School of Medicine, University of Notre Dame, Darlinghurst 2010, Australia; [c] Castlereagh Sports Imaging, 60 Pacific Highway, St Leonards, New South Wales 2065, Australia
* Corresponding author.
E-mail address: jameslinklater@casimaging.com.au

radiologic.theclinics.com

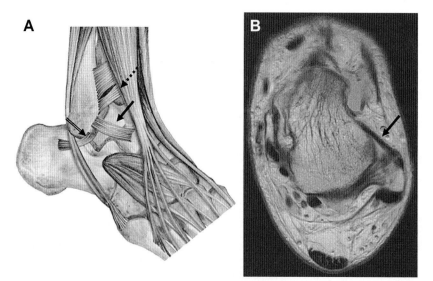

Fig. 1. (*A*) The ALG, which is demarcated superiorly by the inferior fascicle of the AITFL (*dash-tailed arrow*) and inferiorly by the lateral gutter articular facet of the talar dome and anterior border of the lateral malleolus, with the ALG capsule and ATFL (*solid arrow*) at the superficial margin. Note also the CFL (*double-tailed arrow*). (*B*) Axial proton density-weighted MR image through a normal ALG, containing a small amount of synovial fluid, with intact ATFL at the superficial margin (*arrow*).

talar dome during dorsiflexion, causing pain and restriction of dorsiflexion. Over time, the synovitis may become coalescent and undergo hyalinized fibrosis, forming a meniscoid lesion within the ALG,[4,5] which marginates against the inferior fascicle of the AITFL, the anterolateral talar dome, and anterior margin of the lateral malleolus. The term meniscoid lesion is used because of the typically triangular morphology in transverse cross section.[6] Impingement symptoms associated with meniscoid lesions usually relate to compression against the anterolateral talar dome during dorsiflexion.[7] With repetitive abutment, a chondral lesion may form on the anterolateral talar dome.[8]

Posttraumatic synovitis and meniscoid lesions may also occur in the ALG as a result of injury to the AITFL component of the syndesmotic ligament complex. A low-lying fibular attachment of the AITFL may predispose to anterolateral impingement.[9] In addition, laxity of the ATFL and associated increased anterior translation of the talus in relation to the tibial plafond may result in impingement symptoms caused by abutment between the inferior fascicle of the AITFL and the anterolateral talar dome.[10] Capsular scarring or arthrofibrosis may cause anterolateral impingement symptoms[1] and is typically related to previous trauma or surgery.[11–13] Rarely, ganglia may arise from the ALG capsule and cause anterolateral impingement symptoms (**Fig. 2**).[1]

Bony impingement symptoms of the anterolateral ankle usually relate to bony spurs arising from the anterior rim of the tibial plafond, lateral of midline, and inferior to the anterior capsular insertion.[14,15] Such spurs are commonly seen in athletes and do not necessarily indicate underlying osteoarthritis, they are most likely related to a repetitive impaction mechanism.[16,17] It has been hypothesized that the spurs may cause impingement symptoms as a result of entrapment or irritation of the adjacent anterior ankle capsule.[15] Inferior prolongation of an anterior tibial plafond spur may also result in impingement symptoms as a result of impaction on the talar dome articular cartilage during plantar flexion, with complicating sagittally oriented tram-track–type superficial chondral fissures of the talar dome, which may also relate to loose bodies impacting on the articular cartilage (**Fig. 3**). Small chondral delamination lesions are often present at the tibial plafond adjacent to an impingement spur, and may also be a cause of anterolateral ankle pain. Occasionally, fracture of impingement spurs can be a cause of acute anterior ankle pain (**Fig. 4**). Ossicles secondary to a previous avulsion of the ATFL lying in the ALG may rarely cause anterolateral impingement symptoms.

Clinical Features of Anterolateral Impingement

Individuals with anterolateral impingement typically complain of anterolateral ankle pain that is precipitated by supination or pronation of the

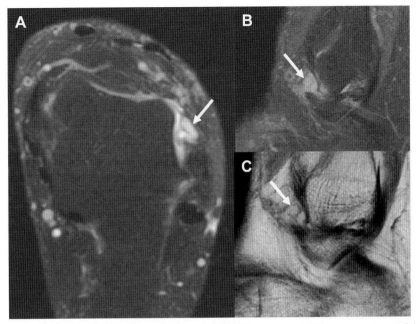

Fig. 2. Oblique axial fat-suppressed T2 (*A*), sagittal proton density-weighted with fat suppression (*B*), and sagittal proton density-weighted without fat suppression (*C*) MR images, showing a small ganglion cyst at the superficial margin of the ALG capsule (*arrows*). The ganglion was aspirated under ultrasound guidance, with resolution of the patient's symptoms.

foot in dorsiflexion.[18] It can be difficult clinically to differentiate anterolateral impingement from a chondral or osteochondral lesion of the anterolateral talar dome.[1] Production or aggravation of pain when an examiner attempts to pinch hypertrophied synovium between the talus and tibia (the positive impingement sign) has been reported to be both sensitive and specific (94.8% and 88%, respectively) for diagnosing anterolateral impingement.[19] Anterolateral tenderness, swelling, pain on

single leg squat, and pain on ankle dorsiflexion and eversion are the clinical findings that correlate most strongly with abnormality at surgery.[20]

Imaging Technique

A routine ankle plain radiograph series may show an anterior bony spur of the tibial plafond in patients with anterolateral impingement symptoms. Lateral radiographs obtained in maximum

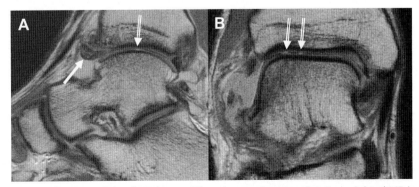

Fig. 3. Sagittal proton density-weighted MR image (*A*) and coronal proton density-weighted MR image (*B*) show an anterior plafond spur and adjacent ossicle (*white arrow*), with complicating superficial sagittally oriented chondral fissures on the talar dome (tram-track lesions), with loss of visualization of the lamina splendens (*double-tailed arrows*).

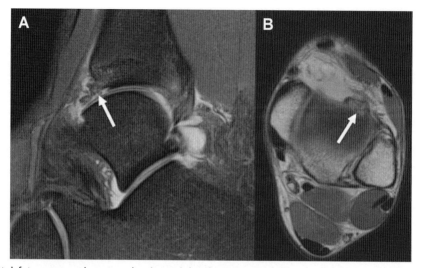

Fig. 4. Sagittal fat-suppressed proton density-weighted MR image (*A*) and axial proton density-weighted MR image (*B*) show a recent fracture of an anterolateral plafond impingement spur (*white arrow*).

dorsiflexion may show abutment of the bony spurs.[21,22] However, it is often not possible to confirm that the spur is anterolateral in position on a routine ankle radiograph series. Multislice helical computed tomography (CT) with sagittal and three-dimensional (3D) reconstructions readily show the site and extent of anterolateral impingement spurs and complicating spur fracture.

The gold standard magnetic resonance (MR) imaging technique for the evaluation of anterolateral impingement is controversial. Some investigators believe that MR imaging is the most useful diagnostic screening test,[23] whereas others state that the diagnostic accuracy of MR imaging is limited in the absence of an ankle joint effusion.[24] One study reported that MR imaging had a sensitivity of 39% and a specificity of 50% for an anterolateral impingement lesion, whereas clinical examination had a sensitivity of 94% and specificity of 75%, using arthroscopy as a gold standard.[18] This finding highlights that disease shown on MR imaging within the ankle may not necessarily be symptomatic.[1] When reporting these studies, it is a reasonable approach to describe the findings and comment that they may predispose the individual to impingement symptoms, rather than making a diagnosis of anterolateral impingement from imaging alone.

The use of intravenous contrast has been advocated as a means of making soft tissue impingement lesions more conspicuous, because posttraumatic synovitis and vascularized scar tissue undergo contrast enhancement. Bagnolesi and colleagues[25] reported mild to moderate contrast enhancement of the abnormal synovium

in 8 of 14 patients with synovial impingement lesions. In patients with a mature meniscoid lesion, the hyalinized fibrosis is relatively avascular and may not enhance. This situation may account for a recent study that found indirect MR arthrography to be less accurate than conventional MR imaging of the ankle for diagnosis of impingement lesions.[26]

Although direct MR arthrography has been reported to have greater levels of accuracy than conventional MR imaging,[27] this technique is not widely practiced, and it is the authors' clinical experience that MR imaging of the ankle using high-resolution nonarthrographic proton density-weighted and fat-suppressed proton density-weighted sequences provides a satisfactory assessment for soft tissue impingement lesions and that a nonarthrographic technique has the advantage of providing an assessment of the extent and distribution of native joint fluid in the ankle.

There have been several reports on the use of ultrasound to assess anterolateral ankle impingement. Cochet and colleagues[28] proposed sonographic diagnostic criteria for synovial thickening in the ALG, which included blood flow on Doppler and the presence of a nonhyperechoic mass measuring a minimum of 4 mm. Using these criteria, sensitivity, specificity, and accuracy of sonography in the diagnosis of anterolateral ankle impingement were 76%, 57%, and 73%, respectively. McCarthy and colleagues[29] described 10 patients with anterolateral impingement who had posttraumatic synovitis detected at sonography and later confirmed with arthroscopy. Hyperemia

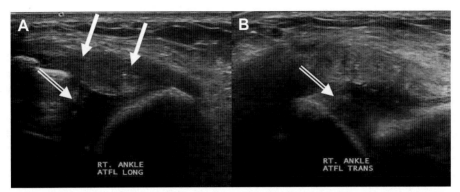

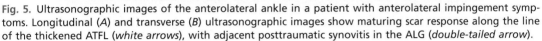

Fig. 5. Ultrasonographic images of the anterolateral ankle in a patient with anterolateral impingement symptoms. Longitudinal (*A*) and transverse (*B*) ultrasonographic images show maturing scar response along the line of the thickened ATFL (*white arrows*), with adjacent posttraumatic synovitis in the ALG (*double-tailed arrow*).

was not shown in the area of synovial thickening in any of their 10 patients. The investigators proposed a 10-mm cutoff size for the synovial thickening and the presence of anterolateral impingement symptoms. Ultrasound-guided injections of the ALG may be helpful in patients with anterolateral impingement symptoms caused by posttraumatic synovitis (**Figs. 5** and **6**).

Imaging Findings in Anterolateral Impingement

Plain radiographs may show an anterior plafond bony spur in patients with anterolateral impingement symptoms. Specific comments on the size, extent of inferior prolongation, and presence of complicating fracture or adjacent long-standing ossicles should be included in the report. CT with sagittal and 3D reconstructions shows anterolateral impingement spurs but does not provide detailed assessment for soft tissue impingement lesions.

Anterolateral tibial plafond impingement spurs, spur fracture, and long-standing ossicles are readily visualized on MR imaging (see **Fig. 3**; **Figs. 7–9**). The adjacent tibial plafond chondral surface should be assessed for associated small basal chondral delamination lesions and subchondral bone marrow edema (**Fig. 10**). When an elongated inferiorly directed tibial plafond spur is present, the adjacent talar dome should be assessed for subtle, sagittally orientated superficial tram-track chondral lesions. The ALG should also be assessed for the presence of synovitis, meniscoid lesions, capsular thickening, and pericapsular edema.

In anterolateral soft tissue impingement, MR imaging may show posttraumatic synovitis within the ALG, which manifests as filiform intermediate signal intensity foci on proton density-weighted and fat-suppressed proton density-weighted or T2-weighted MR sequences (**Figs. 11** and **12**).

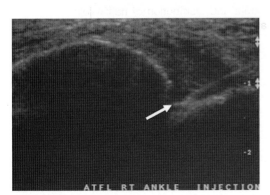

Fig. 6. Ultrasound-guided injection into the ALG. The arrow shows the position of the needle tip in the anterolateral recess of the ankle.

> ### Differential diagnosis in the patient with anterolateral impingement symptoms
>
> *Soft Tissue Lesions*
>
> - Posttraumatic synovitis in the ALG
> - Meniscoid lesion
> - Ganglia arising from the anterolateral capsule
> - Arthrofibrosis
>
> *Bony Lesions*
>
> - Anterolateral plafond spurs and adjacent ossicles, with or without associated chondral lesions involving the tibial plafond or talar dome
> - Loose bodies

Attention should also be directed to the adjacent ATFL and AITFL to assess for evidence of previous injury. As the synovitis becomes more organized and undergoes hyalinized fibrosis, it appears confluent and progressively decreases in signal intensity. A mature meniscoid lesion or fibrous band is of low signal intensity on proton density-weighted or T2-weighted images and is typically triangular in morphology in transverse cross section (**Figs. 13–15**). After arthroscopy, postsurgical scarring of the ALG capsule can mimic a meniscoid lesion on MR imaging.[1] Clinically, however, this scarring is rarely symptomatic (**Fig. 16**).

Arthrofibrosis is visualized as anterior capsular thickening (>3 mm),[30] which may be of intermediate signal on proton density-weighted MR images in the early phase (see **Fig. 16**), and become progressively lower in signal intensity over time (**Fig. 17**).[1] In the early stages, there may be adjacent bone marrow edema in the anterior margin of the tibial plafond at the insertion of the anterior capsule.[30]

Small ganglia arising from the anterolateral ankle capsule may appear inconspicuous on MR imaging (see **Fig. 2**) and may be more readily appreciated on ultrasonography. They may be easily mistaken on MR imaging for joint fluid or a pericapsular vein.[1]

ANTERIOR IMPINGEMENT

Anterior impingement refers to disease at the central anterior aspect of the ankle, either anterolateral or anteromedial, resulting in impingement symptoms. Anterior impingement is less common than anterolateral or anteromedial impingement.

Pathogenesis and Mechanism of Anterior Impingement

Anterior impingement most commonly relates to bone spurs of the anterior tibial plafond, and is typically seen in athletes who subject their ankles to repetitive, forced dorsiflexion (such as ballet dancers and soccer players), or to

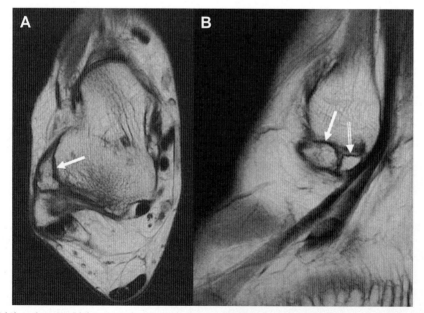

Fig. 7. Axial (*A*) and sagittal (*B*) proton density-weighted MR images showing a large ossicle in the ALG, serving as the point of proximal attachment of the ATFL and related to remote fibular avulsion ATFL, with subsequent growth of a small avulsed fragment and fibrous nonunion (*solid arrows*). The ossicle was causing impingement symptoms. Note the separate avulsion fragment more posteriorly, related to remote avulsive injury at the CFL origin (*double-tailed arrow*).

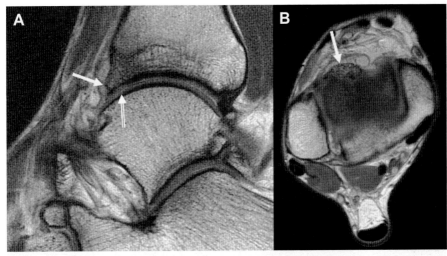

Fig. 8. Sagittal proton density-weighted MR image (*A*) showing an impingement spur of the anterolateral tibial plafond, with moderate inferior prolongation (*solid white arrow*) and adjacent in situ, unstable full-thickness chondral flap of the tibial plafond (*double-tailed white arrow*). Axial proton density-weighted MR image (*B*) shows the anterolateral position of the bony spur (*solid white arrow*).

direct microtrauma (soccer players during ball striking).[31,32] Repeated direct microtrauma leads to bone spur formation. Spurs less commonly form in the superior recess of the talar neck.[33] Although such spurs predispose to anterior impingement, they are commonly asymptomatic.[33–35] It is believed that irritation of the anterior capsule and associated synovitis may be the cause of anterior impingement symptoms (**Fig. 18**).[34] Acute hyperdorsiflexion injuries may also result in anterior impingement symptoms as a result of capsular and pericapsular scar (**Fig. 19**). Loose bodies may lodge in the central aspect of the anterior recess of the ankle and result in anterior impingement (**Fig. 20**).[1]

After an acute ankle sprain, fibrinous debris in the anterior recess of the ankle may undergo hyalinized fibrosis and form fibrous bands (**Fig. 21**). These bands often extend from the medial to lateral margins of the anterior recess and may impinge on the talar dome during dorsiflexion. Traction of the bands on the anterior capsule in plantar flexion may also be a cause of pain (**Fig. 22**).[1]

The talus is a well-recognized site for osteoid osteoma in the hindfoot. Occasionally, these lesions may present with impingementlike symptoms (**Fig. 23**).[1]

Clinical Features of Anterior Impingement

Individuals with anterior impingement typically present with anterior ankle pain and a subjective sensation of blocking on dorsiflexion. Dorsiflexion range of motion is limited and painful. On examination, soft tissue swelling or a bone spur may be palpable over the anterior ankle joint.[36]

Imaging Technique and Findings in Anterior Impingement

Radiographs, preferably when the patient is weight bearing, enable evaluation of anterior

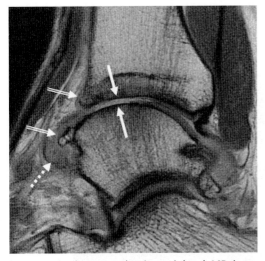

Fig. 9. Sagittal proton density-weighted MR image showing advanced osteoarthritis of the tibiotalar joint, with extensive full-thickness cartilage loss (*solid white arrows*), osteophytes of the anterolateral tibial plafond and talar dome (*double-tailed white arrows*), and degenerative synovitis in the anterior recess of the ankle (*dash-tailed white arrow*).

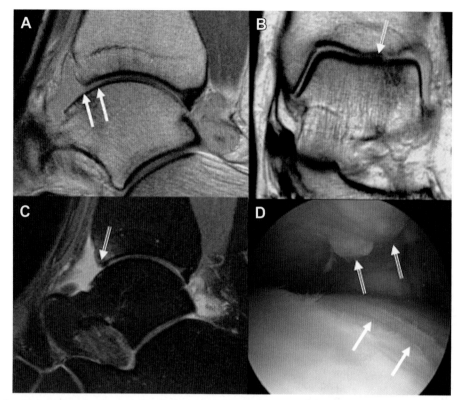

Fig. 10. Sagittal proton density-weighted MR image (*A*) showing a subtle sagittally oriented, tram-track–type superficial chondral lesion of the talar dome (*solid white arrows*), with focal loss of the thin layer of low signal intensity (lamina splendens) at the superficial margin of the chondral surface (*solid white arrows*). A corresponding small anterior tibial plafond spur and loose body are shown on coronal proton density-weighted (*B*) and sagittal fat-suppressed proton density-weighted (*C*) MR images (*double-tailed white arrows*). Arthroscopic image (*D*) from the same patient showing the spur and adjacent loose body (*double-tailed white arrows*), with a tram-track chondral lesion of the talar dome (*solid white arrows*).

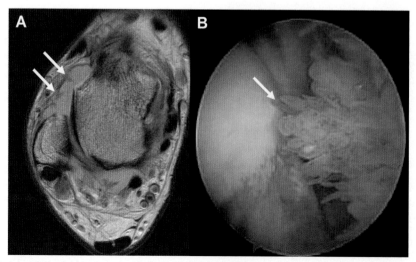

Fig. 11. (*A*) Axial proton density-weighted MR image showing several foci of posttraumatic synovitis in the ALG (*white arrows*). (*B*) Corresponding arthroscopic image showing prominent synovitis in the ALG (*white arrow*).

Differential diagnosis in the patient with anterior impingement symptoms
• Anterior tibial plafond bone spurs
• Synovial thickening/synovitis
• Loose bodies
• Chondral and osteochondral lesions of the anterior tibial plafond and talar dome
• Osteoid osteoma of the talus (mimic)

What the clinician needs to know
• Are there any osseous or soft tissue findings that might predispose to anterior impingement symptoms?
• What is the state of the articular cartilage in the ankle?

bone spurs and the tibiotalar joint space.[37] Fracture of the bone spur and long-standing ossicles may also be shown on plain radiographs. Lateral radiographs obtained in maximal dorsiflexion may show abutment of the bony spurs.[21,22] Assessment of the remainder of the tibiotalar joint for secondary signs of degenerative change using plain radiographs should also be undertaken. Radiographs alone may provide adequate assessment of anterior impingement.[22]

Bony spur formation at the anterior margin of the tibial plafond and dorsal talar neck is usually readily shown on MR imaging on CT (see **Fig. 18**). Acute spur fracture may result in acute impingement symptoms (see **Fig. 4**). MR imaging may be helpful in showing bone marrow edema within the spur, adjacent synovitis in the anterior recess, capsular thickening and edema, and pericapsular edema in patients with symptomatic anterior impingement spurs (see **Fig. 4**). Arthrofibrosis may occasionally involve the anterior ankle capsule in the midline and cause impingement symptoms (see **Fig. 17**).

ANTEROMEDIAL ANKLE IMPINGEMENT
Anatomy of the Anteromedial Gutter

The boundaries of the anteromedial recess or gutter of the ankle include the medial malleolus posteriorly, the anteromedial margin of the talar dome, body, and neck laterally, and the anteromedial ankle capsule superficially. The deltoid ligament complex can be subdivided into deep and superficial components, from its distal insertions. The deep deltoid consists of anterior and posterior tibiotalar components. The fibers of the posterior tibiotalar ligament (PTTL) extend from the medial malleolus to the posterior aspect of the talar body, posteroinferior to the talar articular surface of the medial malleolus (**Fig. 24**). The anterior tibiotalar fascicle of the deltoid ligament lies at the inferior margin of the anteromedial gutter (**Fig. 25**).

Pathogenesis and Mechanism of Anteromedial Impingement

Anteromedial soft tissue impingement is a recognized cause of anteromedial ankle pain and limitation of ankle dorsiflexion and inversion.[31,33,38] The pathogenesis is believed to involve a plantar flexion-inversion injury, with a medial rotational

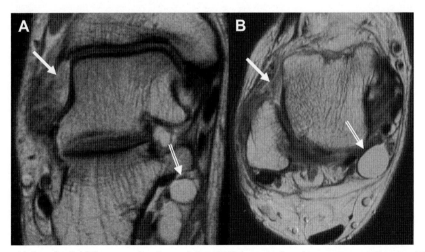

Fig. 12. Coronal (*A*) and axial (*B*) proton density-weighted MR images showing posttraumatic synovitis in the ALG (*solid white arrows*). Note also the ganglion cyst in the tarsal tunnel (*double-tailed white arrows*).

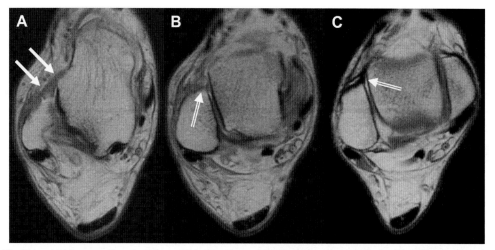

Fig. 13. 39-year-old recreational surfer with anterolateral impingement symptoms. (*A*) Axial proton density-weighted MR image showing a subacute tear of the ATFL with immature scar response (*white arrows*). (*B*) Axial proton density-weighted MR image through the ALG, superior to the ATFL, shows dense posttraumatic synovitis (*double-tailed white arrow*). (*C*) Axial proton density-weighted MR image performed 1 year later shows a meniscoid lesion (*double-tailed white arrow*) formed at the site of the previously shown synovitis.

impaction component.[22,33,39] There is associated contusional injury to the posterior and sometimes anterior tibiotalar components of the deep fibers of the deltoid ligament, and microtrabecular injury to the medial malleolus and medial talar body-neck (medial kissing bone contusions). Posttraumatic synovitis in the anteromedial gutter and immature scarring of the anteromedial capsule and anterior tibiotalar ligament may result in anteromedial impingement symptoms.[40] In time, formation of intra-articular fibrous bands may also result in impingement symptoms.[21,38–40]

Soft tissue disease alone may cause anteromedial impingement in the absence of bony spurs.[1]

Bony spurs are another important cause of anteromedial impingement and may arise from the dorsomedial talar neck, anteromedial tibial plafond, or the anterior margin of the medial malleolus.[1] It is postulated that the pathogenesis of these spurs is secondary to recurrent low-grade impaction associated with sporting activities, such as soccer.[41] Occasionally, anteromedial bony impingement may be caused by a posttraumatic ossicle. The ossicle may be the sequela of

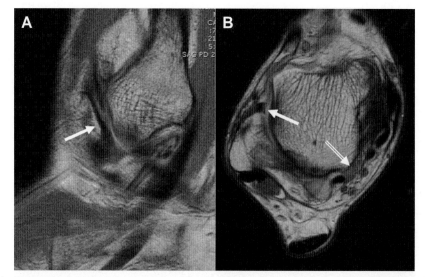

Fig. 14. Sagittal (*A*) and axial (*B*) proton density-weighted MR images through the ALG showing a thick fibrous band in the ALG extending inferiorly from the inferior margin of the inferior fascicle of the AITFL, consistent with a meniscoid lesion (*white arrows*). Note also mild scarring of the posteromedial gutter capsule (*double-tailed white arrow*).

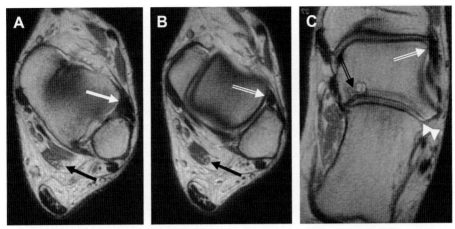

Fig. 15. 27-year-old motorcyclist with anterolateral impingement symptoms. Sequential axial (*A, B*) and coronal (*C*) proton density-weighted MR images. (*A*) Densely scarred, thickened inferior fascicle of the AITFL (*solid white arrow*), reflecting remote syndesmotic injury. This injury is closely related to a mature meniscoid lesion in the ALG, in (*B, C*) (*double-tailed white arrow*). Note also an accessory flexor muscle (*black arrows*), complete longitudinal split tear of the peroneus brevis tendon (*white arrowheads*), and osteochondral lesion of the posterior talar facet (*double-tailed black arrow*).

an avulsion injury involving the insertion of the anterior tibiotalar ligament or anteromedial capsule, may represent dystrophic ossification after ligamentous injury, or be secondary to fracture of a bony spur. The ossicle may become scarred into the deep fibers of the deltoid ligament or into the deep margin of the anteromedial gutter capsule.[1]

Clinical Findings in Anteromedial Impingement

Patients often present with chronic anteromedial ankle pain that is exacerbated by dorsiflexion.

On examination, there is focal anteromedial ankle tenderness and swelling, with limited dorsiflexion and inversion.[39,40] Snapping or popping may also occur with dorsiflexion.[39]

Imaging Technique

Anteromedial impingement spurs at the dorsomedial talar neck, anteromedial tibial plafond, and anterior border of the medial malleolus are best shown on an oblique radiograph of the foot. This projection involves a 45° craniocaudal angulation of the radiograph tube, with the leg positioned in 30° of external rotation (**Fig. 26**).[42] A routine ankle

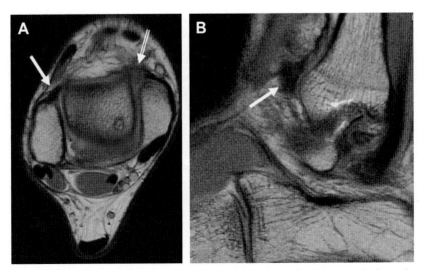

Fig. 16. Axial (*A*) and sagittal (*B*) proton density-weighted MR images show postsurgical scarring of the ALG, mimicking a meniscoid lesion (*white arrows*). Note also postsurgical scarring of the anteromedial ankle capsule at the site of a previous anteromedial arthroscopic portal (*double-tailed white arrow*).

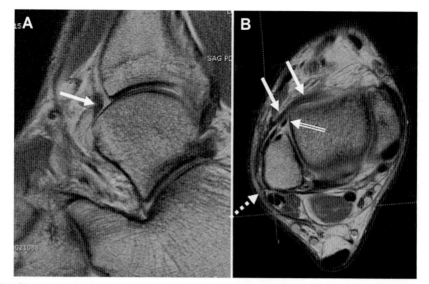

Fig. 17. Arthrofibrotic change of the anterior ankle capsule causing anterior impingement symptoms. Sagittal (*A*) and axial (*B*) proton density-weighted MR images showing thickening and scarring of the anterior ankle capsule lateral of midline (*solid white arrows*). A separate, small fibrous band is seen in the ALG (*double-tailed white arrow*), and there is avulsion of the superior peroneal retinaculum (*dash-tailed white arrow*).

radiograph series often fails to show small anteromedial impingement spurs and does not differentiate anteromedial from centroanterior or anterolateral plafond spurs. Ultrasonography may show synovitis, scar, and loose bodies in the anteromedial gutter (**Figs. 27** and **28**). CT readily shows anteromedial ankle impingement spurs. Some surgeons find 3D reconstructions helpful for preoperative planning in the surgical management of impingement spurs.

Initial reports of anteromedial impingement in the surgical literature suggested that MR imaging had been unhelpful in cases that had been diagnosed at surgery.[39] In the senior author's experience, a combination of high-resolution, nonarthrographic proton density-weighted and fat-suppressed proton density-weighted MR sequences are efficacious in the assessment of patients with anteromedial impingement symptoms (see **Fig. 28**; **Fig. 29**). It has been reported that MR arthrography may improve the conspicuity of medial meniscoid lesions, thickening of the anterior tibiotalar ligament, anteromedial capsular thickening, synovitis, bony spurs, and

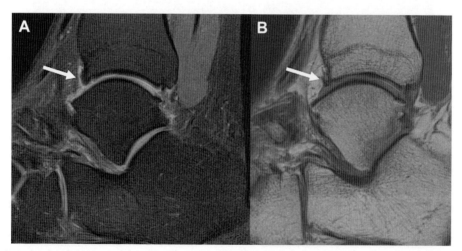

Fig. 18. Anterior impingement. (*A*) Sagittal proton density-weighted MR image with (*A*) and without (*B*) fat suppression show a moderate centroanterior plafond spur (*arrows*) in a patient who presented with anterior impingement symptoms.

chondral or osteochondral lesions; however, it is a technique that is not widely used.[40]

Imaging Findings in Anteromedial Impingement

Anteromedial impingement spurs at the dorsomedial talar neck, anteromedial tibial plafond, and anterior border of the medial malleolus may be evident on a lateral radiograph of the ankle, but are best shown on an oblique radiograph of the foot (see **Fig. 26**).

On MR imaging and CT, anteromedial impingement spurs arising from the dorsomedial aspect of the talar neck and anteromedial tibial plafond are usually best visualized in the sagittal plane (see **Fig. 26**). Dorsomedial talar neck spurs may also be visualized in the oblique coronal plane on MR imaging and CT and in an oblique coronal plane on ultrasonography (see **Fig. 28**). Additional MR imaging findings associated with symptomatic spurs may include bone marrow edema within the spur and adjacent synovitis or capsular thickening in the anteromedial gutter and pericapsular edema (see **Fig. 29**).[43]

Thickening and edema of the anterior tibiotalar ligament may be visualized in the sagittal and sometimes the coronal planes (see **Fig. 25**). Axial and sagittal images may show synovitis and fibrous bands in the anteromedial gutter (**Fig. 30**).

Most MR imaging sequences allow visualization of avulsion fragments and dystrophic ossification secondary to remote deltoid ligament injury, whereas fat-suppressed proton density-weighted or T2-weighted images are important to show associated bone marrow edema (**Figs. 31** and **32**).[1]

MR imaging is also useful in identifying diseases that may mimic anteromedial impingement. These diseases include PTTL contusion, medial kissing bone contusions, osteochondral injuries of the medial talar dome, or injury to the anterior aspect

of the flexor retinacular insertion on the medial malleolus (laciniate ligament) (**Figs. 33–35**).[1]

POSTEROMEDIAL IMPINGEMENT
Anatomy of the Posteromedial Gutter

The boundaries of the posteromedial gutter include the posterior border of the medial malleolus and the PTTL anteriorly, and the posteromedial capsule superficially and posteriorly. The posteromedial border of the talar dome-body and posteromedial process of the talus form the deep margin.

The posteromedial gutter is normally evident as a small recess containing minimal fluid, with a thin overlying capsular layer (see **Fig. 24**). It is readily identified on axial images as the recess lying deep to the interval between the flexor digitorum longus (FDL) and flexor hallucis longus (FHL) tendons (see **Fig. 24**).

Pathogenesis and Mechanism of Posteromedial Impingement

Posteromedial impingement may complicate a plantar flexion, inversion, and medial rotation impaction injury,[1] with resultant contusional injury to the posterior (deep) fibers of the tibiotalar ligament (PTTL) and the posteromedial ankle capsule secondary to compression between the talus and medial malleolus.[33]

Acute edema and immature scar formation involving the deep fibers of the deltoid ligament may evolve into thickening and fibrosis, which may protrude into the posteromedial gutter. There

---

Mimics of anteromedial impingement symptoms

- Posterior tibiotalar (deep deltoid) ligament contusion
- Medial kissing bone contusions
- Osteochondral injuries of the medial talar dome
- Injury to the anterior aspect of the flexor retinacular insertion on the medial malleolus (laciniate ligament)

Differential diagnosis in the patient with anteromedial impingement symptoms

- Synovitis
- Intra-articular fibrous band
- Arthrofibrosis
- Bony impingement spurs: dorsomedial talar neck, anteromedial tibial plafond, or the anterior margin of the medial malleolus
- Spur fracture
- Avulsion fragments

What the clinician needs to know

- Are there bony or soft tissue pathologies that predispose to anteromedial impingement and if so, are they amenable to corticosteroid injection or surgical debridement/excision?
- Are there other diseases that may mimic anteromedial impingement?

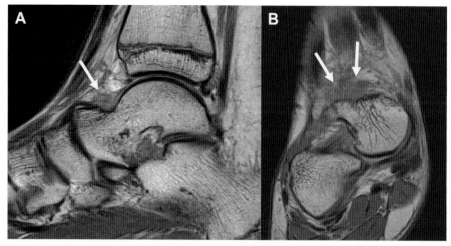

Fig. 19. Subacute anterior impingement in a gymnast after a hyperdorsiflexion injury. Sagittal (*A*) and coronal (*B*) proton density-weighted images show immature pericapsular scar (*white arrows*) adjacent to the neck of the talus.

may also be an overlying posttraumatic synovitis, with thickening and displacement of the posteromedial ankle capsule.[44] This hypertrophic change and fibrosis may protrude between the posteromedial border of the talar dome-body and the posterior margin of the medial malleolus.[44] An avulsion fracture involving the posteromedial process of the talus at the insertion of the PTTL with associated scar tissue can also predispose individuals to posteromedial impingement symptoms.[4]

Clinical Findings of Posteromedial Impingement

Patients usually present with posteromedial pain between the posteromedial border of the talar dome-body and the posterior margin of the medial

malleolus.[44,45] On examination, posteromedial tenderness on inversion with the ankle in plantar flexion helps distinguish posteromedial impingement from posterior tibial tendon dysfunction.[33] With appropriate physiotherapy, sometimes augmented by corticosteroid injection, there may be resolution of the synovitis, and remodeling and thinning of any scar tissue. Recalcitrant symptoms associated with dense mature scar tissue within the posteromedial gutter may require surgical debridement.[44,46]

Imaging Technique

Routine radiographic views of the ankle and hindfoot should be undertaken to screen for bony disease. Although an isotope bone scan has

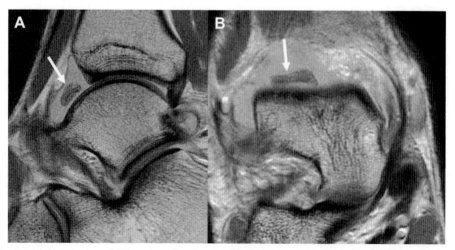

Fig. 20. Sagittal (*A*) and coronal (*B*) proton density-weighted images show an osteochondral joint body in the anterior recess of the ankle (*arrow*), just lateral of midline.

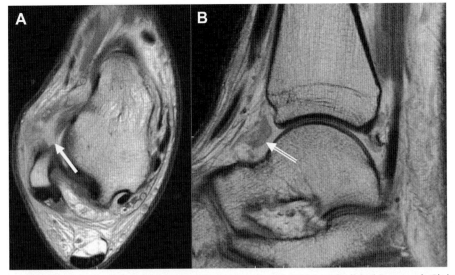

Fig. 21. Axial proton density-weighted MR image (*A*) shows an acute ATFL tear (*solid white arrow*). Globular fibrinous debris are seen in the anterior recess of the ankle (*double-tailed white arrow*) on a midline sagittal proton density-weighted MR image (*B*).

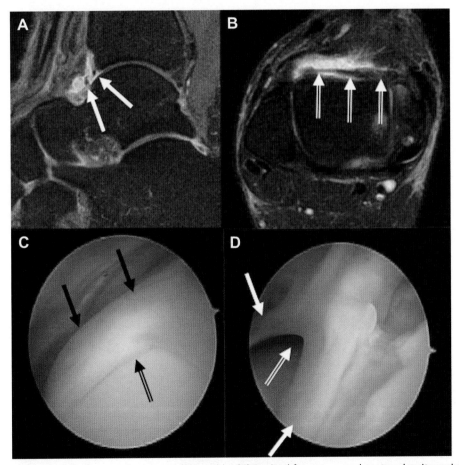

Fig. 22. Fibrous bands in the anterior recess of the ankle. (*A*) Sagittal fat-suppressed proton density-weighted MR image showing 2 transversely oriented fibrous bands in the anterior recess of the ankle manifest as punctate foci of low signal (*solid white arrows*). (*B*) Axial fat-suppressed T2-weighted MR image shows one of the fibrous bands, extending from medial to lateral (*double-tailed white arrows*). (*C*) Arthroscopic image from the same patient with the ankle in dorsiflexion shows the fibrous band (*solid black arrows*) impinging on the talar dome (*double-tailed black arrow*). (*D*) Arthroscopic image with the ankle in plantar flexion shows the fibrous band clear of the talar dome (*double-tailed white arrow*). The fibrous band is partially tethered to the anterior capsule medially and laterally, resulting in the fibrous band being under tension as a result of capsular traction (*white arrows*).

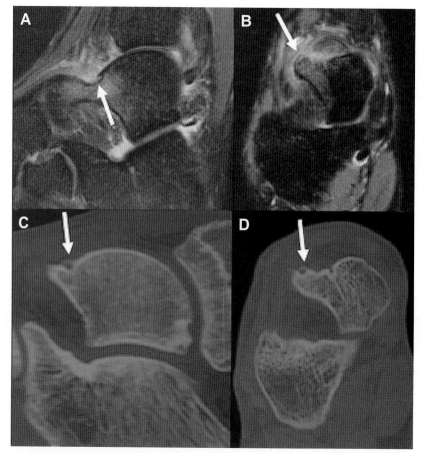

Fig. 23. 26-year-old principal ballerina with persistent anterior impingementlike symptoms, caused by a periosteal osteoid osteoma of the talar neck. (*A*) Sagittal fat-suppressed proton density-weighted and (*B*) coronal fat-suppressed proton density-weighted MR images showing bone marrow edema in the talar neck dorsally, with adjacent soft tissue edema, mild synovitis in the anterior recess of the ankle and focal periosteal deformity (*white arrows*), which was confirmed on multislice CT with sagittal (*C*) and coronal (*D*) reconstructions (*white arrows*). The lesion was excised, with resolution of the patient's symptoms and histopathologic confirmation of the diagnosis.

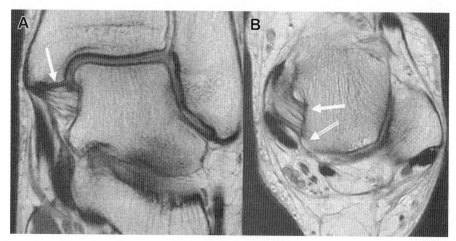

Fig. 24. Normal multifascular appearance of the PTTL shown on coronal (*A*) and axial (*B*) proton density-weighted MR images (*white arrows*). Note also the normal appearance of the posteromedial recess, with a thin capsular layer overlying the posteromedial corner of the talar dome on the axial image, between the level of the FDL and FHL tendons (*double-tailed white arrow*).

been described for the investigation of posteromedial impingement, its lack of specificity limits its clinical usefulness.[44] Ultrasonographic examination in the transverse plane with comparison assessment of the contralateral side usually identifies posteromedial soft tissue impingement lesions (**Fig. 36**).[22] Ultrasound-guided corticosteroid injections may be performed in selected cases.[45] High-resolution sagittal and axial proton density-weighted and fat-suppressed proton density-weighted MR sequences usually provide adequate assessment of the patient with posteromedial impingement symptoms.

Imaging Findings in Posteromedial Impingement

Conventional radiographs are usually negative. Occasionally, they may show an intra-articular ossific loose body or bony spurring or overgrowth at the posteromedial border of the talocrural joint.[44]

Ultrasonography may show hypoechoic thickening of the posterior aspect of the deep fibers of the deltoid ligament, with protrusion into the posteromedial gutter, deep to the posterior tibial tendon, best identified on a transverse view (see **Fig. 36**). In the subacute setting, hyperemia may be shown on color Doppler (**Fig. 37**). With chronicity, the hyperemia may resolve.[45]

MR imaging findings in patients with posteromedial impingement symptoms in the subacute phase after an ankle sprain include edemalike signal in the deep fibers of the deltoid ligament, with loss of the normal striated appearance (see

> **Differential diagnosis in the patient with posteromedial impingement symptoms**
>
> - Injury to the deep fibers of the deltoid ligament with scar response and synovitis protruding into the medial gutter posteriorly, and thickening of the posteromedial ankle capsule
> - Concurrent injury to the flexor retinaculum, with partial scar encasement of the posterior tibial tendon
> - Avulsion fracture of the posteromedial process of the talus
> - Osteochondral lesion of the medial talar dome
> - Isolated flexor retinacular avulsive injury

Fig. 33) and protrusion of scar response and synovitis into the medial gutter posteriorly, with overlying thickening of the posteromedial capsule and loss of the normal clear space in the posteromedial gutter between the levels of the FDL and FHL tendons (see **Figs. 31** and **37**). Occasionally, there may be frank macroscopic tearing of the deep fibers of the deltoid ligament (see **Fig. 34**).[45] There may be adjacent medial kissing bone contusions involving the medial malleolus and medial talar body. Concurrent injury to the flexor retinaculum may result in partial scar encasement of the posterior tibial tendon between the retinaculum and the scarred PTTL.[45,47]

An avulsion fracture fragment derived from the posteromedial process of the talus often consists

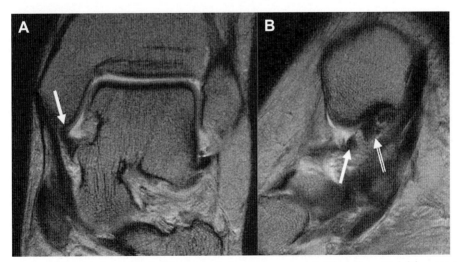

Fig. 25. Anterior tibiotalar ligament (*white arrows*) shown on coronal (*A*) and sagittal (*B*) proton density-weighted cadaveric 3-T MR arthrographic images. The anterior tibiotalar ligament is mildly thickened because of scarring. Note on the sagittal image the relationship to the PTTL (*double-tailed white arrow*).

What the clinician wants to know
• Confirmation of findings predisposing to posteromedial impingement
• Exclude other diseases that may cause posteromedial ankle pain (eg, osteochondral lesions of the talar dome)

of cortical bone only, and may be difficult to identify on MR imaging because of a similar signal intensity to that of the inevitably associated adjacent scar tissue. When MR imaging is inconclusive, a CT scan provides clarification (**Fig. 38**).[1]

POSTERIOR ANKLE IMPINGEMENT AND FHL TENOSYNOVITIS

Posterior ankle impingement has been classically described in ballet dancers who perform in the equinus position.[1] Other athletes such as soccer players, cricket fast bowlers, javelin throwers, divers, figure skaters, and gymnasts may also suffer from this condition.[48] Different names have been given to posterior impingement, including os trigonum syndrome, talar compression syndrome, and posterior block of the ankle.[49,50]

Anatomy of Posterior Impingement

The anatomy of the posterior ankle is a key factor in the occurrence of posterior ankle impingement syndrome.[31] A secondary ossification center forms at the posterolateral aspect of talus between the ages of 8 and 13 years and fuses with the remainder of the talus within 1 year of its appearance.[51] In 7% of the population, failure of fusion results in an os trigonum.[52] The synchondrosis of an os trigonum may vary in orientation from coronal to oblique sagittal.[1] Other osseous anomalies that may predispose an individual to posterior impingement include a prominent posterolateral process of the talus (Stieda process), prominence of the posterior malleolus of the tibia, and prominence of the posterior process of the calcaneus.[53,54]

Injury to soft tissue structures within the posterior aspect of the ankle that may contribute to posterior impingement include the posterior talofibular, posterior intermalleolar, and posterior inferior tibiofibular ligaments, the synovial sheath of

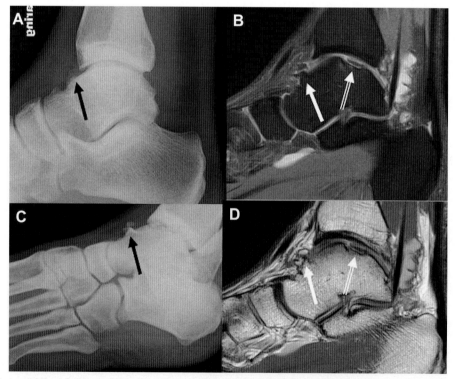

Fig. 26. Lateral (*A*) and oblique (*C*) radiographs show an anteromedial spur arising from the neck of the talus and an adjacent ossicle (*black arrows*). This finding is best appreciated on the oblique projection. Sagittal proton density-weighted images with fat saturation (*B*) and without fat saturation (*D*) also identify the spur and adjacent ossicle (*white arrow*). Note also the medial talar dome osteochondral lesion (*double-tailed white arrows*).

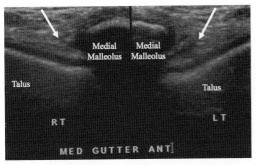

Fig. 27. Ultrasonographic images showing the normal sonographic appearance of the anteromedial gutter (*arrow*).

the FHL tendon, and the posterior synovial recess of the tibiotalar and subtalar joints.[53,54]

Pathogenesis and Mechanism of Posterior Impingement

Posterior ankle impingement may complicate an acute traumatic hyperplantar flexion injury or may be secondary to repetitive low-grade trauma associated with hyperplantar flexion, such as a ballet dancer performing en pointe or in soccer players.[1] The posterior talus and surrounding soft tissues are compressed between the tibial plafond and posterosuperior aspect of the calcaneus during plantar flexion: a so-called nutcracker phenomenon.[54]

Bony anatomic variants of the posterior talus may predispose individuals to posterior impingement.[37] These variants include an os trigonum, prominence of the posterolateral process (Stieda process), or a shelflike superior prominence of the calcaneal tuberosity.[55,56] The presence of an os trigonum in itself is not sufficient to produce impingement; however, when combined with a supination injury, dancing on hard surfaces, or pushing beyond anatomic limits, a posterior ankle impingement syndrome may result.[57]

Destabilization of the cartilaginous synchondrosis between an os trigonum and the talar body may occur as a result of repetitive microtrauma or chronic inflammation and is a potential cause of pain.[37] Compression between the os trigonum and posterior tibia or calcaneus may result in entrapment of the adjacent soft tissues. Synovitis may develop that is centered on the posterior talofibular ligament.[1,43]

Acute fractures of the posterolateral process of the talus (Shepherd fracture) or nonunion of these fractures are potential causes of posterior ankle impingement symptoms.[57,58]

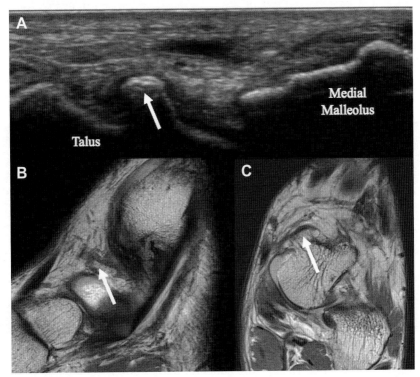

Fig. 28. Ultrasonographic image (*A*) and sagittal (*B*) and coronal (*C*) proton density-weighted MR images show a dorsomedial talar neck spur (*white arrows*) in a patient with anteromedial impingement symptoms.

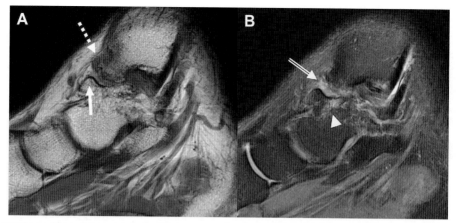

Fig. 29. Anteromedial impingement. Sagittal proton density-weighted (*A*) and fat-saturated proton density-weighted (*B*) MR images showing bony anteromedial impingement, with a dorsomedial talar neck bone spur (*solid white arrow*), anteromedial plafond-medial malleolar bone spur (*dash-tailed white arrow*), with adjacent synovitis and mild capsular thickening in the anteromedial gutter (*double-tailed white arrow*). Note also the bone marrow edema at the base of the talar neck spur (*white arrowhead*).

Bony spurs at the posterior margin of the tibial plafond related to previous syndesmotic injury, and posteroinferiorly directed bony spurs arising from the posterolateral process of the talus, may also contribute to posterior bony ankle impingement.[1]

Loose bodies in the posterior recesses of the ankle or posterior subtalar joint, or a localized synovitis involving the posterior recess of the ankle or subtalar joint, may cause posterior impingement symptoms. In most circumstances, loose bodies are associated with other intra-articular disease.[1]

There are several soft tissue diseases that may predispose individuals to posterior impingement.

These diseases include scarring of the posterior talofibular, intermalleolar, posterior inferior tibiofibular and posterior inferior tibiofibular ligaments, and laxity of the lateral ankle ligament complex.[1,56,59]

Myxoid degenerative change, with or without ganglion formation, may develop in the posterior talofibular ligament (PTFL). Ganglia typically form adjacent to the fibular insertion and decompress posteriorly. Both entities may cause posterior impingement.[1]

A displaced distal tear of the CFL, with protrusion of the ligament stump into the posterior recess of the posterior subtalar joint, is a rare cause of posterior impingement.

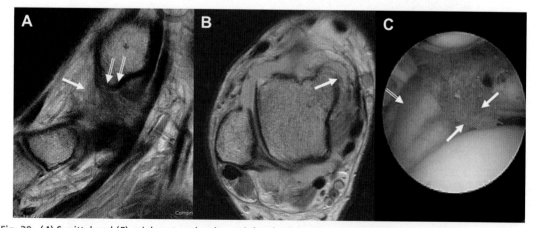

Fig. 30. (*A*) Sagittal and (*B*) axial proton density-weighted MR images showing immature scarring of the anterior tibiotalar ligament (*double-tailed white arrows*), manifest as ligament thickening and hyperintense signal abnormality, with adjacent synovitis in the anteromedial gutter (*solid white arrow*). (*C*) Arthroscopic image from the same patient shows synovitis in the anteromedial gutter (*solid white arrows*), overlying the thickened anterior tibiotalar ligament (*double-tailed white arrow*).

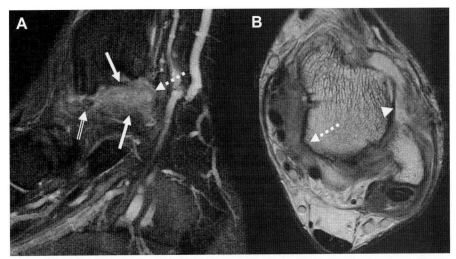

Fig. 31. Sagittal fat-suppressed proton density-weighted (*A*) and axial proton density-weighted (*B*) MR images showing a subacute contusional injury to the PTTL, with resultant ligamentous edema and loss of the normal striated morphology (*solid white arrows*), and protrusion of immature scar response and synovitis into the medial gutter posteriorly (*dash-tailed white arrow*). Note the small rounded ossicle scarred into the medial gutter anteriorly in the region of the anterior tibiotalar ligament (*double-tailed white arrow*) and the posttraumatic synovitis and immature meniscoid lesion in the ALG (*white arrowhead*).

Pathogenesis of FHL Tenosynovitis

In dancers, repetitive overload of the FHL tendon and subsequent tenosynovitis may be secondary to poor en pointe positioning, pronation of the foot, and poor turnout (external rotation) at the hips. Repetitive irritation and thickening of the retinaculum, which forms the roof of the fibro-osseous tunnel for the FHL, may result in focal narrowing of the tunnel and limitation of gliding of the tendon within the tendon sheath. This condition is called stenosing tenosynovitis, and presents clinically as FHL tendon dysfunction.[60] Typically, the

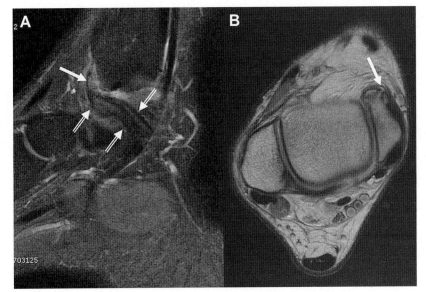

Fig. 32. (*A*) Sagittal fat-suppressed proton density-weighted and (*B*) axial proton density-weighted MR images from a patient presenting with anteromedial impingement symptoms showing a small avulsion fracture fragment at the anterior margin of the medial malleolus (*solid white arrow*). Note the bone marrow edema within the fragment, which serves as the point of attachment of the tibiocalcaneal component of the superficial deltoid ligament (*double-tailed white arrows*).

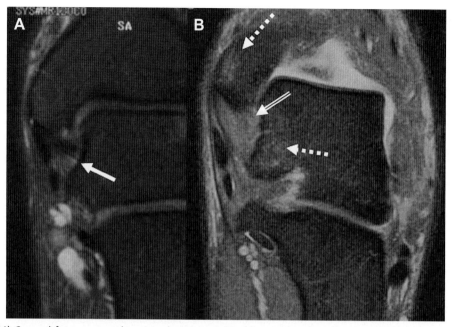

Fig. 33. (*A*) Coronal fat-suppressed proton density-weighted image showing the normal striated appearance of the PTTL, with high-signal fibrovascular tissue interspersed between the ligament fascicles (*solid white arrow*). (*B*) Coronal fat-suppressed proton density-weighted MR image showing contusional injury to the PTTL, manifesting as ligament edema with loss of normal striated morphology (*double-tailed white arrow*). Note adjacent bone marrow edema in the medial talar body and medial malleolus, reflecting medial kissing bone contusions (*dash-tailed arrows*).

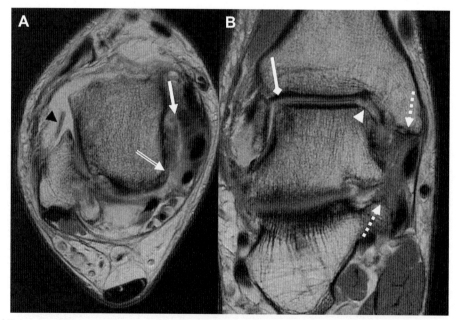

Fig. 34. (*A*) Axial and (*B*) coronal proton density-weighted MR images from a professional rugby league football player, showing a subacute complete tear of the posterior tibiotalar fibers of the deltoid ligament (*solid white arrow*), with moderate adjacent posttraumatic synovitis in the posteromedial gutter (*double-tailed white arrow*). Note also the subacute interstitial tear of the tibiocalcaneal component of the superficial deltoid (*dash-tailed white arrows*), the medial talar dome lesion with a full-thickness chondral defect (*white arrowhead*), displaced chondral fragment in the ALG (*black arrowhead*), and chronic lateral talar dome lesion (*diamond-headed white arrow*). The case highlights the frequently multiple sites of disease in athletes with posttraumatic ankle pain.

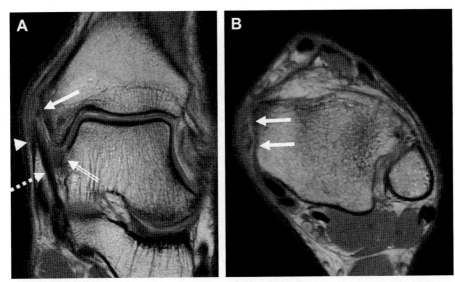

Fig. 35. (A) Coronal and (B) axial proton density-weighted MR images from a professional rugby league player with chronic anteromedial ankle pain related to chronic partial tear at the medial malleolar origin of the tibiocalcaneal component of the superficial fibers of the deltoid ligament and overlying anterior aspect of the flexor retinacular origin (*solid white arrows*). The white arrowhead indicates the more distal aspect of the flexor retinaculum, whereas the dash-tailed white arrow indicates the more distal aspect of the tibiocalcaneal component of the superficial deltoid. Note also the thickened anterior tibiotalar ligament (*double-tailed white arrow*). The findings were confirmed at the time of surgical exploration and repair.

stenosis is over a relatively short segment (5 mm).[61] A low-lying FHL musculotendinous junction and, rarely, an accessory flexor muscle (peroneocalcaneus internus) may cause posterior impingement or FHL tendinitis symptoms. The tendon of the peroneocalcaneus internus courses within the FHL tendon sheath and inserts on the medial aspect of the calcaneus at the level of the sustentaculum, and, when present, is asymptomatic in most individuals.[1]

Clinical Findings of Posterior Impingement

Posterior ankle impingement is typically associated with pain and swelling at the posterolateral aspect of the ankle, which is exacerbated by plantar flexion.[1] Although symptoms may be relieved with rest, recurrence of pain is common on return to activity.[33] The clinical differential diagnosis includes retrocalcaneal bursitis and Achilles or peroneal tendon disease.

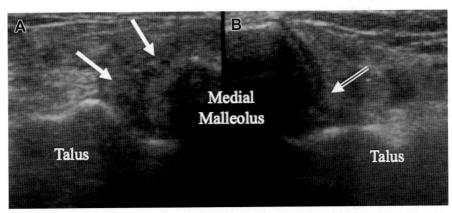

Fig. 36. Posteromedial soft tissue impingement lesion. (A) Transverse ultrasonographic image showing posttraumatic synovitis distending the posteromedial gutter (*solid white arrows*). (B) Comparison image of the contralateral side shows a normal posteromedial gutter (*double-tailed white arrow*).

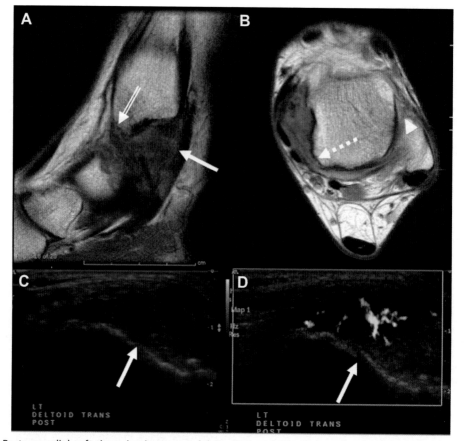

Fig. 37. Posteromedial soft tissue impingement. (*A*) Sagittal and (*B*) axial proton density-weighted MR images show immature scar response within the PTTL (*solid white arrow*) and scarring of the anterior tibiotalar ligament (*double-tailed white arrow*), with protrusion of scar response and synovitis into the posteromedial gutter (*dash-tailed white arrow*), predisposing to posteromedial impingement symptoms. Transverse ultrasonographic images without (*C*) and with color Doppler (*D*) show hyperemic scarring of the PTTL (*solid white arrow*).

FHL tenosynovitis is characterized by postero-medial ankle pain and swelling, pain with passive or active movement of the great toe, limited range of great toe motion, and tenderness over the fibro-osseous tunnel for the FHL. There may be associated palpable crepitus or triggering. The clinical differential diagnosis includes a deltoid ligament sprain, posterior tibial tenosynovitis, posterome-dial tarsal coalition, posteromedial talar dome os-teochondral lesion, plantar fasciitis, and tarsal tunnel syndrome.[1]

Imaging Technique

Conventional radiographs may be used to identify an os trigonum or a Stieda process. If the syn-chondrosis of an os trigonum is oblique in orienta-tion and there is underlying prominence of the posterolateral process of the talus, then an os trig-onum may be superimposed on the posterolateral process of the talus on a straight lateral projection. Augmentation of a routine ankle series with a lazy lateral view in which the ankle is mildly externally rotated, and a lateral view in plantar flexion can help show an os trigonum that remains occult on a standard lateral view and may show bony abut-ment in plantar flexion[62] (**Fig. 39**).

Multidetector CT with multiplanar and 3D recon-structions readily shows the presence of an os trigonum, prominence of the posterolateral process of the talus, and posterolateral talar process fractures; however, soft tissue resolution is poor.[55,59] Isotope bone scans when combined with a CT data set may be positive in cases of posterior impingement but remain relatively insen-sitive for some soft tissue diseases.

Ultrasonography may be a useful modality for the assessment and management of posterior impingement.[22] Injections for posterior impinge-ment associated with an os trigonum may be

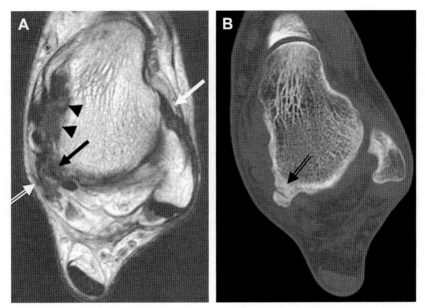

Fig. 38. 34-year-old man with posteromedial impingement symptoms caused by an old avulsion fracture of the posteromedial process of the talus. The avulsion fracture fragment is difficult to appreciate on an axial proton density-weighted MR image (A) because of the similar signal intensity of the fragment (*black arrow*) and the adjacent scarred posteromedial capsule (*double-tailed white arrow*). Note also the scarred PTTL (*black arrowheads*) and the scarred ATFL (*white arrow*). The avulsion fracture fragment was confirmed on CT (B) (*double-tailed black arrow*).

performed under ultrasound or fluoroscopic guidance.[63,64] Injections of this nature may be both diagnostic and therapeutic.

The MR imaging protocol used for investigating posterior ankle impingement should adequately show a small os trigonum, myxoid change in the PTFL, posterior ankle ganglia, FHL tendon disease, and synovitis. The protocols vary according to the MR imaging unit and personal preference. The senior author's preference is to include

sagittal and axial proton density-weighted and fat-suppressed proton density-weighted, and coronal proton density-weighted sequences in the study.

Imaging Findings of Posterior Impingement

Radiographs may identify an os trigonum or Stieda process. A lazy lateral view may be helpful in confirming the presence of an os trigonum

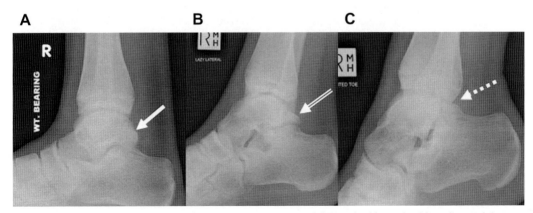

Fig. 39. Plain radiographic assessment of posterior impingement. (A) Standard lateral ankle radiograph in neutral shows a double density projected over the posterior aspect of the talar body (*solid white arrow*), suspicious for the presence of an os trigonum. (B) Lazy lateral projection in mild external rotation confirms the presence of an os trigonum (*double-tailed white arrow*) and profiles the radiolucent synchondrosis. (C) Lateral projection in plantar flexion shows abutment between the posterior malleolus and the os trigonum (*dash-tailed white arrow*).

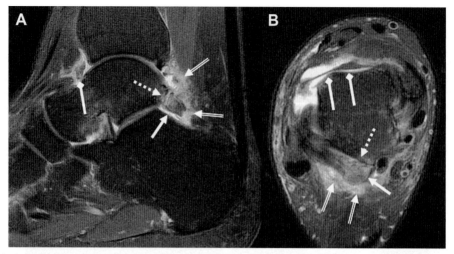

Fig. 40. Active posterior ankle impingement. Sagittal fat-suppressed proton density-weighted (*A*) and oblique axial fat-suppressed T2-weighted (*B*) images show moderate bone marrow edema within a moderate-sized os trigonum (*solid white arrow*), with adjacent signal hyperintensity at the synchondrosis (*dash-tailed white arrows*), indicating at least partial destabilization. Moderate synovitis in the posterior recesses of the ankle and subtalar joint and adjacent pericapsular edema is consistent with a degree of active posterior impingement (*double-tailed white arrows*). Note the thick intra-articular fibrous band in the anterior recess of the ankle (*diamond-headed arrows*).

(see **Fig. 39**). Radiographs may also show cystic and sclerotic changes along the synchondrosis.[65] An os trigonum must be differentiated from an acute fracture of the posterolateral process of the talus. Radiographs with the foot in plantar flexion may show bony abutment of the os trigonum or lateral talar tubercle between the posterior medial malleolus and calcaneal tuberosity (see **Fig. 39**).

The size of an os trigonum or degree of prominence of the posterolateral process of the talus is not strongly correlated with the severity of posterior impingement symptoms.[59]

An os trigonum can usually be identified on ultrasonography. Ultrasonography may show myxoid change in the posterior talofibular ligament and complicating ganglion cyst formation in some

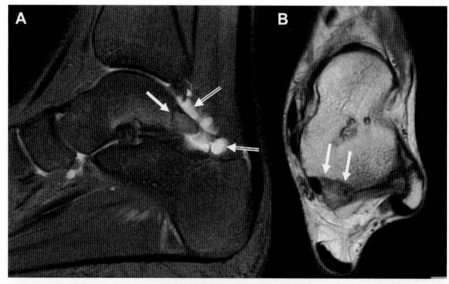

Fig. 41. Sagittal fat-saturated proton density-weighted (*A*) and axial proton density-weighted (*B*) MR images in an athlete with posterior ankle impingement symptoms. There is a subacute nondisplaced fracture of the posterolateral process of the talus (*solid white arrows*), with extensive bone marrow edema at the margins, adjacent fluid distension of the posterior recesses of the ankle and subtalar joints, and associated mild synovitis (*double-tailed white arrows*) Note the underlying prominence of the posterolateral process of the talus, which extends posterior to the arc of curvature of the talar dome in the sagittal plane.

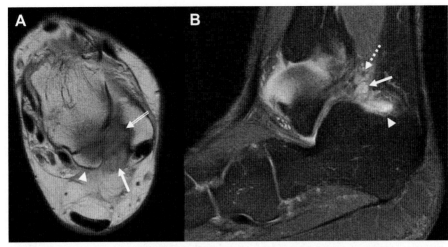

Fig. 42. Posterior ankle impingement. Axial proton density-weighted (*A*) and sagittal fat-suppressed proton density-weighted (*B*) MR images show thickening of the posterior talofibular ligament and signal hyperintensity (*double-tailed white arrow*), consistent with myxoid change. Complicating ganglion cystic change is evident, decompressing posteriorly (*solid white arrows*). Note the adjacent pericapsular edema at the superior margin (*dash-tailed white arrow*) and the fluid distension of the posterior recess of the subtalar joint and mild synovitis (*white arrowhead* in *B*). Note also the moderate-sized os trigonum (*white arrowhead* in *A*).

patients with posterior impingement.[33] There is usually no increase in blood flow within the abnormal soft tissues on color Doppler examination.[37] Dynamic ultrasonographic assessment of the posterolateral aspect of the ankle during forced plantar flexion may be helpful in distinguishing between a ganglion cyst and fluid-distended recess of the ankle or subtalar joint.

CT is able to characterize pathologic changes at the interface between the os trigonum and talus, including cystic change and sclerosis at the synchondrosis margins and widening of the synchondrosis.[55]

An os trigonum is usually readily identified on MR images, although a small os may be extremely subtle, at times being evident on a single axial or sagittal image. On T1-weighted or proton density-weighted sequences, an os trigonum usually shows fatty marrow signal intensity and corticated margins. Bone marrow edema within the os may occur in active posterior impingement (**Fig. 40**). Sclerosis within the os is less common. Occasionally, pericapsular fat may mimic an os trigonum. Conventional MR imaging can accurately identify disease at the synchondrosis. Signal hyperintensity at the synchondrosis on proton

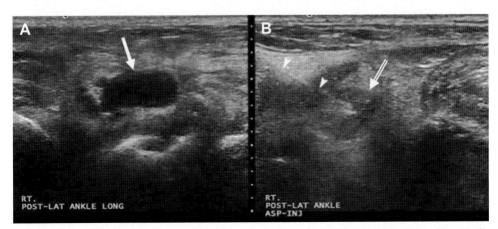

Fig. 43. Posterior ankle ganglion. (*A*) Sagittal ultrasonographic image shows a posterior ankle ganglion cyst (*white arrow*). (*B*) Ultrasound-guided aspiration of the ganglion. The arrowheads indicate the needle. The double-tailed white arrow indicates the collapsed ganglion.

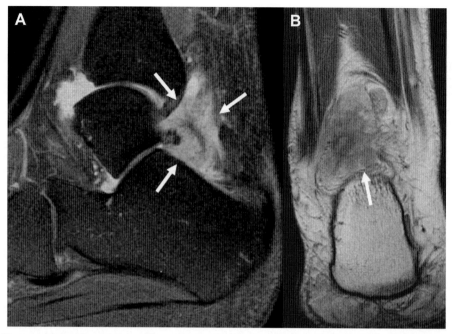

Fig. 44. 25-year-old beach sprinter with posterior impingement symptoms. Sagittal fat-suppressed proton density-weighted (A) and coronal proton density-weighted (B) MR images showing a proliferative synovial mass (*arrows*) in the posterior recesses of the talocrural and subtalar joints,. The patient underwent surgical excision. The histopathologic diagnosis was granulomatous synovitis.

density-weighted or T2-weighted MR images with fat suppression usually indicates a degree of stress across the synchondrosis and is often associated with bone marrow edema at the

synchondrosis margins (see **Fig. 40**). Frank fluid signal at the synchondrosis indicates destabilization. Findings that are likely to be associated with posterior ankle impingement symptoms (but are

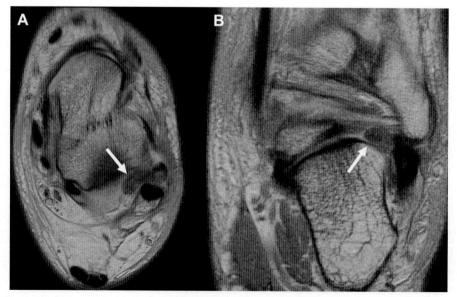

Fig. 45. Elite rugby league player with posterior impingement symptoms caused by a displaced tear of the CFL, with the ligament stump displaced into the posterior recess of the subtalar joint (*solid white arrows*), shown on axial (A) and coronal (B) proton density-weighted MR images.

A B

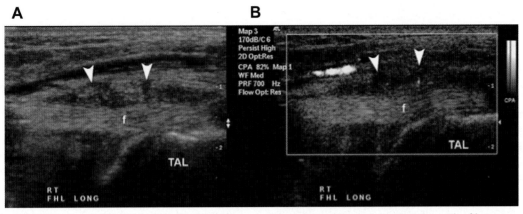

Fig. 46. FHL tenosynovitis. (*A*) Longitudinal ultrasonographic images of the FHL tendon above the fibro-osseous tunnel show hypoechoic tenosynovial thickening (*arrowheads*). Note the fibrillar echotexture of the FHL tendon (f). (*B*) Color Doppler image shows mild hyperemia within the tenosynovial thickening.

not specific) include bone marrow edema at the margins of the synchondrosis, synovitis involving the posterior recesses of the ankle and posterior subtalar joint, and pericapsular edema (see **Fig. 40**). Sclerosis and cystic change at the margins of the synchondrosis indicate chronic stress across the synchondrosis.[1] Bone marrow edema may be seen in a prominent posterolateral talar process in the setting of active posterior impingement.

Sagittal MR images are used to assess the posterolateral process of the talus. The posterolateral process is considered prominent if it extends posterior to the arc of curvature of the talar dome in the sagittal plane (**Fig. 41**).[1] Recent fractures of the posterolateral process show bone marrow edema and linear T1 hypointensity at the fracture line (see **Fig. 41**).

The PTFL should be assessed for myxoid change and ganglion formation. Tears of the PTFL are uncommon. When present, myxoid change shows mild signal hyperintensity and thickening of the PTFL on all pulse sequences. Ganglion cysts manifest as a discrete area of fluid signal intensity on MR sequencing, often decompressing posteriorly (**Fig. 42**). Intraosseous extension into the lateral malleolus or talar body may occasionally be seen. A fluid-distended recess of the ankle or subtalar joint may mimic a posterior ganglion cyst. Ultrasonography can be helpful in differentiating between a ganglion and a fluid-distended recess and can be used to guide aspiration and injection of the ganglion (**Fig. 43**).

The posterior intermalleolar ligament is best assessed on coronal and axial scans with the ankle in a neutral position.[1] Thickening and intermediate signal intensity tissue, with ill-defined margins on proton density-weighted or fat-suppressed proton

density-weighted sequences, and adjacent synovial thickening may be identified in posterior impingement.

Fluid distension of the posterior recesses of the ankle and subtalar joints is nonspecific. Synovial thickening and adjacent edema should also be present in posterior impingement. Administration of intravenous gadolinium may improve detection of localized foci of synovitis.[54] A focal proliferative synovitis in the posterior recess of the ankle or subtalar joint is a less common cause of posterior impingement (**Fig. 44**).

Intra-articular loose bodies are usually small and should be confirmed in 3 planes on MR imaging. Mimics of loose bodies include the deep fibers of the posteroinferior tibiofibular ligament in sagittal cross section, fibrous bands, or pericapsular fat.[1]

A rare cause of posterior impingement is a displaced distal tear of the CFL, with protrusion of the ligament stump into the posterior recess of the posterior subtalar joint (**Fig. 45**).

FHL tendon disease may mimic or accompany posterior impingement symptoms. MR imaging is of limited sensitivity for the diagnosis of FHL

Differential diagnosis
• Os trigonum
• Prominent posterolateral process of the talus
• Posterior intermalleolar ligament disease
• Myxoid change in the PTFL
• Posterior ankle ganglia
• FHL tendon disease
• Synovitis/synovial thickening

What the clinician wants to know

- Presence of an os trigonum: are there features of active posterior impingement?
- Presence of a prominent posterolateral process of the talus: this may predispose to impingement symptoms.
- Is there soft tissue disease that may predispose the patient to impingement symptoms?
- Is there disease that may be amenable to injection therapy?

tendinosis.[1] Fluid distension of the FHL tendon sheath may be present in asymptomatic ankles, and in isolation is not pathologic. An FHL tendon sheath effusion in the absence of an ankle or posterior subtalar joint effusion is more suggestive of FHL tenosynovitis, but is still nonspecific. Ultrasonography can be helpful in differentiating an inert FHL tendon sheath effusion from a tenosynovitis (**Fig. 46**). The ultrasonographic and MR imaging features of FHL tenosynovitis include tenosynovial thickening within the tendon sheath, thickening of the retinaculum for the FHL at the level of the fibro-osseous tunnel, tendon thickening, and intratendinous signal abnormality/echotextural change and edema in the fat plane adjacent to the tendon sheath.[1] Magic angle phenomenon on low echo time (TE) sequences (T1 or proton density) can mimic tendinosis. Enhancement within the tendon sheath may be identified after the administration of intravenous contrast. Ganglionic change within the FHL tendon sheath can also mimic posterior impingement. Internal septation and mass affect on the distal FHL muscle support the diagnosis of a ganglion.

SUMMARY

There are several impingement syndromes within the ankle. In most circumstances, impingement lesions are secondary to posttraumatic synovitis and intra-articular fibrous bands/scar tissue, capsular scarring, or bony prominences. A multimodality approach to imaging patients with impingement symptoms has been outlined, commencing with appropriate use of plain radiographs, including specific views for anteromedial, anterior, and posterior impingement. Cross-sectional imaging most commonly consists of MR imaging, if it is readily available. MR imaging is able to characterize the soft tissue and bony diseases that may predispose to impingement and can show features that may suggest a degree of active impingement at the time of the MR

imaging. Ultrasonography can be helpful in the diagnosis of impingement syndromes and provides image guidance for concurrent corticosteroid injection. CT can be helpful in characterizing bony disease in patients with osseous impingement.

REFERENCES

1. Linklater J. MR imaging of ankle impingement lesions. Magn Reson Imaging Clin North Am 2009; 17:775–800.
2. De Berardino TM, Arciero RA, Taylor DC. Arthroscopic treatment of soft-tissue impingement of the ankle in athletes. Arthroscopy 1997;13(4):492–8.
3. Guhl JF. Soft tissue (synovial) pathology. In: Ankle arthroscopy: pathology and surgical techniques. 2nd edition. Thorofare (NJ): Slack; 1993. p. 93–135.
4. Brostrom L, Sundelin P. Histologic changes in recent and "chronic" ligament ruptures. Acta Chir Scand 1966;132(3):248–53.
5. Meislin RJ, Rose DJ, Parisien JS, et al. Arthroscopic treatment of synovial impingement of the ankle. Am J Sports Med 1993;21(2):186–9.
6. Wolin I, Glassman F, Sideman S, et al. Internal derangement of the talo-fibular component of the ankle. Surg Gynecol Obstet 1950;91:193–200.
7. Lahm A, Erggelet C, Steinwachs M, et al. Arthroscopic management of osteochondral lesions of the talus: results of drilling and usefulness of magnetic resonance imaging before and after treatment. Arthroscopy 2000;16(3):299–304.
8. Bassett F, Gates H, Billys J, et al. Talar impingement by the anteroinferior tibiofibular ligament. J Bone Joint Surg Am 1990;72:55–9.
9. Akseki D, Pinar H, Yaldiz K, et al. The anterior inferior tibiofibular ligament and talar impingement: a cadaveric study. Knee Surg Sports Traumatol Arthrosc 2002;10:321–6.
10. Golano P, Vega J, Pérez-Carro L, et al. Ankle anatomy for the arthroscopist. Part II: role of the ankle ligaments in soft tissue impingement. Foot Ankle Clin 2006;11:275–96.
11. Lindenfeld TN, Wojtys EM, Husain A. Operative treatment of arthrofibrosis of the knee. J Bone Joint Surg Am 1999;81(12):1772–84.
12. Enneking WF, Horowitz M. The intra-articular effects of immobilization on the human knee. J Bone Joint Surg Am 1972;54(5):973–85.
13. Noyes FR, Barber-Westin SD. Reconstruction of the anterior and posterior cruciate ligaments after knee dislocation: use of early protected postoperative motion to decrease arthrofibrosis. Am J Sports Med 1997;25(6):769–78.
14. Van Dijk CN, Tol JL, Verheyen CC. A prospective study of prognostic factors concerning the outcome

of arthroscopic surgery for anterior ankle impingement. Am J Sports Med 1997;25:737–45.

15. Tol JL, Verheyen CP, van Dijk CN. Arthroscopic treatment of anterior impingement in the ankle. J Bone Joint Surg Br 2001;83:9–13.

16. O'Donoghue DH. Impingement exostoses of the talus and tibia. J Bone Joint Surg Am 1957;39:835–52.

17. Hawkins RB. Arthroscopic treatment of sports-related anterior osteophytes in the ankle. Foot Ankle 1988;9:87–90.

18. Liu SH, Nuccion SL, Finerman G. Diagnosis of anterolateral ankle impingement. Comparison between magnetic resonance imaging and clinical examination. Am J Sports Med 1997;25(3):389–93.

19. Molloy S, Solan MC, Bendall SP. Synovial impingement in the ankle: a new physical sign. J Bone Joint Surg Br 2003;85:330–3.

20. Liu SH, Raskin A, Osti L, et al. Arthroscopic treatment of anterolateral ankle impingement. Arthroscopy 1994;10:215–8.

21. Umans H. Ankle impingement syndromes. Semin Musculoskelet Radiol 2002;6:133–9.

22. Robinson P. Impingement syndromes of the ankle. Eur Radiol 2007;17:3056–65.

23. Ferkel RD, Karzel RP, Del Pizzo W, et al. Arthroscopic treatment of anterolateral impingement of the ankle. Am J Sports Med 1991;19(5):440–6.

24. Rubin DA, Tishkoff NW, Britton CA, et al. Anterolateral soft-tissue impingement in the ankle: diagnosis using MR imaging. AJR Am J Roentgenol 1997; 169(3):829–35.

25. Bagnolesi P, Carafoli D, Ortori S, et al. Anterolateral fibrous impingement of the ankle: discrepancy between MRI findings and arthroscopy (Ab). Eur Radiol 1998;8:1295.

26. Haller J, Bernt R, Seeger T, et al. MR-imaging of anterior tibiotalar impingement syndrome: agreement, sensitivity and specificity of MR-imaging and indirect MR-arthrography. Eur J Radiol 2006;58:450–60.

27. Robinson P, White LM, Salonen DC, et al. Anterolateral ankle impingement: MR arthrographic assessment of the anterolateral recess. Radiology 2001; 221(1):186–90.

28. Cochet H, Pelé E, Amoretti N, et al. Anterolateral ankle impingement: diagnostic performance of MDCT arthrography and sonography. AJR Am J Roentgenol 2010;194:1575–80.

29. McCarthy CL, Wilson DJ, Coltman TP. Anterolateral ankle impingement: findings and diagnostic accuracy with ultrasound imaging. Skeletal Radiol 2008; 37:209–16.

30. Linklater JM, Fessa CK. Imaging findings in arthrofibrosis of the ankle and foot. Semin Musculoskelet Radiol 2012;16:185–91.

31. Cerezal L, Abascal F, Canga A, et al. MR imaging of ankle impingement syndromes. AJR Am J Roentgenol 2003;181:551–9.

32. O'Kane JW, Kadel N. Anterior impingement syndrome in dancers. Curr Rev Musculoskelet Med 2008;1:12–6.

33. Datir A, Connell D. Imaging of impingement lesions in the ankle. Tech Foot Ankle Surg 2008;7(3):152–61.

34. Cheng JC, Ferkel RD. The role of arthroscopy in ankle and subtalar degenerative joint disease. Clin Orthop 1998;349:65–72.

35. Massada JL. Ankle overuse injuries in soccer players: morphological adaptation of the talus in the anterior impingement. J Sports Med Phys Fitness 1991;31(3):447–51.

36. Tol JL, Verheyen CP, van Dijk CN. Arthroscopic treatment of anterior impingement in the ankle: a prospective study with a five- to eight-year follow-up. J Bone Joint Surg Br 2001;83:9–13.

37. Donovan A, Rosenberg ZS. MRI of ankle and lateral hindfoot impingement syndromes. AJR Am J Roentgenol 2010;195:595–604.

38. Egol KA, Parisien JS. Impingement syndrome of the ankle caused by a medial meniscoid lesion. Arthroscopy 1997;13:522–5.

39. Mosier-La Clair SM, Monroe MT, Manoli A. Medial impingement syndrome of the anterior tibiotalar fascicle of the deltoid ligament on the talus. Foot Ankle Int 2000;21:385–91.

40. Robinson P, White LM, Salonen D, et al. Anteromedial impingement of the ankle: MR arthrography assessment of the anteromedial recess. AJR Am J Roentgenol 2002;178:601–4.

41. Tol JL, van Dijk CN. Etiology of the anterior ankle impingement syndrome: a descriptive anatomical study. Foot Ankle Int 2004;25:382–6.

42. van Dijk CN, Wessel RN, Tol JL, et al. Oblique radiograph for the detection of bone spurs in anterior ankle impingement. Skeletal Radiol 2002;31:214–21.

43. van Dijk CN. Anterior and posterior ankle impingement. Foot Ankle Clin 2006;11:663–83.

44. Paterson RS, Brown JN. The posteromedial impingement lesion of the ankle. A series of six cases. Am J Sports Med 2001;29(5):550–7.

45. Messiou C, Robinson P, O'Connor PJ, et al. Subacute posteromedial impingement of the ankle in athletes: MR imaging evaluation and ultrasound-guided therapy. Skeletal Radiol 2006;35:88–94.

46. Liu SH, Mirzayan R. Postero-medial impingement. Arthroscopy 1993;9(6):709–11.

47. Koulouris G, Connell D, Schneider T, et al. Posterior tibiotalar ligament injury resulting in the posteromedial impingement. Foot Ankle Int 2003;24:575–83.

48. De Asla R, O'Malley M, Hamilton WG. Flexor hallucis tendonitis and posterior ankle impingement in the athlete. Tech Foot Ankle Surg 2002;1(2):123–30.

49. Howse AJG. Posterior block of the ankle joint in dancers. Foot Ankle 1982;3:81–3.

50. Brodsky AE, Khalil MA. Talar compression syndrome. Am J Sports Med 1986;14:472–6.

51. McDougall A. The os trigonum. J Bone Joint Surg Br 1955;37:257–65.

52. Quirk R. Common foot and ankle injuries in dance. Orthop Clin North Am 1994;25:123–33.

53. Bureau NJ, Cardinal E, Hobden R, et al. Posterior ankle impingement syndrome: MR imaging findings in seven patients. Radiology 2000;215:497–503.

54. Robinson P, White LM. Soft-tissue and osseous impingement syndromes of the ankle: role of imaging in diagnosis and management. Radiographics 2002; 22:1457–71.

55. Karasick D, Schweitzer ME. The os trigonum syndrome: imaging features. AJR Am J Roentgenol 1996;166:125–9.

56. Rosenberg ZS, Cheung YY, Beltran J, et al. Posterior intermalleolar ligament of the ankle: normal anatomy and MR imaging features. AJR Am J Roentgenol 1995;165:387–90.

57. van Dijk CN, Lim LS, Poortman A, et al. Degenerative joint disease in female ballet dancers. Am J Sports Med 1995;23:295–300.

58. Sarrafian SH. Anatomy of the ankle: descriptive, topographic and functional. Philadelphia: JB Lippincott; 1993.

59. Hamilton WG, Geppert MJ, Thompson FM. Pain in the posterior aspect of the ankle in dancers. Differential diagnosis and operative treatment. J Bone Joint Surg Am 1996;78(10):1491–500.

60. Hamilton WG. Stenosing tenosynovitis of the flexor hallucis longus tendon and posterior impingement upon the os trigonum in ballet dancers. Foot Ankle 1982;3(2):74–80.

61. Na JB, Bergman AG, Oloff LM, et al. The flexor hallucis longus: tenographic technique and correlation of imaging findings with surgery in 39 ankles. Radiology 2005;236(3):974–82.

62. Linklater JM, Anderson IF, Read JW. The ankle and foot. In: Atlas of imaging in sports medicine. 2nd edition. Sydney (Australia): McGraw-Hill; 2008. p. 540.

63. Mouhsine E, Crevoisier X, Leyvraz PF, et al. Post-traumatic overload or acute syndrome of the os trigonum: a possible cause of posterior ankle impingement. Knee Surg Sports Traumatol Arthrosc 2004;12:250–3.

64. Jaffee NW, Gilula LA, Wissman RD, et al. Diagnostic and therapeutic ankle tenography: outcomes and complications. AJR Am J Roentgenol 2001;176: 365–71.

65. Karasick D, Schweitzer ME. Tear of the posterior tibial tendon causing asymmetric flatfoot: radiologic findings. AJR Am J Roentgenol 1993;161:1237–40.

Overuse Injuries of the Lower Extremity

Howard R. Galloway, BM, BS, FRANZCR

KEYWORDS

- Stress fracture • Stress injury • Chronic compartment syndrome • Tendinopathy • Grading system

KEY POINTS

- The clinical and imaging findings of overuse injuries reflect a pathologic condition that is more often dominated by an incomplete or maladaptive repair process rather than the findings of acute injury.
- Although imaging can accurately depict different stages and severity of bone stress injury, there is an inconsistent relationship between imaging and clinical severity. Imaging findings may persist following complete clinical resolution. In the developing skeleton, increased stress may lead to abnormalities in ossification in the physis, resulting in avulsion or chronic nonunion particularly around the pelvis.
- Chronic compartment syndromes may demonstrate increased T2 signal intensity in the affected compartment on exercise. However, there is no clear consensus on either imaging or pressure criteria for diagnosis; the clinical picture remains the most important diagnostic factor.
- Tendon volume and vascularity on ultrasound and high signal intensity on magnetic resonance imaging correlate with the clinical severity on presentation but do not predict clinical outcome at 12 months.
- Image-guided injection therapies are an important and generally safe adjunct to the treatment of tendinopathy; but the relative effectiveness on various injectates, including growth factor-containing preparations, is yet to be determined.

INTRODUCTION

Overuse injuries have been an important part of sports medicine practice for many years. However, they are increasingly recognized in not only the physically active general population but also in groups whose underlying conditions mean that their musculoskeletal systems are unable to cope with the normal daily activities. The clinical and imaging findings of overuse injuries reflect the pathologic condition that is more often dominated by an incomplete or maladaptive repair process rather than the findings of acute injury. It is, therefore, useful to consider and review the process of injury and repair in the major musculoskeletal tissues.

This article reviews the underlying imaging and pathologic correlates of overuse injuries and deals specifically with osseous stress injuries, friction syndromes, compartment syndromes, and tendinopathy. Image-guided injections play an important part in therapy, particularly for tendinopathy, whereby the emphasis is now on healing of the underlying pathologic condition rather than pain relief alone. The current status of image-guided injection therapy for tendinopathy is also reviewed.

OSSEOUS STRESS INJURIES

Osseous stress injuries occur when the normal adaptive response of bone resorption and new bone formation is unable to keep pace with increased loading. The histology of acute bone stress injury follows a predictable pattern. During the first week of increased activity, there is osteoclastic resorption of the cortex but no decalcification, microfracture, microcallus, or osteocyte death. Callus formation begins in the second

12 Roe Street, Griffith ACT 2603, Australia
E-mail address: galloway.howard@gmail.com

Radiol Clin N Am 51 (2013) 511–528
http://dx.doi.org/10.1016/j.rcl.2012.11.007

week. If activity ceases, a fracture does not occur; but if activity persists, then a cortical crack appears near the end of the second week. Bone resorption is maximal at the end of the third week, and callus is maximal by 6 weeks. In clinical practice, the findings may represent a mix of these features, reflecting recurrent episodes of injury and partial recovery.

Magnetic resonance (MR) imaging demonstrates a spectrum of findings in osseous stress injury, reflecting the underlying histology. These findings range from the presence of the bone marrow edema pattern in response to increased bone stress from focal striations or resorption cavities within the cortex through the presence of localized periosteal or endosteal high T2 signal to a frank fracture line and/or periosteal reaction.

In 2005, Gaeta and colleagues[1] examined the computed tomography (CT) and MR imaging findings in athletes with tibial stress injuries and compared these with bone scintigraphy. In their study, 63 patients with clinically suspected tibial stress injury, verified by clinical consensus among 3 sports physicians, and supported by pressure measurements and ultrasound when appropriate, were examined within 1 month of symptom onset. In the earliest phases, imaging demonstrated the presence of resorption cavities and localized osteopenia; there was often uptake of radionuclide in the opposite tibia on bone scan. The CT and MR imaging findings reflected the histologic findings of bone resorption, with multiple parallel striations in the anterior tibial cortex and small resorption cavities in the posterior cortex (**Figs. 1** and **2**). In their series, bone scintigraphy failed to detect 8 cortical stress injuries seen with MR, CT, or both. Their findings are summarized in **Table 1**.

Imaging is able to reflect the earliest stages of bony response to stress, and it is important to appreciate this to not overinterpret findings that represent the normal adaptive response of bone to increased activity. Schweitzer and White[2] have elegantly demonstrated the presence of increased bone marrow edema with a change in biomechanics.

Stress fractures in the lower limb may occur at any site, usually along the weight-bearing axis. However, the exact site differs with the age of the patient, the nature of the activity, the individual biomechanics of the patient, and any underlying condition affecting the health of the bone (**Fig. 3**). Clinically, some stress fractures in the lower limb have been regarded as critical because of a high rate of nonunion. These fractures include the anterior tibia, medial malleolus, talus, navicular, fifth metatarsal, and sesamoid bones. In contrast, stress fractures in the medial tibia, fibula, and second, third, or fourth metatarsals are regarded

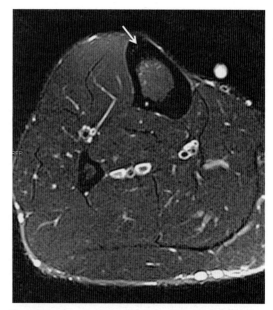

Fig. 1. Axial T2 fat-saturated MR image demonstrating an early stress fracture of the tibia, demonstrating multiple striations and early resorption cavities in the anterior cortex (*arrow*).

as noncritical; the treatment of the stress fractures usually involves only relative rest.

Stress fracture locations that are more common in an older population, or in individuals with absolute or relative osteoporosis, include subcortical

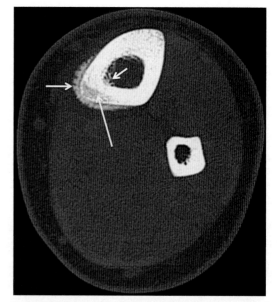

Fig. 2. Axial CT scan of an established posteromedial stress fracture demonstrating a cortical resorption cavity (*arrow*) with prominent overlying periosteal and endosteal reaction (*short arrows*).

Table 1
CT and MR imaging criteria of tibial stress injuries after Gaeta and colleagues

Type of Lesion	CT Finding	MR Imaging Finding
Fracture	Hypoattenuating line	Low-signal-intensity line in all sequences
Cortical abnormality		
Osteopenia	Increased hypoattenuation	Loss of cortical signal void
Resorption cavity	Round or oval intracortical hypoattenuation	Round or oval intracortical area of increased signal intensity
Striation	Subtle intracortical linear hypoattenuation	Subtle intracortical linear hyperintensity
Bone marrow edema	Increased attenuation of yellow marrow	Increased bone marrow signal intensity on T2-weighted images and decreased bone marrow signal intensity on T1-weighted images
Periosteal edema	Soft tissue mass adjacent to periosteal surface of bone	Hyperintensity along periosteal surface on T2-weighted images, and tissue with low to intermediate signal intensity along periosteal surface on T1-weighted images

Data from Gaeta M, Minutoli F, Scribano E, et al. CT and MR imaging findings in athletes with early tibial stress injuries: comparison with bone scintigraphy findings and emphasis on cortical abnormalities. Radiology 2005;235:553–61.

insufficiency fractures of the femoral head (**Fig. 4**)[3]; subcortical insufficiency fractures of the femoral condyle (previously thought to represent spontaneous osteonecrosis of the knee)[4]; insufficiency fractures of the proximal tibia, particularly the medial tibial plateau; linear stress fractures of the tibial shaft[5]; and stress fractures of the calcaneal tuberosity (**Fig. 5**).

Given the importance of stress injury in high-level sport, there has been considerable ongoing interest in the ability of imaging to accurately and reliably determine injury severity and estimate time to healing. Beck and colleagues[6] examined the comparative performance of radiographic, nuclear

medicine bone scanning, MR imaging, and CT severity grades against the clinical severity and time to healing in tibial stress injuries. They found that intra-assessor reliability was high to very high for bone scintigraphy, CT, and nuclear medicine. The severity grades from one imaging modality were not consistently or strongly related to grades from another imaging modality. They also found no significant relationship between time to healing and severity score for any imaging modality, although a positive trend existed for MR imaging. **Table 2** summarizes the imaging findings. Interestingly, the relationship between clinical severity and time to healing was negative, as was the relationship

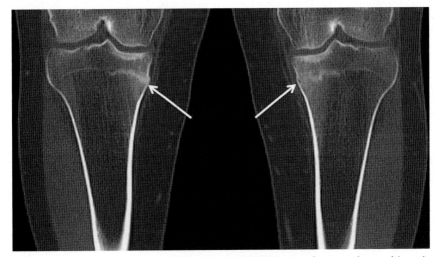

Fig. 3. Coronal CT reformations demonstrating bilateral medial tibial stress fractures (*arrows*) in a vitamin D–deficient, but otherwise normal, patient who had recently commenced an exercise program.

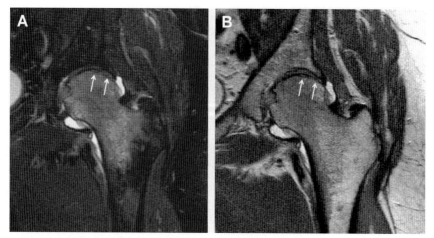

Fig. 4. Coronal (*A*) T2 fat-saturated and (*B*) proton density–weighted MR images of the left hip in a 57-year-old patient with a subtle low signal intensity line (*arrows*) paralleling the articular surface, compatible with a subchondral insufficiency fracture (*arrows*). Extensive bone marrow edema is seen in the femoral head and neck. (*Courtesy of* Kathryn Stevens, MD.)

between clinical severity and imaging severity. They suggest that pain is an unreliable marker of healing and suggest that follow-up MR imaging at symptom resolution may have some role in guiding recommendations for the return to training, although this is yet to be established. The author has seen several patients with persistent imaging findings of anterior tibial and navicular stress fractures who have not only become asymptomatic but have returned to Olympic competition (**Figs. 6** and **7**).

Imaging Grading Systems

Attempts have been made over many years to produce clinically meaningful grading systems for stress injury and these are well summarized in Beck and colleagues' article (see **Table 2**).[6]

Kijowski and colleagues[7] have recently attempted to validate the Fredericson classification and suggested an abbreviated classification that may be more clinically relevant. This proposed classification is summarized in **Table 3**.

Medial Tibial Stress Syndrome

Medial tibial stress syndrome (MTSS), or shin splints, may be described as a clinical entity characterized by diffuse tenderness over the posteromedial aspect of the distal third of the tibia. Shin splints have been reported to account for 12% to 18% of running injuries, and women seem more frequently affected than men. All aspects of this syndrome have been the subject of a comprehensive review by Moen and colleagues.[8] The clinical challenge is often to differentiate medial tibial stress syndrome from stress fracture or exertional compartment syndrome. Histologic studies[8] have failed to provide evidence that MTSS is caused

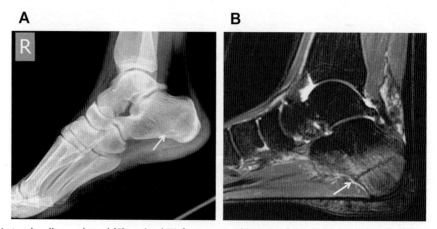

Fig. 5. (*A*) Lateral radiograph and (*B*) sagittal T2 fat-saturated image of the right foot in a runner demonstrating a typical stress fracture of the calcaneal tuberosity (*arrows*). (*Courtesy of* Kathryn Stevens, MD.)

Table 2
Tibial stress injury grading criteria after Beck and colleagues

Grade	Radiography[1]	Bone Scintigraphy[2]	MR Imaging[3]	CT Scanning[4]
0	No abnormality	No abnormality	No abnormality	No abnormality
I	Gray cortex sign: margin is indistinct and of decreased density	Linear increased activity in cortical region	Mild to moderate periosteal edema on T2-weighted images only, with no focal bone marrow abnormality	Soft tissue mass adjacent to periosteal surface
II	Acute periosteal reaction, and density differs from rest of cortex showing incomplete mineralization	Small focal area of increased activity	Periosteal edema and bone marrow edema seen only T2-weighted images only	Increased attenuation of yellow marrow
III	Lucent areas in cortex, ill-defined foci at site of pain	Larger focal lesions with markedly increased activity in the cortical region	Bone marrow edema on T1- and T2- weighted images, with or without periosteal edema on T1- or T2- weighted images, and loss of cortical signal void, intracortical increased intensity and intracortical linear hyperintensity	Increased hypoattenuation (osteopenia), intracortical hypoattenuation (resorption cavity), and subtle intracortical linear hypoattenuation (striation)
IV	Fracture line present	Very large focal region of highly increased activity	Low-signal-intensity fracture line with all sequences, moderate to severe periosteal edema on T1- and T2- weighted images, bone marrow edema on both T1- and T2-weighted images, may also show severe periosteal edema and moderate muscle edema	Hypoattenuating line

Data from Beck BR, Bergman AG, Miner M, et al. Tibial stress injury: relationship of radiographic, nuclear medicine bone scanning, MR imaging, and CT severity grades to clinical severity and time to healing. Radiology 2012;263(3):811–18.

by traction injury to the periosteum but have shown the same response as seen in stress fracture with cortical resorption exceeding new bone formation in response to stress. Radiographs and CT are negative in MTSS. Scintigraphy will demonstrate characteristic diffuse linear increased activity along the periosteum, which is distinct from the more focal cortical uptake seen in stress fractures. MR imaging shows a linear abnormality with a high signal along the posteromedial border of the tibia (**Fig. 8**). In the series of Aoki and colleagues,[9] this signal diminished in 5 out of

14 patients with continuing exercise, presumably reflecting adaptation to the increased loading. However, some patients with MTSS will go on to develop frank stress fractures (**Fig. 9**).

Epiphyseal and Apophyseal Stress Injury

In addition to stress injury of the cancellous and cortical bone, the epiphyses and apophyses are also subject to stress injury in the developing skeleton. The zone of apoptosis and reduced cartilage hydration at the tidemark is the weakest portion of

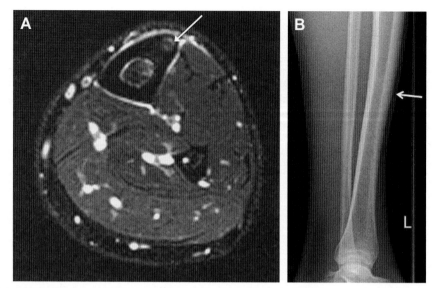

Fig. 6. (A) Axial T2 fat-saturated MR image demonstrating an anterior tibial cortex stress fracture with a focal anterior cortex resorption cavity (*arrow*) and associated periosteal and bone marrow edema. (B) Lateral radiograph of the same patient at 12 months with persistent cortical lucency (*arrow*). The patient was asymptomatic and had returned to Olympic competition.

the bone and is vulnerable to separation. Lysis of the apophysis results from disruption of metaphyseal perfusion and impaired chondrocyte ossification in the zone of provisional calcification. The physis widens as chondrocytes accumulate but cannot calcify. During the rapid phase of growth, these changes may lead to avulsion or chronic nonunion at the apophysis.[10] The most clinically relevant sites are around the pelvis at the anterior inferior iliac spine at the origin of the rectus femoris

(Fig. 10), the common hamstring origin at the ischial tuberosity (Fig. 11), and the pubic apophysis.

Osteitis Pubis

The presence of bone marrow edema at the pubic symphysis on MR imaging has been described as part of the spectrum of imaging findings associated with athletic pubalgia. Verrall and colleagues[11] showed that this pattern histologically represented

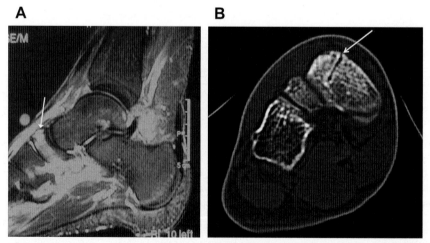

Fig. 7. (A) Sagittal T2 fat-saturated MR image of a middle-distance runner who presented with bilateral midfoot pain and marked bone marrow edema in the tarsal navicular bones bilaterally. Note that the edema is most intense in the dorsal aspect of the navicular (*arrow*). (B) Coronal CT scan of a middle-distance runner (different patient than in Fig. 7A) 12 months after presentation who was asymptomatic and had returned to competition demonstrating a fibrous nonunion of a navicular stress fracture (*arrow*).

Table 3	
Revised Fredericson classification proposed by Kijowski and colleagues	
Grade	Imaging Findings
0	No abnormality
1	Periosteal edema with no associated bone marrow signal abnormalities
2	(Fredericson grades 2, 3, and 4a) Periosteal edema and bone marrow edema visible on T1 and T2 images with or without multiple areas of intracortical signal abnormality.
3	(Fredricson grade 4b) Linear intracortical signal abnormality and bone marrow edema on both T1 and T2 images

Data from Kijowski R, Choi J, Shinki K, et al. Validation of MRI classification system for tibial stress injuries. Am J Roentgenol 2012;198(4):878–84.

a maladaptive healing pattern with a predominance of woven bone. Lovell and colleagues[12] performed a longitudinal study of soccer players and showed that bone marrow edema was a marker of increased stress at the pubic symphysis and was a predictor of clinical injury, although the major risk factor was the increase in training load (**Fig. 12**).

FRICTION SYNDROMES

Numerous factors and mechanical forces play a substantial role in adapting connective tissue at any given site. Connective tissue is capable of

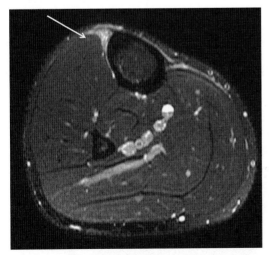

Fig. 8. Axial T2 fat-saturated MR image demonstrating prominent anterolateral periosteal high signal (*arrow*) in a patient with recent onset of anterior pain following an increased training load.

metaplasia from loose connective tissue through bursa formation and cartilaginous or osseous metaplasia, and the forces placed on it regulate connective tissue differentiation. When loose connective tissue is placed under compression, it is typical for signs of inflammation and metaplasia to develop. The most well-known friction syndrome in the lower limb is the iliotibial band friction syndrome on the lateral aspect of the distal femur. Histologically, the iliotibial band contacts the lateral femoral epicondyle and the proximal fibers of the lateral collateral ligament; with suboptimal biomechanics, a friction syndrome can develop at the site. A study by Muhle and colleagues[13] demonstrated that there is only a thin layer of fibrofatty connective tissue between the iliotibial band and the lateral femoral epicondyle in normal individuals, with no evidence of a bursa.[13] In patients with iliotibial band friction syndrome, ill-defined edema is seen between the iliotibial band and lateral femoral condyle (**Fig. 13**); in some cases, an adventitial bursa may develop. Histologic examination of tissue taken from this site shows macroscopic inflammation over and around the lateral femoral epicondyle, with synovial-like fibrous tissue and cystlike areas of mucoid degeneration and fibrinoid necrosis.[14]

A similar process can occur at other sites around the knee, including the insertion of the pes anserine tendons and the medial collateral ligament. The presence of an adventitial bursa as a result of a friction syndrome should be considered when patients present with localized high signal intensity on MR imaging in the subcutaneous or sometimes deeper tissues overlying a possible friction point. On ultrasound, this is seen as hypoechoic clefts within the fat and loose connective tissue (**Fig. 14**). The diagnosis can often be established by correlation with the patient's specific history.

CHRONIC EXERTIONAL COMPARTMENT SYNDROME

Chronic exertional compartment syndrome (CECS) of the lower limb is a group of overuse lower limb injuries with common presenting features, including pain on activity.

CECS is defined as reversible ischemia occurring when a noncompliant osteofascial compartment is unable to respond to the expansion of muscle volume that occurs with exercise.[15] The pathophysiology of the condition is poorly understood, and the criteria used to make the diagnosis have yet to be standardized. In the lower leg, CECS is most commonly seen in the anterior compartment but may also be present in the lateral

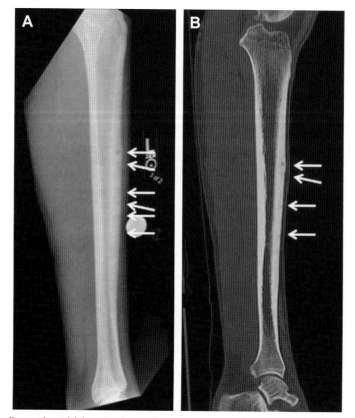

Fig. 9. (A) Lateral radiograph and (B) sagittal CT reformat in a long-distance runner with long-standing anterior shin pain demonstrates multiple lucent lines (dreaded black lines) through the anterior cortex of the midtibia (arrows), corresponding to incomplete stress fractures. (Courtesy of Kathryn Stevens, MD.)

or posterior compartments. In addition, compartment syndromes can present in unusual locations, such the foot and the medial compartment of the thigh.[16] It is conventionally diagnosed by the invasive measurement of raised intramuscular pressures in the compartments of the lower limb. Aweld and colleagues[17] reviewed the relevant published evidence on diagnostic criteria commonly in use for CECS. They found that there was no currently agreed test protocol, that current

pressure criteria for diagnosis are unreliable, and that the emphasis on diagnosis should remain on clinical history. They suggest that intracompartmental pressure measurements are best taken at 1 minute after exercise because the mean pressures at this time interval only did not overlap between patients and controls in the studies that were analyzed. Intracompartmental pressure measurements more than the highest reported value for controls (27.5 mm Hg), along with

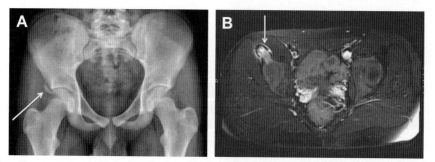

Fig. 10. (A) Anteroposterior radiograph and (B) axial T2 fat-saturated axial MR image demonstrating an acute avulsion injury of the anterior inferior iliac spine (arrow) in an adolescent athlete.

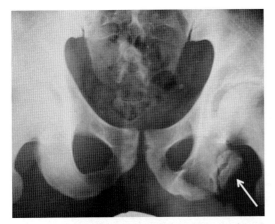

Fig. 11. Pelvic radiograph demonstrating a chronic avulsion injury at the hamstring tendon origin on the ischial tuberosity (*arrow*) in an older patient with minimal symptoms.

a good history, were regarded as highly suggestive of CECS.

A recent review by Roberts and Miller[15] also concluded that with the exception of relaxation pressure, the current criteria for diagnosing CECS, considered to be the gold standard, overlapped the range found in normal healthy subjects. This lack of certainty over the clinical and pressure criteria for diagnosis makes evaluation by noninvasive imaging methods more attractive.

The major role of imaging in the investigation of patients with suspected CECS is to exclude other causes of symptoms, such as stress fractures, stress reaction, periostitis, claudication, popliteal artery entrapment, ganglia, and peripheral nerve entrapment.

Nevertheless, considerable interest has been shown in noninvasive imaging methods for the

diagnosis of compartment syndrome; however, these do not yet have a firmly established place in the diagnosis. Diagnostic criteria for MR have included increased signal intensity on T2-weighted images in the involved compartment. However, increased signal may be seen in asymptomatic compartments after normal exercise. Proposed criteria have included a failure of the signal intensity within the compartment to return to normal within 25 minutes of exercise[16,17] and, more recently, increased signal intensity in the affected compartment (usually the anterior) compared with the unaffected compartment. George and Hutchinson[18] showed a statistically significant increase in T2 signal intensity within the affected anterior compartment during exercise in patients with a chronic compartment syndrome compared with both the unaffected superficial posterior compartment and the anterior compartment of normal controls. This effect disappeared after fasciotomy. Recently, Ringler and colleagues[19] have described an MR imaging methodology for the diagnosis of CECS, based on quantitative T2 estimates validated against compartmental pressure measurements, using a diagnostic T2-weighted intensity threshold of 1.54. They showed a sensitivity and specificity of 87% and 62%, respectively, relative to intracompartmental pressure measurements. In the subset of 36 patients who also had intramuscular pressure measurements, 23 patients met the clinical criteria for CECS; only 19 patients met both intramuscular pressure measurements and clinical criteria for CECS.

Other modalities, including methoxyisobutylisonitrile (MIBI) scanning,[20] near infrared spectroscopy,[21] and MR imaging blood-oxygen-level-dependent (BOLD) imaging,[22] have shown promise but have not yet been validated for routine clinical use.

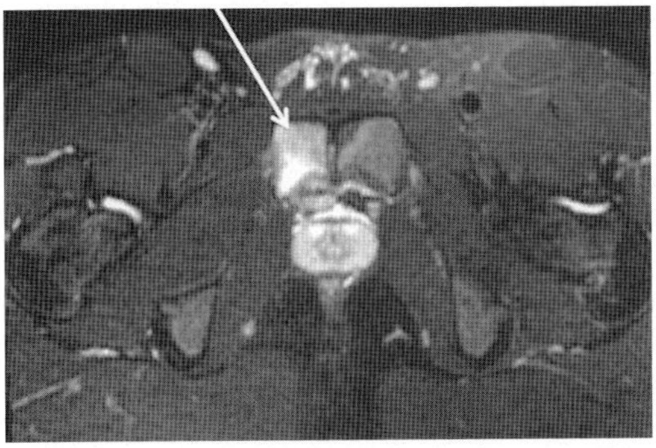

TENDINOPATHY

Chronic tendon injuries, particularly of the patellar and Achilles tendons, are a common and important source of morbidity in athletes of all levels. They are often associated with performance-limiting disability in elite athletes. Knowledge of the normal anatomy and histology of the tendon is important in understanding the pathophysiology and imaging characteristics of these disorders. The tendon is comprised of fibrils, fibers, subfascicles, fascicles, and tertiary fiber bundles. This structure is supported by the epitenon and surrounded by the loose areolar connective tissues, forming the paratenon. There are specialized adaptations of the tendon at the myotendinous and osteotendinous junctions. Histologically, basic elements of the

Fig. 12. Axial T2 fat-saturated MR image demonstrating unilateral bone marrow edema in the pubic bone (*arrow*) on the right in a soccer player who was asymptomatic at the time but who developed groin pain subsequently with increased training load.

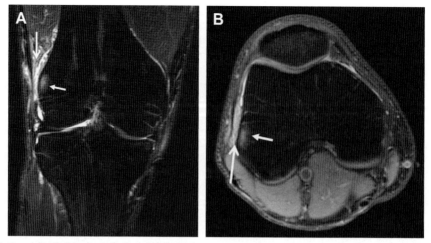

Fig. 13. (*A*) Coronal T2 fat-saturated and (*B*) axial proton fat-saturated MR images in a 24-year-old woman training for a marathon demonstrates focal high T2 signal (*arrow*) deep to a mildly thickened iliotibial band. Focal bone marrow edema is also seen within the adjacent lateral femoral condyle (*short arrow*). (*Courtesy of Kathryn Stevens, MD.*)

tendon are the helical tropocollagen bundles, the supporting tenocytes, and the associated ground substance.

Normal Imaging Appearances of Tendons

The normal imaging appearance of tendons reflects this anatomic organization. On ultrasound, there are dense, clearly defined, parallel, and slightly wavy collagen bundles (see **Fig. 14**). Little cellular material is seen, and there is an absence of ground substance between the collagen bundles. Small arteries are noted parallel to the collagen fibers in the end tendon. On ultrasound, it is important to be aware of the effect of anisotropy, which may mimic changes of tendinopathy (**Fig. 15**). The strongest echoes on ultrasound are found when the reflecting surfaces are perpendicular to the beam.

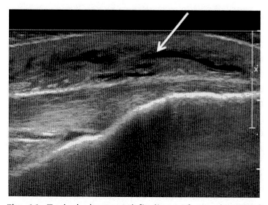

Fig. 14. Typical ultrasound findings of an adventitial bursa secondary to friction with hypoechoic clefts in the fat and loose connective tissue (*arrow*), in this case in the prepatellar region.

As the reflecting surfaces in the tendon curve away from the beam, there is an associated loss of returned echoes and an apparent hypoechoic area in the tendon. This artifact can be minimized by careful positioning of the transducer and, more recently, by the use of beam steering or compound imaging.

On MR imaging, normal tendons are usually dark on all imaging sequences (**Fig. 16**). However, it is important to be aware of the magic angle effect on T1 and proton density (PD) images. The normal Achilles tendon has a normal fascicle on T1-weighted images. This normal fascicle is seen as a single line in the substance of the tendon and relates to the blending of the 2 major bundles of the Achilles tendon (see **Fig. 16**).

Pathology and Pathogenesis

The pathogenesis of tendinopathy has been well reviewed by Fu and colleagues[23] and is best thought of as a failed healing process. Imaging of tendinopathy reflects the underlying histopathology of mucoid degeneration, with thinning of collagen fibers, and mucoid pouches and vacuoles between the fibers. Neovascularization is a prominent feature of tendinopathy (**Fig. 17**). Mucoid degeneration, fibrosis, and vascular proliferation occur in the paratenon, with only a mild inflammatory infiltrate (**Fig. 18**). Current theories in the pathogenesis of tendinosis place emphasis on metaplasia or stress shielding caused by compression. Compression is thought to explain the occurrence of tendinosis in the midsubstance of the Achilles tendon and at the distal insertion. The occurrence of tendinosis in

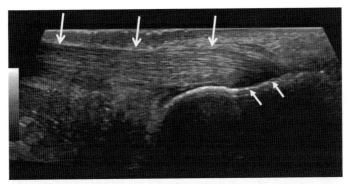

Fig. 15. Longitudinal ultrasound image of normal Achilles tendon demonstrating parallel echogenic fibers (*arrows*). Anisotropy is seen in the insertional fibers, which are no longer perpendicular to the ultrasound beam (*small arrows*). (*Courtesy of* Kathryn Stevens, MD.)

the deep one-third of the patellar tendon at its insertion is thought to be caused by stress shielding.[23,24]

Terminology and Classification

Following proposals by Maffuli and colleagues[25] in 1998, the term *tendinopathy* has been generally used for overuse injuries of tendons without tendon sheaths, such as the patella and Achilles tendons. In 2011, van Dijk and colleagues[26] proposed a classification taking account of

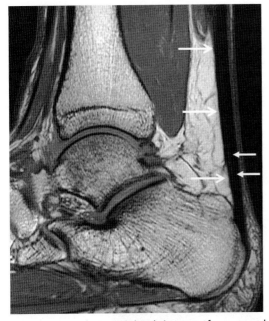

Fig. 16. Sagittal T1-weighted image of a normal Achilles tendon demonstrating a low-signal-intensity band of uniform thickness (*arrows*). A thin linear area of slightly higher signal intensity is seen within the tendon (*small arrows*), corresponding to a normal fascicle where the 2 major bundles of the Achilles merge.

anatomic location, signs and symptoms, clinical findings, and histopathology in the Achilles tendon, which provides a guide for the evaluation of tendons elsewhere. Their classification is summarized in **Table 4** and the imaging correlates in **Table 5**.

Clinical Correlates of Tendon Imaging

Tendinopathy is a common and clinically important condition. There has been a lot of interest in the correlation of imaging findings with symptoms and in the predictive value of imaging. It has generally been thought that the size of the tendon and the degree of increased vascularity are the most closely correlated with the clinical findings. The extent of the vascularity is generally assessed by using the Victorian Institute of Sport Assessment (VISA) scoring system, which measures the length of the abnormal vessels and has been validated for use in both the patellar and Achilles tendons.[27,28] Khan and colleagues[29] showed that the total volume of hypoechogenicity on ultrasound and/ or high signal intensity on MR imaging correlated with the severity of tendinopathy at presentation and the Victorian Institute of Sport Assessment Achilles (VISA-A) score. However, baseline ultrasound with power and color Doppler did not predict the outcome at 12 months. MR imaging and ultrasound showed only a moderate correlation with the clinical assessment of chronic Achilles tendinopathy. There is an overlap between abnormal signal on MR imaging in symptomatic and asymptomatic cases, and imaging abnormalities tend to persist following the resolution of symptoms. Although abnormal vessels seen on power Doppler are broadly related to the size of the tendon, they are not always symptomatic. Particularly in young athletes, neovascularization is seen in normal volume asymptomatic tendons, presumably related to increased but

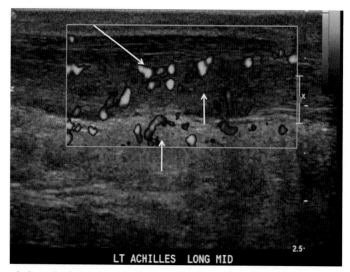

LT ACHILLES LONG MID

Fig. 17. Thickening and altered echo texture in the mid substance of the Achilles (*arrow*), with typical dorsal and intrasubstance neovascularization in an acutely symptomatic runner (*short arrows*).

adapted mechanical load. Exercise has been shown to result in increased vessel length in abnormal patellar tendons.[30]

Image-Guided Treatment of Tendinopathy

The common factor in symptomatic tendinopathy is a painful abnormal healing response. Treatments should ideally interrupt this and result in a more normal, painless healing of the tendon. Image guidance, particularly ultrasound, has proved to be a practical and effective way of delivery injection therapy, enabling precise placement of the injectate and monitoring of response to therapy, particularly the presence of abnormal vascularity (**Fig. 19**).[31]

Conservative treatment measures, such as rest, ice, and nonsteroidal antiinflammatories, have substantial failure rates in the treatment of patellar and Achilles tendinopathy.[32] Further measures, such as heavy load eccentric exercise,[33] topical nitrous oxide,[34] prolotherapy[35] and injection therapy with dry needling,[36] corticosteroids,[37] sclerosants,[38–40] autologous blood,[41] platelet-rich plasma (PRP),[42] matrix metalloproteinase (MMP) inhibitor aprotinin,[43] and hyaluronate,[44] have been individually investigated and have been the subject of evidence-based reviews.[45–47]

Current management strategies for chronic Achilles tendinopathy have advanced substantially during the past decade, and efforts now focus on comprehensive treatment algorithms aimed at restoring function and normalizing structure as well as reducing pain. One such algorithm proposed by Alfredson and Cooke[48] commences with 6 to 12 weeks of heavy-load eccentric training, then suggests training modifications and treatment alternatives (topical glycerol trinitrate, extracorporeal

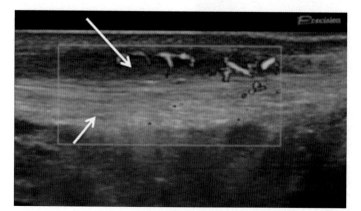

Fig. 18. Longitudinal ultrasound image of the Achilles tendon of an acutely symptomatic athlete demonstrating marked vascularity in the hypoechoic, thickened paratenon (*arrow*). The Achilles tendon itself seems relatively normal (*short arrow*).

Table 4
Terminology for Achilles tendon–related disorders, including the anatomic location, symptoms, clinical findings, and histopathology after Van Dijk

Term	Anatomic Location	Symptoms	Clinical Findings	Histopathology
Midportion Achilles tendinopathy	2–7 cm from the insertion into the calcaneus	A combination of pain, swelling, and impaired performance	Diffuse or localized swelling	Includes but is not limited to the histopathologically diagnosis of tendinosis: implies histopathologic diagnosis of tendon degeneration without clinical or histologic signs of intratendinous inflammation, not necessarily symptomatic
Paratendinopathy				
Acute	Around the midportion Achilles tendon	Edema and hyperemia	Palpable crepitations and swelling	Edema and hyperemia of paratenon with infiltration of inflammatory cells, possibly with production of a fibrinous exudate that fills the spaces between the tendon sheath and tendon
Chronic	Around the midportion Achilles tendon	Exercise-induced pain	Crepitations and swelling less pronounced	Paratenon thickened as a result of fibrinous exudate; prominent and widespread proliferation of myofibroblasts; formation of new connective tissue; and adhesions between tendon, paratenon, and crural fascia
Insertional Achilles tendinopathy	Insertion of Achilles tendon onto calcaneus, most often with formation of bone spurs and calcifications in tendon at insertion site	Pain, stiffness, sometimes swelling	Painful tendon insertion at the midportion of the posterior aspect of the calcaneus	Ossification of entheseal fibrocartilage and sometimes small tendon tears at the tendon-bone interface
Retrocalcaneal bursitis	Bursa in the retrocalcaneal recess	Painful swelling superior to calcaneus	Painful swelling medial and lateral to the Achilles tendon at the level of the posterosuperior calcaneus	Fibrocartilaginous bursal walls show degeneration and or calcification with synovial hypertrophy and bursal fluid
Superficial calcaneal bursitis	Bursa between calcaneal prominence or Achilles tendon and skin	Visible, painful, solid swelling posterolateral calcaneus	Visible, painful, solid swelling and discoloration of skin	Acquired adventitial bursa developing in response to friction

Data from van Dijk CN, Van Sterkenburg MN, Wiegerinck JI, et al. Terminology for Achilles tendon related disorders. Knee Surg Sports Traumatol Arthrosc 2011;19:835–41.

Table 5
Imaging findings in Achilles tendon disorders after Van Dijk

Term/Imaging	Plain Radiography	Ultrasound	CT	MR Imaging
Midportion Achilles tendinopathy	Deviation of soft tissue contours is usually present; in rare cases, calcifications can be found	Tendon larger than normal in both cross-sectional area and anteroposterior diameter; hypoechoic areas within the tendon, disruption of fibrillar pattern, increase in tendon vascularity (echo-Doppler) mainly in ventral peritendinous area	In case (massive) calcification is seen on plain radiography; CT imaging can be helpful in preoperative planning, showing the exact size and location of the calcifications	Fat-saturated T1- or T2-weighted images; fusiform expansion, central enhancement consistent with intratendinous neovascularization
Paratendinopathy				
Acute		A normal Achilles tendon with circumferential hypoechogenic halo		Peripheral enhancement on fat-saturated T1- or on T2-weighted images
Chronic		A thickened hypoechoic paratenon with poorly defined borders may show as a sign of peritendinous adhesions; increase in tendon vascularity (echo-Doppler) mainly in ventral peritendinous area		
Insertional Achilles tendinopathy	May show ossification or a bone spur at the tendon's insertion; possibly a deviation of soft tissue contours	Calcaneal bony abnormalities	Bone formation at insertion; CT scan indicated mainly for preoperative planning; shows the exact location and size of the calcifications and spurs	Bone formation and/or high T2 signal at tendon insertion
Retrocalcaneal bursitis	Posterosuperior calcaneal prominence can be identified; increased density of the retrocalcaneal recess; possible deviation of soft tissue contours	Fluid in retrocalcaneal area/bursa (hyperechoic)		Hyperintense signal in retrocalcaneal recess on T2-weighted images
Superficial calcaneal bursitis	Possible deviation in soft tissue contours	Fluid between skin and Achilles tendon		Hyperintense signal between Achilles tendon and subcutaneous tissues on T2-weighted images

Data from van Dijk CN, Van Sterkenburg MN, Wiegerinck JI, et al. Terminology for Achilles tendon related disorders. Knee Surg Sports Traumatol Arthrosc 2011;19:835–41.

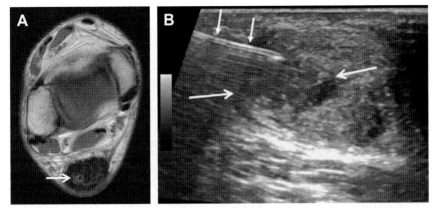

Fig. 19. (A) Axial proton density–weighted image of a patient with severe tendinopathy of the Achilles tendon. The Achilles tendon is markedly thickened, with areas of high T2 signal intensity (arrow). (B) Transverse ultrasound image demonstrates an echogenic needle (small arrows) positioned in corresponding areas of hypoechogenicity within the tendon before the injection of platelet-rich plasma. (Courtesy of Dr Kathryn Stevens, MD.)

shock wave therapy, corticosteroid or other injection) in those who do not initially respond to the training protocol. The question of the optimal injection therapy remains unresolved. The types of injection therapy may, however, be divided into several general classes.

Injection Technique and Dry Needling

The injection technique is often not specified in articles but may be peritendinous, direct single injection into the tendon or multiple injections through the tendon (fenestration). Needling of the tendon has been shown experimentally to increase blood flow and oxygenation[36] and may well have a substantial healing effect independent of the injectate. The dry needling technique may be a useful alternative when injectates are otherwise contraindicated.

Corticosteroids

Corticosteroids in combination with long-acting local anesthetic injections are the most commonly used in routine practice. In systematic reviews, these have been shown to be effective for short- to medium-term pain relief.[45] The perceived risk of tendon rupture injection means that most clinicians will not directly inject tendons with corticosteroid.[49] Experimental studies do show weakening of tendons from both intratendinous and retrocalcaneal bursal injections.[50] Although injection-associated tendon rupture is reported,[51] it seems to be uncommon; a small series has demonstrated the safety of image-guided peritendinous injection.[52] Tendon rupture has also been associated with systemic steroid use and fluoroquinolone antibiotic therapy.[53]

Sclerosants

Alfredssohn and Ohberg[54] demonstrated neurovascular ingrowth in painful tendons and a reduction in pain with sclerosis of the neovessels in both the patellar and Achilles tendons.[38,39] Polidocanol and dextrose have been used and seems generally safe and successful in reducing the neovascularization and pain,[55] although tendon rupture has been reported following multiple sclerosant injections.[56]

Growth Factors

Recent research has begun to elucidate the role of growth factors in tendon healing, and there is much interest in their use as therapeutic agents. Autologous blood was used initially, and more recently platelet-enriched plasma has emerged as a treatment option; both have become popular adjuncts to therapy. Their use in elite sport has prompted reviews sponsored by the International Olympic Committee into the molecular basis of connective tissue and muscle injuries in sport[57] and the use of PRP in sports medicine,[58] providing comprehensive reviews of the theoretical and practical aspects. The use of PRP is relatively expensive; despite numerous small trials with favorable results, randomized trials have not yet proven the benefit of PRP.[59,60]

High-Volume Tendon Injection

High-volume injections of 10 mL of 0.5% bupivacaine hydrochloride, 25 mg of hydrocortisone acetate, and 40 mL of 0.9% sodium chloride saline solution have been performed under ultrasound guidance at the interface between the Achilles tendon and paratenon and the interface between the deep aspect of the patellar tendon and

Hoffa's fat pad in an effort to disrupt the neovascularity. These injections have shown promising results in patients resistant to other conservative measures.[61,62] However, the role of this technique in management has yet to be determined, and adequately controlled randomized trials have yet to be published.

Achilles Insertional Tendinopathy

The subgroup of patients with insertional Achilles tendinopathy is more difficult to manage and respond less well to the treatment algorithm for midsubstance tendinopathy. A systematic review concluded that conservative methods should be used before loading and shock wave therapy, although there is limited evidence by which to judge their effectiveness.[47] Preliminary studies whereby injection of sclerosants and disruption of neovascularity showed a favorable response have not been followed with randomized studies; therefore, the role of sclerosant injection in insertional tendinopathy remains unclear.[63]

Image-guided injection therapy for tendinopathy has an important role; it is hoped that over the next few years, important issues regarding the optimization of therapy will be clarified with high-quality randomized trials that control for measures such as injection technique and use optimized conservative treatment in the control groups.

In conclusion, overuse syndromes occur when increased and persistent load exceeds the tissues ability to adapt, which results in a consistent and predictable pattern of pathologic change in bone, loose connective tissue, and tendon that is reflected in the imaging appearances. However, there is a variable correlation between the imaging appearances and patient signs and symptoms. Although the imaging appearances can be graded, their ability to reliably predict prognosis is not yet established; imaging remains only one part of a comprehensive clinical workup. Image-guided injection therapy for tendinopathy is an important and rapidly progressing area; although these therapies seem safe, their overall and relative effectiveness remains to be established.

REFERENCES

1. Gaeta M, Minutoli F, Scribano E, et al. CT and MR imaging findings in athletes with early tibial stress injuries: comparison with bone scintigraphy findings and emphasis on cortical abnormalities. Radiology 2005;235:553–61.
2. Schweitzer ME, White L. Does altered biomechanics cause marrow edema? Radiology 1996;198:851–3.
3. Legroux Gerot I, Demondion X, Louville AB, et al. Subchondral fractures of the femoral head: a review of seven cases. Joint Bone Spine 2004;71(2):131–5.
4. Yao L, Stanczak J, Boutin RD. Presumptive subarticular stress reactions of the knee: MRI detection and association with meniscal tear patterns. Skeletal Radiol 2004;33(5):260–4.
5. Craig JG, Widman D, van Holsbeeck M. Longitudinal stress fracture: patterns of edema and the importance of the nutrient foramen. Skeletal Radiol 2003;32(1):22–7.
6. Beck BR, Bergman AG, Miner M, et al. Tibial stress injury: relationship of radiographic, nuclear medicine bone scanning, MR imaging, and CT severity grades to clinical severity and time to healing. Radiology 2012;263(3):811–8.
7. Kijowski R, Choi J, Shinki K, et al. Validation of MRI classification system for tibial stress injuries. Am J Roentgenol 2012;198(4):878–84.
8. Moen M, Tol JL, Weir A, et al. Medial tibial stress syndrome: a critical review. Sports Med 2009; 39(7):523–46.
9. Aoki Y, Yasuda K, Tohyama H, et al. Magnetic resonance imaging in stress fractures and shin splints. Clin Orthop Relat Res 2004;421:260–7.
10. Martin TA, Pipkin G. Treatment of avulsion of the ischial tuberosity. Clin Orthop Relat Res 1957;10:108.
11. Verrall GM, Henry L, Fazzalari NL. Bone biopsy of the parasymphyseal pubic bone region in athletes with chronic groin injury demonstrates new woven bone formation consistent with a diagnosis of pubic bone stress injury. Am J Sports Med 2008;36(12):2425–31.
12. Lovell G, Galloway H, Hopkins W, et al. Osteitis pubis and assessment of bone marrow edema at the pubic symphysis with MRI in an elite junior male soccer squad. Clin J Sport Med 2006;16(2): 117–22.
13. Muhle C, Ahn JM, Yeh L, et al. Iliotibial band friction syndrome: MR imaging findings in 16 patients and MR arthrographic study of six cadaveric knees. Radiology 1999;212(1):103–10.
14. Martens M, Libbrecht P, Burssens A. Surgical treatment of the iliotibial band friction syndrome. Am J Sports Med 1989;17(5):651–4.
15. Roberts A, Franklyn-Miller A. The validity of the diagnostic criteria used in chronic exertional compartment syndrome: a systematic review. Scand J Med Sci Sports 2012;22(5):585–95.
16. Amendola A, Rorabeck CH, Vellett D, et al. The use of magnetic resonance imaging in exertional compartment syndromes. Am J Sports Med 1990; 1891:29–34.
17. Aweid O, Del Buono A, Malliaras P, et al. Systematic review and recommendations for intracompartmental pressure monitoring in diagnosing chronic exertional compartment syndrome of the leg. Clin J Sport Med 2012;22(4):356–70.

18. George CA, Hutchinson MR. Chronic exertional compartment syndrome. Clin Sports Med 2012; 31(2):307–12.

19. Ringler MD, Litwiller DV, Felmlee JP, et al. MRI accurately detects chronic exertional compartment syndrome: a validation study. Skeletal Radiol 2012. [Epub ahead of print].

20. Owens S, Edwards P, Miles K, et al. Chronic compartment syndrome affecting the lower limb: MIBI perfusion imaging as an alternative to pressure monitoring: two case reports. Br J Sports Med 1999; 33(1):49–51.

21. Van den Brand JG, Nelson T, Verleisdonk EJ, et al. The diagnostic value of intracompartmental pressure measurement, magnetic resonance imaging, and near-infrared spectroscopy in chronic exertional compartment syndrome: a prospective study in 50 patients. Am J Sports Med 2005;33(5): 699–704.

22. Noseworthy MD, Davis AD, Elzibak AH. Advanced MR imaging technique for skeletal muscle evaluation. Semin Musculoskelet Radiol 2010;14(2):257–67.

23. Fu SC, Rolf C, Cheuk YC, et al. Deciphering the pathogenesis of tendinopathy: a three-stages process. Sports Med Arthrosc Rehabil Ther Technol 2010;2:30.

24. Almekinders LC, Weinhold PS, Maffulli N. Compression etiology in tendinopathy. Clin Sports Med 2003; 22(4):703–10.

25. Maffulli N, Khan KM, Puddu G. Overuse tendon conditions: time to change a confusing terminology. Arthroscopy 1998;14(8):840–3.

26. van Dijk CN, Van Sterkenburg MN, Wiegerinck JI, et al. Terminology for Achilles tendon related disorders. Knee Surg Sports Traumatol Arthrosc 2011; 19:835–41.

27. Visentini PJ, Khan KM, Cook JL, et al. The VISA score: an index of severity of symptoms in patients with jumper's knee (patellar tendinosis). Victorian Institute of Sport Tendon Study Group. J Sci Med Sport 1998;1(1):22–8.

28. Robinson JM, Cook JL, Purdam C, et al. The VISA-A questionnaire: a valid and reliable index of the clinical severity of Achilles tendinopathy. Victorian Institute Of Sport Tendon Study Group. Br J Sports Med 2001;35(5):335–41.

29. Khan KM, Forster BB, Robinson J, et al. Are ultrasound and magnetic resonance imaging of value in the assessment of Achilles tendon disorders? A two year prospective study. Br J Sports Med 2003; 37:149–53.

30. Richards PJ, McCall IW, Day C, et al. Longitudinal microvascularity in Achilles tendinopathy (power Doppler ultrasound, magnetic resonance imaging time–intensity curves and the Victorian Institute of Sport Assessment–Achilles questionnaire): a pilot study. Skeletal Radiol 2010;39:509–21.

31. Fredberg U, Bolvig L, Pfeiffer-Jensen M, et al. Ultrasonography as a tool for diagnosis, guidance of local steroid injection and, together with pressure algometry, monitoring of the treatment of athletes with chronic jumper's knee and Achilles tendinitis: a randomized, double-blind, placebo-controlled study. Scand J Rheumatol 2004;33(2):94–101.

32. Maffulli N, Sharma P, Luscombe KL. Achilles tendinopathy: aetiology and management. J R Soc Med 2004;97(10):472–6.

33. Fahlström M, Jonsson P, Lorentzon R, et al. Chronic Achilles tendon pain treated with eccentric calf-muscle training. Knee Surg Sports Traumatol Arthrosc 2003;11(5):327–33.

34. Bokhari AR, Murrell GA. The role of nitric oxide in tendon healing. J Shoulder Elbow Surg 2012;21(2): 238–44.

35. Yelland MJ, Sweeting KR, Lyftogt JA, et al. Prolotherapy injections and eccentric loading exercises for painful Achilles tendinosis: a randomised trial. Br J Sports Med 2011;45(5):421–8.

36. Kubo K, Yajima H, Takayama M, et al. Effects of acupuncture and heating on blood volume and oxygen saturation of human Achilles tendon in vivo. Eur J Appl Physiol 2010;109(3):545–50.

37. Shrier I, Matheson GO, Kohl HW 3rd. Achilles tendonitis: are corticosteroid injections useful or harmful? Clin J Sport Med 1996;6(4):245–50.

38. Alfredson H, Öhberg L. Sclerosing injections to areas of neo-vascularisation reduce pain in chronic Achilles tendinopathy: a double-blind randomised controlled trial. Knee Surg Sports Traumatol Arthrosc 2005;13(4):338–44.

39. Alfredson H, Öhberg L. Neovascularisation in chronic painful patellar tendinosis – promising results after sclerosing neovessels outside the tendon challenge the need for surgery. Knee Surg Sports Traumatol Arthrosc 2005;13(2):74–80.

40. Maxwell NJ, Ryan MB, Taunton JE, et al. Sonographically guided intratendinous injection of hyperosmolar dextrose to treat chronic tendinosis of the Achilles tendon: a pilot study. Am J Roentgenol 2007;189(4):W215–20.

41. Rabago D, Best TM, Zgierska AE, et al. A systematic review of four injection therapies for lateral epicondylosis: prolotherapy, polidocanol, whole blood and platelet rich plasma. Br J Sports Med 2009; 43(7):471–81.

42. Owens RF Jr, Ginnetti J, Conti SF, et al. Clinical and magnetic resonance imaging outcomes following platelet rich plasma injection for chronic midsubstance Achilles tendinopathy. Foot Ankle Int 2011; 32(11):1032–9.

43. Orchard J, Massey A, Brown R, et al. Successful management of tendinopathy with injections of the MMP-inhibitor aprotinin. Clin Orthop Relat Res 2008;466(7):1625–32.

44. Oryan A, Moshiri A, Meimandi Parizi AH, et al. Repeated administration of exogenous sodium-hyaluronate improved tendon healing in an in vivo transection model. J Tissue Viability 2012; 21(3):88–102.

45. Coombes BK, Bisset L, Vicenzino B. Efficacy and safety of corticosteroid injections and other injections for management of tendinopathy: a systematic review of randomised controlled trials. Lancet 2010; 376:1751–67.

46. van Ark M, Zwerver J, van den Akker-Scheek I. Injection treatments for patellar tendinopathy. Br J Sports Med 2011;45(13):1068–76.

47. Kearney R, Costa ML. Insertional Achilles tendinopathy management: a systematic review. Foot Ankle Int 2010;31(8):689–94.

48. Alfredson H, Cook JL. A treatment algorithm for managing Achilles tendinopathy: new treatment options. Br J Sports Med 2007;41(4):211–6.

49. Johnson JE, Klein SE, Putnam RM. Corticosteroid injections in the treatment of foot & ankle disorders: an AOFAS survey. Foot Ankle Int 2011; 32(4):394–9.

50. Hugate R, Pennypacker J, Saunders M, et al. The effects of intratendinous and retrocalcaneal intrabursal injections of corticosteroid on the biomechanical properties of rabbit Achilles tendons. J Bone Joint Surg Am 2004;86(4):794–801.

51. Csizy M, Hintermann B. Rupture of the Achilles tendon after local steroid injection. Case reports and consequences for treatment. Swiss Surg 2001; 7(4):184–9 [in German].

52. Gill SS, Gelbke MK, Mattson SL. Fluoroscopically guided low-volume peritendinous corticosteroid injection for Achilles tendinopathy. A safety study. J Bone Joint Surg Am 2004;86(4):802–6.

53. Blanco I, Krähenbühl S, Schlienger RG. Corticosteroid-associated tendinopathies: an analysis of the published literature and spontaneous pharmacovigilance data. Drug Saf 2005;28(7):633–43.

54. Alfredson H, Öhberg L, Forsgren S. Is vasculo-neural ingrowth the cause of pain in chronic Achilles tendinosis? An investigation using ultrasonography and colour Doppler, immunohistochemistry, and diagnostic injections. Knee Surg Sports Traumatol Arthrosc 2003;11(5):334–8.

55. Hart L. Corticosteroid and other injections in the management of tendinopathies: a review. Clin J Sport Med 2011;21(6):540–1.

56. Hamilton B, Remedios D, Loosemore M, et al. Achilles tendon rupture in an elite athlete following multiple injection therapies. J Sci Med Sport 2008; 11(6):566–8.

57. Ljungqvist A, Schwellnus MP, Bachl N, et al. International Olympic Committee consensus statement: molecular basis of connective tissue and muscle injuries in sport. Clin Sports Med 2008;27:231–9.

58. Engebretsen L, Steffen K, Alsousou J, et al. IOC consensus paper on the use of platelet-rich plasma in sports medicine. Br J Sports Med 2010;44:1072–81.

59. Mishra A, Woodall J Jr, Vieira A. Treatment of tendon and muscle using platelet-rich plasma. Clin Sports Med 2009;28(1):113–25.

60. de Vos RJ, van Veldhoven PL, Moen MH, et al. Autologous growth factor injections in chronic tendinopathy: a systematic review. Br Med Bull 2010; 95:63–77.

61. Humphrey J, Chan O, Crisp T, et al. The short-term effects of high volume image guided injections in resistant non-insertional Achilles tendinopathy. J Sci Med Sport 2010;13(3):295–8.

62. Crisp T, Khan F, Padhiar N, et al. High volume ultrasound guided injections at the interface between the patellar tendon and Hoffa's body are effective in chronic patellar tendinopathy: a pilot study. Disabil Rehabil 2008;30(20–22):1625–34.

63. Ohberg L, Alfredson H. Sclerosing therapy in chronic Achilles tendon insertional pain-results of a pilot study. Knee Surg Sports Traumatol Arthrosc 2003;11(5):339–43.

Application of Advanced Magnetic Resonance Imaging Techniques in Evaluation of the Lower Extremity

Hillary J. Braun, BA[a,b], Jason L. Dragoo, MD[b],
Brian A. Hargreaves, PhD[a,c], Marc E. Levenston, PhD[d],
Garry E. Gold, MD, MSEE[a,b,c],*

KEYWORDS

- Magnetic resonance imaging • Lower extremity • Cartilage • Joints

KEY POINTS

- Magnetic resonance imaging (MR imaging) is the most promising modality for evaluation of the lower extremity, particularly the hip, knee, and ankle joints.
- The structural composition of musculoskeletal tissues such as ligaments, cartilage, or muscle is variable. Tissue-specific MR imaging techniques are therefore crucial for optimal visualization and assessment of these structures.
- The most recent advancements in MR imaging of the lower extremity include imaging with higher magnetic field strengths and a greater number of receiver channels, imaging using T2*, and imaging around metal.

INTRODUCTION

Imaging of the lower extremity provides important information about musculoskeletal tissues in both the healthy and disease states. The hip, knee, and ankle joints are frequently subjected to both acute traumatic injuries and chronic debilitating diseases such as rheumatoid arthritis or osteoarthritis (OA). The identification and evaluation of these structures is crucial for treating patients with musculoskeletal pathology; in the United States alone, more than 27 million Americans are affected by OA. Arthroscopy is regarded as the gold standard for joint assessment, permitting direct visualization of intra-articular structures. However, arthroscopy is invasive and requires a surgical procedure; therefore, it is typically reserved for confirmation of the cross-sectional imaging diagnosis and treatment of the underlying pathology. Imaging of a joint may also be performed following arthroscopy if symptoms fail to improve or recur.

MAGNETIC RESONANCE IMAGING

Magnetic resonance imaging (MR imaging) is perhaps the most promising imaging modality for evaluation of the lower extremity, as it provides

Conflicts of Interest: Drs Gold and Hargreaves receive research support from GE Healthcare. Dr Gold also serves as a consultant for Zimmer, Arthrocare, and Isto Inc and receives funding support from the Arthritis Foundation, NIH EB002524, and NIH K24 AR062068. Dr Dragoo receives funding from Genzyme, Linvatec, Ossur, and Smith & Nephew.
[a] Department of Radiology, Stanford University, 1201 Welch Road P271, Stanford, CA 94305, USA;
[b] Department of Orthopaedic Surgery, Stanford University, CA 94305, USA; [c] Department of Bioengineering, Stanford University, CA 94305, USA; [d] Department of Mechanical Engineering and (by courtesy) Bioengineering, Stanford University, CA 94305, USA
* Corresponding author. Department of Radiology, Stanford University, 1201 Welch Road P271, Stanford, CA 94305.
E-mail address: gold@stanford.edu

radiologic.theclinics.com

detailed anatomic visualization of the joint, but is noninvasive and does not require the use of radiation. Therefore, this article focuses on advanced MR imaging techniques used to evaluate the lower extremity, particularly with regard to imaging of joints. Many studies have documented the strong correlation between arthroscopy and MR imaging of the knee,[1] hip,[2,3] and ankle (**Fig. 1**). These studies encourage the use of MR imaging as a noninvasive means of assessing the musculoskeletal system.

Conventional MR Imaging

Common MR imaging methods include 2-dimensional (2D) or multislice T1-weighted, proton density (PD), and T2-weighted imaging.[4] Spin echo (SE) and fast-spin echo (FSE) imaging techniques are useful in the evaluation of focal cartilage defects. Recent improvements in hardware, software, gradients, and radiofrequency (RF) coils have led to the use of FSE or turbo-spin echo (TSE) imaging, fat saturation, and water excitation[4] to improve tissue contrast.

ADVANCED TISSUE-SPECIFIC MR IMAGING TECHNIQUES

The soft tissues of the lower extremity include bone, tendons, ligaments, articular cartilage, fibrocartilage, and synovium. Each of these tissues can be visualized using MR imaging, but optimal visualization and evaluation requires careful attention to technique.

Bone

Radiography and computed tomography scanning remain the imaging modalities of choice for evaluation of cortical bone. However, MR imaging plays a crucial role in the evaluation of musculoskeletal tumors and bone marrow composition in oncology patients. MR imaging is increasingly being used to detect subtle changes in subchondral bone composition in early OA. Features such as bone marrow edema–like lesions, subchondral cyst–like lesions, and subchondral bone attrition indicate disease progression.[5,6] These types of cancellous bone abnormalities are best visualized on MR imaging using PD-weighted, intermediate-weighted, T2-weighted, or short tau inversion recovery and are seen as hypointense regions on T1-weighted SE images.[7–10]

Qualitative and quantitative MR assessment of cortical bone is now possible using ultrashort echo time (uTE) imaging. A variety of different approaches have been used, including basic uTE sequences with TEs as low as 8 μs, adiabatic inversion recovery prepared uTE sequences, and saturation recovery uTE sequences (**Fig. 2**).[11]

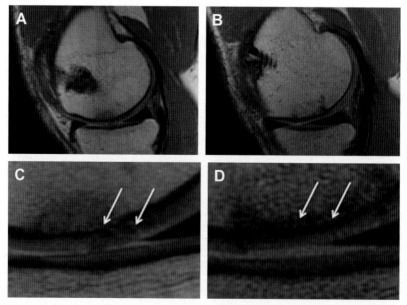

Fig. 1. Arthroscopy remains the gold standard for direct imaging of the joint but has been well correlated with noninvasive MR imaging techniques. This figure depicts a cartilage defect before (*A*) and after (*B*) osteochondral allograft transplant using a sagittal intermediate-weighted PD MR imaging. The femoral articular cartilage is frayed and textured (*arrows*) before the allograft procedure (*C*). Post-operatively, normal and uniform cartilage morphology (*arrows*) is largely restored (*D*).

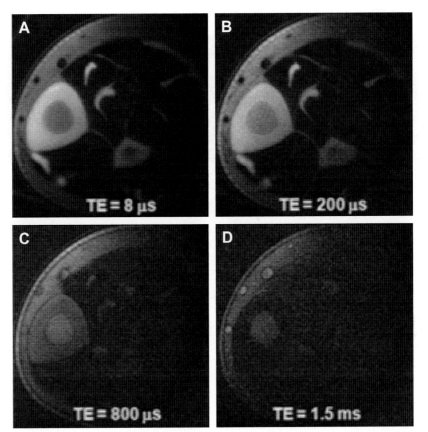

Fig. 2. uTE imaging can enhance visualization of cortical bone. Axial images (*A–D*) depict the middiaphyseal tibia of a 31-year-old healthy volunteer with TE delays of 8 μs, 200 μs, 800 μs, and 1.5 ms. The tibial cortex demonstrates high signal intensity at uTEs of 8 μs and μ 200 us. (*From* Du J, Takahashi AM, Bae WC, et al. Dual inversion recovery, ultrashort echo time (DIR UTE) imaging: creating high contrast for short-T(2) species. Magn Reson Med 2010;63:447–55; with permission.)

Muscle

Muscle is well vascularized and has the ability to repair itself, so it is rarely imaged with the idea of surgical intervention in mind. MR imaging can provide a detailed depiction of skeletal musculature and is useful in the detection of muscle pathology. Muscle typically demonstrates intermediate T1 and T2 relaxation times similar to articular cartilage. Acute muscle strains with edema manifest as high signal on T2-weighted images. Occasionally there may also be corresponding high signal on T1-weighted images, reflecting hemorrhage. Muscle atrophy often occurs in chronic disease and may be seen as decreased muscle bulk or fatty replacement of muscle tissue. T2 mapping[12] and assessment of the apparent diffusion coefficient may also be useful in the evaluation of muscle function and activity (Fig. 3).

Tendons and Ligaments

Tendons connect bone to muscle and facilitate joint motion by transmitting large forces from muscle to bone. Ligaments connect bone to bone, thus guiding joint motion and maintaining stability. Both fibrous tissues are composed of dense, parallel collagen fibers. The ordered collagen structure and the high concentration of both free and bound water in these tissues afford unique imaging properties, particularly with regard to MR imaging.

Because of their highly ordered collagen structures, tendons and ligaments are characterized on MR imaging by short T2 relaxation times. Imaging techniques such as uTE are therefore necessary to shorten the TE and acquire visible signal in tissues of interest. Compared with conventional MR imaging, uTE uses TEs 20 to 50 times shorter in length[13–15] and measures free induction decay as soon as possible after the RF pulse. One approach to uTE uses half-sinc pulses, nonselective pulses, selective pulses, and discrete pulses and acquires readouts in radial or spiral methods.[16] Two-dimensional acquisitions obtain a single slice or multiple slices with in-plane resolutions ranging from 0.5 to

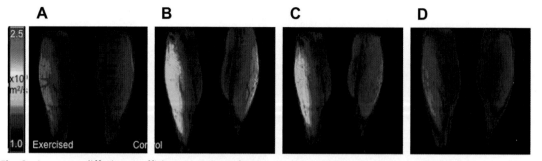

Fig. 3. Apparent diffusion coefficient mapping of gastrocnemius muscle using a quantitative dual echo steady state technique. Coronal images acquired preexercise (A) and immediately post-exercise (B), and at 8 minutes (C), and 16 minutes post-exercise (D) depict a transient increase in muscle diffusion in the exercised calf. (*Courtesy of* Lauren Shapiro, Stanford University School of Medicine.)

0.8 mm; 3D acquisitions obtain isotropic resolutions of 0.28 to 0.9 mm.

In the knee, uTE has permitted evaluation of the anterior cruciate ligament (ACL), posterior cruciate ligament (PCL), lateral collateral ligament, and patellar tendon. In 2009, Rahmer and colleagues[17] described the potential of uTE for assessing tissue grafts in ACL reconstruction. Imaging of graft material and the graft-implant interface was markedly improved in uTE images compared with conventional 3D gradient-recalled echoes (GREs) and T1-weighted TSE images obtained at 1.5 T (Fig. 4). More recently, Qian and colleagues[18] demonstrated the technical feasibility of imaging the human knee using uTE imaging (0.28–0.14 mm) with the acquisition-weighted stack of spirals sequence at 3.0 T. In the ACL and PCL, the ligaments appeared hyperintense, with clinically visible bundles and entheses. Similarly, the patellar tendon showed collagen bundle hyperintensity; however, it was also subject to the magic angle effect resulting from the orientation of the collagen bundles with respect to the main magnetic field.

In the ankle, uTE is frequently used to improve visualization of the Achilles tendon. Du and colleagues[11] used a uTE T1rho sequence and obtained images of the Achilles tendon in healthy subjects at 3.0 T. Compared with the 3D angle-modulated partitioned k-space spoiled gradient echo snapshots sequence, the uTE T1rho scan improved signal and spatial resolution and signal-to-noise ratio (SNR) in the Achilles tendon (Fig. 5). Additional investigations have used a combination of uTE and pointwise encoding time reduction with radial acquisition (PETRA)[19] or magnetization transfer[20] to image the Achilles tendon in vivo.

Fibrocartilage

Knee-menisci

Despite the short T2 relaxation times in the menisci, MR imaging is quite sensitive for meniscal tears, because tears appear of intermediate or high signal against the low-signal background of the meniscus. The sagittal plane is most frequently used to evaluate meniscal pathology, but recent studies have shown that imaging in the coronal[21,22] or axial planes[23,24] may improve diagnosis of specific tear types. A variety of sequences are used for diagnostic imaging, but TEs must remain short to reduce scan time, improve SNR,

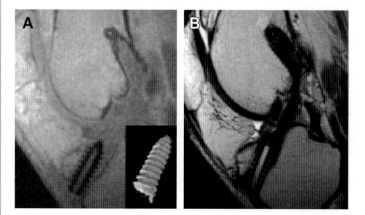

Fig. 4. (A) uTE imaging (TR/TE: 8.6/0.06 msec) improves visualization of the anterior cruciate ligament graft interference screw compared with (B) standard T1-weighted turbo spin echo images (TR/TE: 500/21 ms). (*From* Rahmer J, Bornert P, Dries SP. Assessment of anterior cruciate ligament reconstruction using 3D ultrashort echo-time MR imaging. J Magn Reson Imaging 2009;29(2):443–8; with permission.)

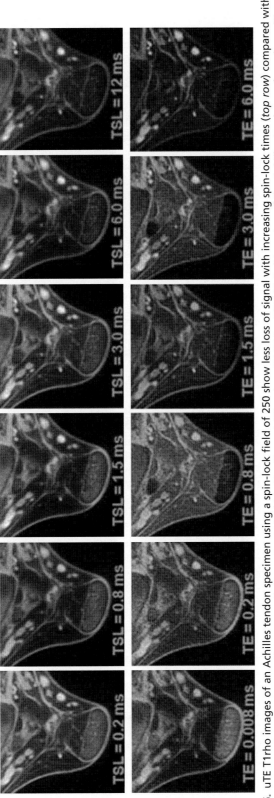
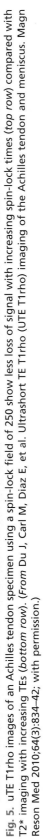

Fig. 5. uTE T1rho images of an Achilles tendon specimen using a spin-lock field of 250 show less loss of signal with increasing spin-lock times (*top row*) compared with T2* imaging with increasing TEs (*bottom row*). (*From* Du J, Carl M, Diaz E, et al. Ultrashort TE T1rho (UTE T1rho) imaging of the Achilles tendon and meniscus. Magn Reson Med 2010;64(3):834–42; with permission.)

acquire more slices per scan, and decrease susceptibility and artifact.[25,26] Commonly used sequences include PD-weighted SE or FSE with or without fat saturation, T1-weighting, and GREs.[25] PD-weighted imaging is ideal for diagnostic imaging of the menisci because it has a short TE and optimizes SNR.[16] The addition of fat saturation to PD sequences is increasingly common in clinical practice.[25,27] In 2005, Blackmon and colleagues[28] reported 93% sensitivity and 97% specificity for diagnosing meniscal tears using a fat-saturated conventional SE PD–weighted sequence.

Recent advancements in MR imaging have improved structural visualization of the intact meniscus. Higher field strengths (1.5 and 3.0 T) improve SNR while maintaining comparable sensitivity and specificity.[21,29,30] Parallel imaging methods use multiple channels to extend the imaging field of view without increasing scan time by exploiting the spatially varying sensitivity profiles of the phased array coil elements. These techniques have been shown to reduce scan time by nearly 50%,[31] while retaining diagnostic sensitivity, specificity, and accuracy.[32] As is the case with tendons and ligaments, uTE imaging has also significantly improved MR imaging of the menisci. In particular, uTE imaging sequences permit identification of different zones within the meniscus.

In addition to structural assessment, quantitative MR imaging techniques such as T2 and T1rho mapping have been recently used to evaluate the physiology of the meniscus. Son and colleagues[33] evaluated the spatial distribution of T2 and T1rho relaxation times and correlated these findings with biochemical, histologic, and biomechanical analyses of cadaveric meniscus specimens. The investigators found that T1rho and T2 relaxation times varied significantly across meniscal regions and that both T1rho and T2 correlated significantly with each other and with the tissue water content.

Hip labrum

Femoroacetabular impingement has been increasingly implicated in the development of early hip OA in young patients.[34–36] Surgical repair or debridement of the labrum can halt these disease processes, but detection of early tissue pathology is essential. Imaging of the acetabular labrum usually consists of MR arthrography using 2D fat-saturated T1-weighted FSE sequences. Noncontrast MR imaging with 2D-FSE and 3D-dimensional spoiled gradient recalled echo imaging with fat suppression (3D-SPGR) sequences and the combination of 3D sequences and arthrography have been used for imaging of the labrum. However, no studies to date have directly compared 3D sequences with arthrography to standard 2D fat-saturated T1-weighted FSE imaging of the labrum.

Articular Cartilage

Knee

The bulk of current literature focuses on the assessment of articular cartilage in the knee. MR imaging provides exquisite contrast and enables morphologic and physiologic imaging of articular cartilage. The most commonly used MR imaging techniques in morphologic imaging of cartilage include SE and GRE sequences, 2D-FSE, and 3D-FSE and GRE. Physiologic imaging techniques such as T_2 mapping, delayed gadolinium–enhanced MR imaging of cartilage (dGEMRIC), T1rho mapping, sodium MR imaging, and diffusion-weighted imaging provide insight into the molecular composition of the tissue.

Knee morphology

Information about tissue structure is acquired using morphologic assessment of cartilage. Many techniques enable imaging of fraying, fissuring, and focal or diffuse cartilage loss. Three-dimensional-SPGR is the current standard for morphologic imaging of cartilage.[37,38] In 3D-SPGR, contrast similar to T1-weighted sequences is obtained by spoiling the transverse steady state with semirandom RF phase alterations. SPGR acquires nearly isotropic voxels, yielding high-resolution images with high cartilage signal and low signal from adjacent joint fluid (Fig. 6). Driven equilibrium Fourier transform (DEFT) is another high-quality imaging technique. Instead of using T1-weighted contrast, DEFT imaging generates contrast by exploiting the T2/T1 ratio of tissues. DEFT returns magnetization to the z-axis with a 90-degree pulse that results in enhanced signal in tissues with long T1 relaxation times. In cartilage imaging, DEFT increases synovial fluid signal and preserves cartilage signal, resulting in bright synovial fluid at a short repetition time, high cartilage SNR, and improved imaging of the full cartilage thickness (Fig. 7).[39] Similarly, 3D dual-echo steady-state (DESS) imaging results in high signal intensity in both cartilage and synovial fluid, which enables morphologic assessment of cartilage. 3D-DESS acquires 2 or more gradient echoes, separates each pair of echoes with a refocusing pulse, and combines image data to obtain higher T2* weighting. 3D-DESS has been validated for clinical use[40,41] and affords advantages such as high SNR, high cartilage-to-fluid contrast, near-isotropic sections, and reduced scan time

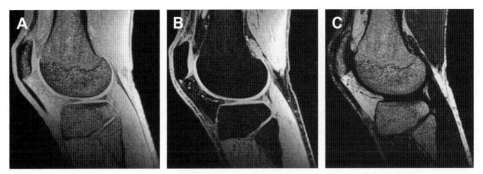

Fig. 6. Sagittal IDEAL-SPGR images obtained from a healthy 36-year-old man. IDEAL-SPGR acquisition can generate combined water-fat (*A*), water-only (*B*), and fat-only (*C*) images. (*From* Siepmann DB, McGovern J, Brittain JH, et al. High-resolution 3D cartilage imaging with IDEAL SPGR at 3 T. AJR Am J Roentgenol 2007;189:1510–5; with permission.)

when compared with 3D-SPGR (Fig. 8). This is the sequence of choice for the Osteoarthritis Initiative.[42]

Another group of methods with synovial fluid-cartilage contrast is steady-state free precession (SSFP) MR imaging techniques. Balanced SSFP (bSSFP) is otherwise known as true fast imaging with steady-state precession (true FISP), fast imaging employing steady-state acquisition (FIESTA), and balanced fast field echo imaging. In all of these techniques, fluid is depicted with increased signal while cartilage signal intensity is preserved, resulting in excellent contrast and diagnostic utility. Several derivatives of SSFP exist. Fluctuating equilibrium MR (FEMR) is used for morphologic assessment of cartilage of the knee.[43] FEMR generates contrast based on the ratio of T1/T2 in tissues. In the knee, FEMR produces bright synovial fluid signal and high signal in cartilage while maintaining high SNR. Another SSFP derivative, vastly undersampled isotropic projection (VIPR) imaging, combines bSSFP imaging with 3D radial k-space acquisition using isotropic spatial resolution and T2/T1 weighted contrast.[44] VIPR reduces banding artifacts, obtains high SNR and tissue contrast, and afford short acquisition times (Fig. 9).[44] Finally, 3D-FSE techniques obtain isotropic images with PD or T2-weighted contrast. 3D-FSE (Cube by GE Health care, VISTA by Philips, and SPACE by Siemens) uses a restore pulse and variable flip angle RF pulses applied along an echo train to produce a pseudo steady state. 3D-FSE has demonstrated improved SNR and better SNR efficiency.[45–47]

Knee cartilage physiology

MR technology has evolved to enable quantitative assessment of articular cartilage physiology. These developments have been useful in identifying early damage and breakdown in conditions such as OA, where proteoglycan and collagen content are reduced.[48] Osteoarthritis disrupts the collagen network and results in increased water

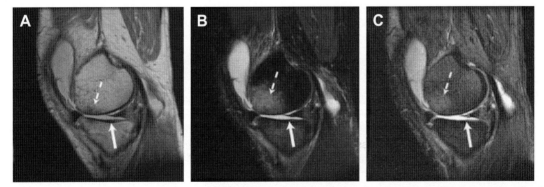

Fig. 7. Sagittal images acquired with PD weighting (*A*), T2 weighting (*B*), and 3D-DEFT (*C*) from the knee of a patient with a full thickness cartilage defect in the medial femoral condyle (*dashed arrow*). The DEFT images (*C*) allow superior visualization of the defect and adjacent tibial cartilage (*solid arrow*). (*From* Gold GE, Fuller SE, Hargreaves BA, et al. Driven equilibrium magnetic resonance imaging of articular cartilage: initial clinical experience. J Magn Reson Imaging 2005;21(4):476–81; with permission.)

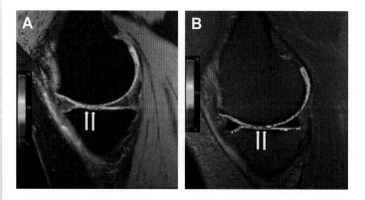

Fig. 8. T2 maps overlaid on quantitative DESS (*A*) and 2D-FSE (*B*) sagittal images of the medial compartment in a patient with OA. Arrows indicate regions of elevated T2 signal. qDESS imaging affords higher resolution and shorter scan times versus 2D-FSE acquisitions.

content and matrix degradation. Newer methods of MR imaging exploit these macromolecule changes to provide a quantitative understanding of the breakdown process.

In cartilage, changes in T2 are dependent up on the quantity of water and the integrity of the proteoglycan-collagen matrix. By measuring the spatial distribution of T2 relaxation times throughout articular cartilage, areas of increased or decreased water content (which generally correlate with cartilage damage) are identified. Generally, a multi-echo SE is used to shorten scan time, and signal levels are fitted to one or more decaying exponentials, depending up on whether more than one T2 distribution is anticipated in the tissue.[49] T2 mapping software is currently commercially available, allowing for simple implementation on most imaging systems (**Fig. 10**).

T1rho mapping is sensitive to the macromolecule content of tissue and is therefore effective in visualizing early changes in OA.[50,51] In T1rho, magnetization is tipped into the transverse plane and "spin-locked" by a constant RF field. When proteoglycan depletion occurs in articular cartilage, physical and chemical interactions in the macromolecule environment are disrupted. T1rho allows measurement of the interaction between motion-restricted water molecules and their extracellular environment.[52] Elevated T1rho relaxation times have been measured in osteoarthritic knee cartilage compared with normal cartilage.[53–55]

Sodium MR imaing is based on the concept of negative fixed charged density within the extracellular matrix of cartilage. In healthy cartilage, high concentrations of positively charged ^{23}Na are associated with the negatively charged glycosaminoglycan (GAG) side chains, which contain negatively charged carboxyl and sulfate groups. When proteoglycan depletion occurs in cartilage breakdown, GAGs are damaged and sodium signals decline (**Fig. 11**).[51,56,57] ^{23}Na imaging, therefore, represents a potentially useful means of differentiating early stage degenerate cartilage and normal tissue.[56]

Like sodium imaging, dGEMRIC also relies on the principle of fixed charge density. Ions in the extracellular fluid are distributed in relation to the concentration of negatively charged GAGs, which is a reflection of the quantity of proteoglycan content in cartilage. The negatively charged Gd(DTPA)$^{2-}$ molecules accumulate in high concentration in areas lacking in GAG and in low concentrations in GAG-rich regions. Subsequent imaging using 3D-SPGR pulse

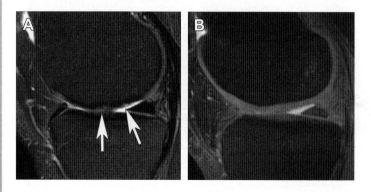

Fig. 9. Sagittal images of a knee with cartilage lesions on the medial femoral condyle (*arrows*) obtained using routine 2D-FSE sequence (*A*) and 3D-VIPR (*B*), an SSFP sequence derivative. VIPR obtains images with greater SNR and tissue contrast and uses shorter scan times. (*From* Kijowski R, Blankenbaker DG, Klaers JL, et al. Vastly undersampled isotropic projection steady-state free precession imaging of the knee: diagnostic performance compared with conventional MR. Radiology 2009; 251(1):185–94; with permission.)

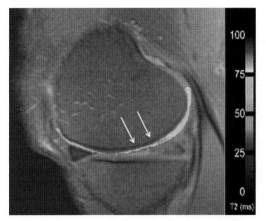

Fig. 10. T2 mapping in the articular cartilage of the medial femur in a patient with moderate OA. The T2 relaxation time is elevated in the weight-bearing region of the medial femoral condyle (*arrows*). (*Adapted from* Braun HJ, Gold GE. Diagnosis of osteoarthritis: imaging. Bone 2012;51:278–88; with permission.)

sequences with variable flip angles,[58] bSSFP, or T1 generates a GAG distribution. This T1 measurement is referred to as the dGEMRIC index. Regions with low T1 signal correspond to a low dGEMRIC index, which indicates high

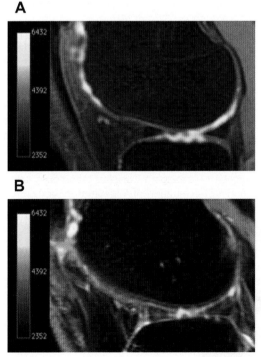

Fig. 11. The increased sodium signal in A (*top row*) correlates with higher GAG concentration. (*From* Braun HJ, Gold GE. Diagnosis of osteoarthritis: imaging. Bone 2012;51:278–88; with permission.)

$Gd(DTPA)^{2-}$ penetration and greater GAG depletion (**Fig. 12**).

Hip cartilage

Imaging of the articular cartilage in the hip is less straightforward than the knee because of the spherical geometry of the femoral head and acetabulum, and the thinner cartilage layer.[59] A recent study examined using fat-water separation MRI combined with spoiled gradient echo at 3T to evaluate hip cartilage.[60] Two-dimensional and 3D MR arthrography have also been compared in the imaging of articular cartilage of the hip. In 2004, Knuesel and colleagues[61] evaluated the ability of a sagittal water excitation DESS sequence and a sagittal fat-saturated T1-weighted FSE sequence to detect surgically confirmed cartilage lesions at 1.5 T. The DESS sequence had significant lesion conspicuity, but both sequences were found to have similar sensitivity and specificity for lesion detection. More recently in 2009, Ullrick and colleagues[62] conducted a similar study at 3.0 T comparing an IDEAL-SPGR sequence with a multiplanar, fat-saturated T1-weighted FSE sequence. IDEAL-SPGR had significantly greater sensitivity but significantly lower specificity and accuracy than T1-weighted FSE sequences for cartilage detection. Three-dimensional sequences allow higher in-plane spatial resolution and may improve detection of articular chondropathies due to decreased slice thickness.

Similar to the knee, although less widespread, methods of cartilage evaluation such as dGEMRIC, T2 mapping, and T1p mapping have been used to quantify physiologic changes in the articular cartilage of the hip (**Fig. 13**).[63]

Ankle cartilage

Unlike the hip and the knee, the articular cartilage of the ankle is less often involved in primary OA but more frequently undergoes changes as a result of post-traumatic tissue damage.[64] The incongruent surfaces of the tibia and talar dome complicate the detection of cartilage lesions,[65,66] but the thin continuous slices and high resolution characteristics of 3D sequences make these techniques attractive for the imaging of the articular cartilage in the ankle.

Bauer and colleagues[65] compared 2D fat-saturated intermediate-weighted FSE, fat-saturated SPGR, and fat-saturated FIESTA sequences for the detection of artificial chondral defects in human cadaver joints at both 1.5 and 3.0 T. Overall, the 3D sequences demonstrated lower diagnostic performance at both field strengths. However, 2 studies have suggested that 3D isotropic imaging may prove useful in the

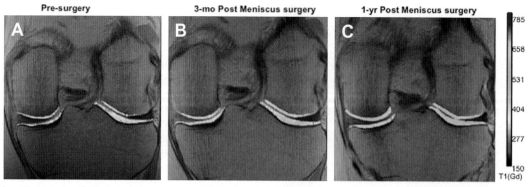

Fig. 12. Images of the menisci presurgery (A) and at 2 follow-up time points (B, C). dGEMRIC imaging permits quantitative assessment of cartilage integrity, which appears to improve following surgical intervention. (*From* Braun HJ, Gold GE. Diagnosis of osteoarthritis: imaging. Bone 2012;51:278–88; with permission.)

imaging of ankle cartilage morphology. Welsch and colleagues[67] recently used a water excitation true-FISP sequence with 0.3-mm isotropic resolution to image ankle cartilage at 3.0 T and observed sustained image quality with the use of this balanced SSFP sequence. Stevens and colleagues[46] also established that an isotropic resolution intermediate-weighted FSE-Cube sequence demonstrated significantly higher SNR efficiency in cartilage, synovial fluid, and muscle compared with a 2D-FSE sequence. These recent findings suggest that 3D-FSE sequences may aid the detection of joint pathology in this complex anatomic region.

Quantitative assessment of ankle articular cartilage physiology in the ankle through mapping methods such as dGEMRIC, T2, and T1rho is possible but technically challenging, as the talar and tibial cartilage can often be difficult to separate.[64]

Synovium

The synovial membrane is a thin, connective tissue lining the inside of fibrous joint capsules. It is composed of an intimal layer 1 to 3 cells thick, consisting of macrophage-like (Type A) and fibroblast-like (Type B) synoviocytes, and

a subintimal layer consisting of nerve endings, vasculature, and lymphatics. The role of healthy synovium is to lubricate the joint and nourish the articular cartilage. However, inflammation of the synovium (synovitis) has been implicated in many joint pathologies including rheumatoid arthritis, hemophilic arthropathy, and OA. Because the synovium is a potent source of degradative enzymes, proinflammatory mediators, and angiogenic growth factors, improving the visualization and characterization of this tissue may lead to important insights in disease initiation and progression. The synovium is typically imaged using ultrasound (US) or MR imaging.

In the knee, the most commonly imaged sites of synovial hypertrophy are the suprapatellar pouch and the medial and lateral recesses.[68] Current US technology acquires images with wide fields of view using high-resolution probes operating at frequencies of up to 20 MHz.[69] This technology has allowed the detection of synovial pathologies including hypertrophy, vascularity, and presence of synovial fluid[69,70] and the detection of synovitis in joints that appear otherwise clinically quiescent.[69] Doppler techniques allow an indirect evaluation of inflammatory activity via

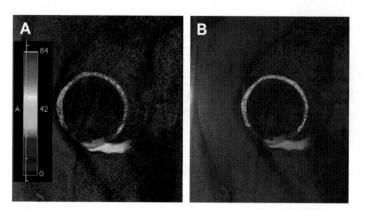

Fig. 13. T2 (A) and T1 rho (B) mapping of the articular cartilage of the hip. Images taken from a patient with a tear of the anterior labrum and pincer femoracetabular impingement. (*Courtesy of* Stephen Matzat, Stanford University.)

the assessment of vascularity.[71,72] Recently, contrast enhanced (CE)-US has been proposed as a novel technique aimed at quantifying synovial vascularization.[68] CE-US showed higher sensitivity (95%) in imaging synovitis than CE-MR imaging (82%), power Doppler US (64%), or grayscale US (58%).[68]

MR imaging is also used for assessment of the synovium. Unlike US, MR imaging is able to visualize synovium located deep within joints such as the hip without being obscured by bony structures. The 2 primary methods for MR detection of synovitis are the use of non-CE–MR imaging and gadolinium (Gd)-based CE-MR imaging. Synovitis was first correlated with hypointense signal alterations in Hoffa's fat pad on sagittal, non-CE T1-weighted SE images.[73] Since then, hyperintense signal changes in Hoffa's fat pad on fat-suppressed PD or T2-weighted SE sequences have been suggested as surrogate markers for joint-wide synovitis.[74,75]

Non-CE–MR imaging has been a common and effective tool for imaging of synovitis, but CE-MR imaging generally improves tissue visualization. Alhough the administration of intravenous Gd is suboptimal, CE-MR imaging more clearly differentiates inflamed synovium from joint effusion. In CE-MR imaging, synovium with inflammatory activity is enhanced, whereas effusion remains hypointense; on non-CE–MR imaging, both synovium and effusion are often depicted as signal hyperintensity. Recent studies have shown that signal changes in Hoffa's fat pad on non-CE–MR imaging were less specific for peripatellar synovitis than CE sequences[76] and that microscopic synovitis is not correlated with non-CE–MR imaging.[77] Additional investigations have shown that CE-MR imaging–detected synovitis correlates with histology[77,78] and is more sensitive[68] and specific[76] than non-CE–MR imaging. These studies further the belief that Gd-based CE-MR imaging improves imaging of the synovium. However, obvious drawbacks to intravenous Gd administration exist, including prolonged scan time, increased cost, possible allergic reactions, and a risk of nephrogenic systemic fibrosis.

TECHNICAL ADVANCES IN MR IMAGING

Recent advancements in MR imaging have paved the way for several exciting applications, including imaging at high field strengths, imaging using multiple RF channels, and T2* imaging.

High Field Strengths

Many clinical systems continue to use 1.5 T magnets for routine imaging. However, imaging at 3 T is becoming increasingly more common for clinical patients, and optimizing imaging at 7 T is a subject of much current research.[79] Higher field strengths such as 3.0 T improve SNR, allowing for greater temporal and spatial resolution and decreased scan time.[79] These advantages are also achieved at higher field strengths. However, B1 inhomogeneities, increased chemical shift differences between water and fat, RF power deposition, and changes in tissue relaxation characteristics significantly influence musculoskeletal MR imaging at 7.0 T.[79] A recent investigation by Jordan and colleagues[80] found that the T1 relaxation times of cartilage, muscle, synovial fluid, bone marrow, and subcutaneous fat were significantly greater at 7.0 T compared with 3.0 T. The opposite trend was observed for T2 values at these field strengths. However, although higher field strengths introduce new challenges to musculoskeletal MR imaging, their advantages may prove more valuable. The knee and ankle joints have been successfully evaluated in vivo at 7 T; the hip joint has been evaluated in cadaveric specimens.[81,82]

Most high field studies have been conducted in the knee. Most recently, multiple channel array coils[83] and sodium imaging[84] have been explored in the knee in vivo at 7 T. In the ankle, Juras and colleagues[85] compared SNR and contrast-to-noise (CNR) at 3 T and 7 T in 3 routine clinical imaging sequences: (1) 3D-GRE, (2) 2D PD-weighted FSE, and (3) 2D T1-weighted SE. SNR was calculated for cartilage, bone, muscle, synovial fluid, Achilles tendon, and Kager's fat pad, whereas CNR was measured for cartilage/bone, cartilage/fluid, cartilage/muscle, and muscle/fat pad. Significant increases in SNR were observed in the 3D-GRE and T1-weighted 2D-FSE sequences at 7 T, whereas an increase in CNR was observed in T1-weighted 2D-FSE sequences and most 3D-GRE sequences (**Fig. 14**). The PD-weighted 2D-FSE sequences showed a decreased SNR at 7 T.

Multiple Receiver Channels

Improvements in RF coil technology are being developed to keep pace with higher field strengths. Phased array coils have a higher intrinsic surface SNR than quadrature coils at the cost of some loss of intensity uniformity of MR images. Parallel imaging methods use multiple channels to extend the imaging field of view without increasing scan time, by exploiting the spatially varying sensitivity profiles of the phased array coil elements. These techniques reduce scan time and required RF pulses while also shortening TEs; parallel imaging compromises image

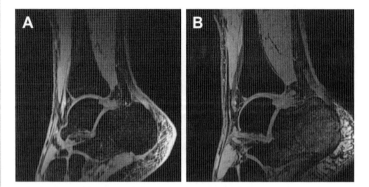

Fig. 14. Three dimensional T1-weighted, GRE sequences obtained from a healthy ankle in the sagittal plane at 3 T (*A*) and 7 T (*B*). Compared with 3 T, higher SNR and CNR were observed at 7 T. (*From* Juras V, Apprich S, Pressl C, et al. Histological correlation of 7T multi-parametric MRI performed in ex-vivo Achilles tendon. Eur J Radiol 2011 Dec 15. [Epub ahead of print]; with permission.)

uniformity and SNR, but phased array coils with as many as 32 channels may be able to offset these shortcomings. A recent in vivo study conducted at 7.0 T by Chang and colleagues[83] demonstrated that a 28-channel receive array coil increased SNR and CNR for evaluating morphology and mapping T2 relaxation times in articular cartilage in comparison to a quadrature volume coil. Furthermore, the 28-channel coil afforded a 40% to 48% reduction in scan time. These results lend support for the use of high field MR imaging to improve soft tissue contrast. However, the cartilage T2 relaxation times obtained by the 28-channel coil were 20% less than those obtained by the quadrature coil, leading the investigators to advise coil consistency in longitudinal imaging studies.

T2* Imaging

Like T2, T2* describes the transverse relaxation of tissue. However, in addition to spin-spin dephasing, T2* accounts for magnetic field inhomogeneity and gradient susceptibility, both factors that affect dephasing. Consequently, T2* is always shorter than T2, as these additional factors cause the signal to decay more rapidly. Two-dimensional UTE, 3D-UTE, and 2D-UTE spectroscopy have been used to measure T2* in the menisci, ligaments, tendons, and articular cartilage (**Fig. 15**). Average T2* relaxation times have been reported

as 22.6 to 24.1 ms for articular cartilage,[59] 4 to 10 ms for the meniscus (with zonal variation), 3 ms for ligaments,[86] and 2 ms for tendons.[86] Like T2, measurements of voxel-by-voxel T2* relaxation times are generated by acquiring a series of images at different TEs and fitting the values to a monoexponential decay curve. Although T2* is well correlated with T2,[59] T2* may provide additional information regarding tissue health and structure. Future studies are necessary to better understand the T2* measurement and to apply this imaging technique to other anatomic sites of the lower extremity.

Imaging Around Metal

The number of primary and revision total hip and knee arthroplasties continues to increase. Between 1990 and 2002, hip replacements and revisions increased by 62% and 79%; knee replacements and revisions saw even more dramatic changes, increasing by 192% and 195%, respectively.[87] Complications of total joint replacements include soft tissue irritation, periprosthetic osteolysis, loosening, malposition, instability, and infection.[88] MR imaging is normally preferred for the noninvasive evaluation of soft tissues. However, in the presence of metal, the main magnetic field is disrupted and strong; spatially varying local gradients are induced.[89]

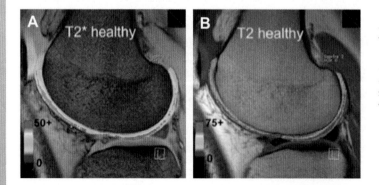

Fig. 15. T2* (*A*) and T2 (*B*) mapping of articular cartilage in healthy medial femoral condyle. (*From* Mamisch TC, Hughes T, Mosher TJ, et al. T2 star relaxation times for assessment of articular cartilage at 3 T: a feasibility study. Skeletal Radiol 2012;41:287–92; with permission.)

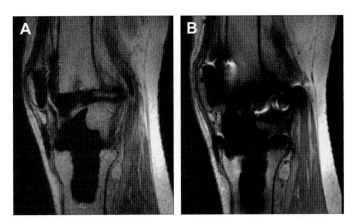

Fig. 16. (*A*) Sagittal MR images through the knee obtained using SEMAC, which corrects for spatial distortions by performing extra slice encoding and VAT and (*B*) conventional PD-weighted sequence. Compared with the spin echo PD image (*B*), SEMAC affords improved visualization of tissues around metallic implants.

Accordingly, MR image quality is disrupted due primarily to the presence of signal loss and distortion artifacts.[89] A pressing need to improve the ability to noninvasively image around metal has accompanied the growth in total joint procedures.

View angle tilting (VAT) was first used to correct in plane distortion; however it failed to correct for through plane distortion.[90,91] Two 3D-MR imaging techniques were developed within the past few years to further improve the correction of metal-induced artifacts: slice encoding for metal artifact correction (SEMAC)[92] and multiacquisition variable-resonance image combination (MAVRIC).[93] SEMAC builds on earlier techniques for imaging around metal, using a SE to prevent signal loss from dephasing and a VAT compensation gradient to minimize in plane distortion. In addition, SEMAC acquires signal using a 3D SE, which resolves through plane distortion by allowing all slice profiles to be resolved and aligned to

their actual voxel location (**Fig. 16**). MAVRIC does not use a 2D multislice excitation approach, but instead excites a series of limited spectral bandwidths to restrict in plane distortion. A 2011 study by Chen and colleagues[88] compared SEMAC and MAVRIC techniques in patients with total knee replacements and a knee replacement model. Both techniques corrected for the metal artifact, and allowed PD, T1, and T2 contrast with inversion-recovery for fat suppression. Both techniques showed accurate measurement of implant alignment and delivered high-resolution images. Most recently, MAVRIC-SL (Multi-Acquisition with Variable Resonance Image Combination – Slice Selective), a hybrid of SEMAC and MAVRIC, has been proposed to combine the advantages of each individual technique.[94] This acquisition uses the z-selectivity of SEMAC and the spectral properties of MAVRIC and has been shown to decrease the metallic artifacts

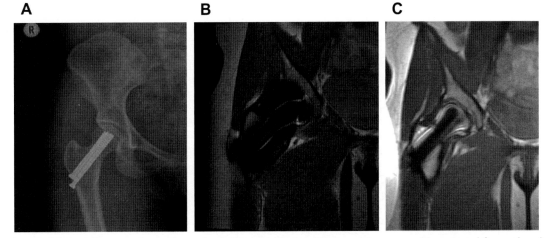

Fig. 17. (*A*) Anterior-posterior radiograph of the right hip in a 22-year-old woman with a pinned femoral neck fracture. The hardware and surrounding soft tissue are obscured on the coronal PD-weighted acquisition (*B*) but are well visualized with the MAVRIC-SL sequence (*C*). (*Courtesy of* Dr Kathryn Stevens, Stanford University.)

around implants at field strengths up to 3.0 T (**Fig. 17**).[94]

SUMMARY

MR imaging of the lower extremity provides a comprehensive, noninvasive and nonionizing evaluation of pathology. Traditional MR imaging methods provide excellent and reliable depictions of anatomy and internal derangements. New MR imaging methods are providing insight into tissue physiology and function, including inflammation. MR imaging of the lower extremity is an evolving, exciting field that continues to push the envelope using new MR technology.

REFERENCES

1. Quatman CE, Hettrich CM, Schmitt LC, et al. The clinical utility and diagnostic performance of magnetic resonance imaging for identification of early and advanced knee osteoarthritis: a systematic review. Am J Sports Med 2011;39(7):1557–68.
2. Katz LD, Haims A, Medvecky M, et al. Symptomatic hip plica: MR arthrographic and arthroscopic correlation. Skeletal Radiol 2010;39(12):1255–8.
3. Zlatkin MB, Pevsner D, Sanders TG, et al. Acetabular labral tears and cartilage lesions of the hip: indirect MR arthrographic correlation with arthroscopy–a preliminary study. AJR Am J Roentgenol 2010;194(3):709–14.
4. Gold GE, Mosher TJ. Arthritis in color: advanced imaging of osteoarthritis. Philadelphia: Elsevier Saunders; 2009. p. 153–92.
5. Carrino JA, Blum J, Parellada JA, et al. MRI of bone marrow edema-like signal in the pathogenesis of subchondral cysts. Osteoarthritis Cartilage 2006; 14(10):1081–5.
6. Crema MD, Roemer FW, Marra MD, et al. MRI-detected bone marrow edema-like lesions are strongly associated with subchondral cysts in patients with or at risk for knee osteoarthritis: the MOST study. Osteoarthritis Cartilage 2008;14:1033–40.
7. Bergman AG, Willen HK, Lindstrand AL, et al. Osteoarthritis of the knee: correlation of subchondral MR signal abnormalities with histopathologic and radiographic features. Skeletal Radiol 1994;23(6):445–8.
8. Roemer FW, Hunter DJ, Guermazi A. MRI-based semiquantitative assessment of subchondral bone marrow lesions in osteoarthritis research. Osteoarthritis Cartilage 2009;17(3):414–5 [author reply: 416–7].
9. Yu JS, Cook PA. Magnetic resonance imaging (MRI) of the knee: a pattern approach for evaluating bone marrow edema. Crit Rev Diagn Imaging 1996;37(4): 261–303.
10. Zanetti M, Bruder E, Romero J, et al. Bone marrow edema pattern in osteoarthritic knees: correlation between MR imaging and histologic findings. Radiology 2000;215(3):835–40.
11. Du J, Carl M, Diaz E, et al. Ultrashort TE T1rho (UTE T1rho) imaging of the Achilles tendon and meniscus. Magn Reson Med 2010;64(3):834–42.
12. Patten C, Meyer RA, Fleckenstein JL. T2 mapping of muscle. Semin Musculoskelet Radiol 2003;7(4): 297–305.
13. Gatehouse PD, He T, Puri BK, et al. Contrast-enhanced MRI of the menisci of the knee using ultrashort echo time (UTE) pulse sequences: imaging of the red and white zones. Br J Radiol 2004;77(920): 641–7.
14. Gold GE, Bergman AG, Pauly JM, et al. Magnetic resonance imaging of knee cartilage repair. Top Magn Reson Imaging 1998;9(6):377–92.
15. Robson MD, Gatehouse PD, Bydder M, et al. Magnetic resonance: an introduction to ultrashort TE (UTE) imaging. J Comput Assist Tomogr 2003; 27(6):825–46.
16. Gold GE, Pauly JM, Macovski A, et al. MR spectroscopic imaging of collagen: tendons and knee menisci. Magn Reson Med 1995;34(5):647–54.
17. Rahmer J, Bornert P, Dries SP. Assessment of anterior cruciate ligament reconstruction using 3D ultrashort echo-time MR imaging. J Magn Reson Imaging 2009;29(2):443–8.
18. Qian Y, Williams AA, Chu CR, et al. High-resolution ultrashort echo time (UTE) imaging on human knee with AWSOS sequence at 3.0 T. J Magn Reson Imaging 2012;35(1):204–10.
19. Grodzki DM, Jakob PM, Heismann B. Ultrashort echo time imaging using pointwise encoding time reduction with radial acquisition (PETRA). Magn Reson Med 2012;67(2):510–8.
20. Syha R, Martirosian P, Ketelsen D, et al. Magnetization transfer in human Achilles tendon assessed by a 3D ultrashort echo time sequence: quantitative examinations in healthy volunteers at 3T. Rofo 2011;183(11):1043–50.
21. Magee T, Williams D. Detection of meniscal tears and marrow lesions using coronal MRI. AJR Am J Roentgenol 2004;183(5):1469–73.
22. Magee TH, Hinson GW. MRI of meniscal bucket-handle tears. Skeletal Radiol 1998;27(9):495–9.
23. Lee JH, Singh TT, Bolton G. Axial fat-saturated FSE imaging of knee: appearance of meniscal tears. Skeletal Radiol 2002;31(7):384–95.
24. Tarhan NC, Chung CB, Mohana-Borges AV, et al. Meniscal tears: role of axial MRI alone and in combination with other imaging planes. AJR Am J Roentgenol 2004;183(1):9–15.
25. Helms CA. The meniscus: recent advances in MR imaging of the knee. AJR Am J Roentgenol 2002; 179(5):1115–22.

26. Fox MG. MR imaging of the meniscus: review, current trends, and clinical implications. Radiol Clin North Am 2007;45(6):1033–53, vii.

27. De Smet AA, Tuite MJ. Use of the "two-slice-touch" rule for the MRI diagnosis of meniscal tears. AJR Am J Roentgenol 2006;187(4):911–4.

28. Blackmon GB, Major NM, Helms CA. Comparison of fast spin-echo versus conventional spin-echo MRI for evaluating meniscal tears. AJR Am J Roentgenol 2005;184(6):1740–3.

29. Craig JG, Go L, Blechinger J, et al. Three-tesla imaging of the knee: initial experience. Skeletal Radiol 2005;34(8):453–61.

30. Ramnath RR, Magee T, Wasudev N, et al. Accuracy of 3-T MRI using fast spin-echo technique to detect meniscal tears of the knee. AJR Am J Roentgenol 2006;187(1):221–5.

31. Kreitner KF, Romaneehsen B, Krummenauer F, et al. Fast magnetic resonance imaging of the knee using a parallel acquisition technique (mSENSE): a prospective performance evaluation. Eur Radiol 2006;16(8):1659–66.

32. Niitsu M, Ikeda K. Routine MR examination of the knee using parallel imaging. Clin Radiol 2003; 58(10):801–7.

33. Son MS, Levenston ME, Hargreaves BA, et al. T1ρ and T2 show regional variation in degenerate human menisci: correlation with biomechanics and matrix composition. international society for magnetic resonance in medicine. Melbourne (Australia): Wiley, Inc; 2012.

34. Clohisy JC, Beaule PE, O'Malley A, et al. AOA symposium. Hip disease in the young adult: current concepts of etiology and surgical treatment. J Bone Joint Surg Am 2008;90(10):2267–81.

35. Ganz R, Parvizi J, Beck M, et al. Femoroacetabular impingement: a cause for osteoarthritis of the hip. Clin Orthop Relat Res 2003;(417):112–20.

36. Leunig M, Beaule PE, Ganz R. The concept of femoroacetabular impingement: current status and future perspectives. Clin Orthop Relat Res 2009; 467(3):616–22.

37. Cicuttini F, Forbes A, Asbeutah A, et al. Comparison and reproducibility of fast and conventional spoiled gradient-echo magnetic resonance sequences in the determination of knee cartilage volume. J Orthop Res 2000;18(4):580–4.

38. Eckstein F, Westhoff J, Sittek H, et al. In vivo reproducibility of three-dimensional cartilage volume and thickness measurements with MR imaging. AJR Am J Roentgenol 1998;170(3):593–7.

39. Gold GE, Fuller SE, Hargreaves BA, et al. Driven equilibrium magnetic resonance imaging of articular cartilage: initial clinical experience. J Magn Reson Imaging 2005;21(4):476–81.

40. Duc SR, Pfirrmann CW, Schmid MR, et al. Articular cartilage defects detected with 3D water-excitation true FISP: prospective comparison with sequences commonly used for knee imaging. Radiology 2007; 245(1):216–23.

41. Eckstein F, Hudelmaier M, Wirth W, et al. Double echo steady state magnetic resonance imaging of knee articular cartilage at 3 Tesla: a pilot study for the Osteoarthritis Initiative. Ann Rheum Dis 2006; 65(4):433–41.

42. Peterfy CG, Schneider E, Nevitt M. The osteoarthritis initiative: report on the design rationale for the magnetic resonance imaging protocol for the knee. Osteoarthritis Cartilage 2008;16(12):1433–41.

43. Vasanawala SS, Pauly JM, Nishimura DG. Fluctuating equilibrium MRI. Magn Reson Med 1999; 42(5):876–83.

44. Kijowski R, Blankenbaker DG, Klaers JL, et al. Vastly undersampled isotropic projection steady-state free precession imaging of the knee: diagnostic performance compared with conventional MR. Radiology 2009;251(1):185–94.

45. Friedrich KM, Reiter G, Kaiser B, et al. High-resolution cartilage imaging of the knee at 3T: basic evaluation of modern isotropic 3D MR-sequences. Eur J Radiol 2011;78(3):398–405.

46. Stevens KJ, Busse RF, Han E, et al. Ankle: isotropic MR imaging with 3D-FSE-cube–initial experience in healthy volunteers. Radiology 2008; 249(3):1026–33.

47. Stevens KJ, Wallace CG, Chen W, et al. Imaging of the wrist at 1.5 Tesla using isotropic three-dimensional fast spin echo cube. J Magn Reson Imaging 2011;33(4):908–15.

48. Dijkgraaf LC, de Bont LG, Boering G, et al. The structure, biochemistry, and metabolism of osteoarthritic cartilage: a review of the literature. J Oral Maxillofac Surg 1995;53(10):1182–92.

49. Smith HE, Mosher TJ, Dardzinski BJ, et al. Spatial variation in cartilage T2 of the knee. J Magn Reson Imaging 2001;14(1):50–5.

50. Mosher TJ, Zhang Z, Reddy R, et al. Knee articular cartilage damage in osteoarthritis: analysis of MR image biomarker reproducibility in ACRIN-PA 4001 multicenter trial. Radiology 2011;258(3): 832–42.

51. Wheaton AJ, Casey FL, Gougoutas AJ, et al. Correlation of T1rho with fixed charge density in cartilage. J Magn Reson Imaging 2004;20(3):519–25.

52. Blumenkrantz G, Majumdar S. Quantitative magnetic resonance imaging of articular cartilage in osteoarthritis. Eur Cell Mater 2007;13:76–86.

53. Li X, Han E, Crane JC. Development of in vivo multislice spiral T1 rho mapping in cartilage at 3T and its application to osteoarthritis. Annual Meeting International Society of Magnetic Resonance in Medicine. Miami (FL), May 7-13, 2005.

54. Regatte RR, Akella SV, Wheaton AJ, et al. 3D-T1rho-relaxation mapping of articular cartilage: in vivo

assessment of early degenerative changes in symptomatic osteoarthritic subjects. Acad Radiol 2004; 11(7):741–9.

55. Stahl R, Luke A, Li X, et al. T1rho, T2 and focal knee cartilage abnormalities in physically active and sedentary healthy subjects versus early OA patients–a 3.0-Tesla MRI study. Eur Radiol 2009; 19(1):132–43.

56. Borthakur A, Shapiro EM, Beers J, et al. Sensitivity of MRI to proteoglycan depletion in cartilage: comparison of sodium and proton MRI. Osteoarthritis Cartilage 2000;8(4):288–93.

57. Wang L, Wu Y, Chang G, et al. Rapid isotropic 3D-sodium MRI of the knee joint in vivo at 7T. J Magn Reson Imaging 2009;30(3):606–14.

58. McKenzie CA, Williams A, Prasad PV, et al. Three-dimensional delayed gadolinium-enhanced MRI of cartilage (dGEMRIC) at 1.5T and 3.0T. J Magn Reson Imaging 2006;24(4):928–33.

59. Mamisch TC, Hughes T, Mosher TJ, et al. T2 star relaxation times for assessment of articular cartilage at 3 T: a feasibility study. Skeletal Radiol 2012;41(3): 287–92.

60. Blankenbaker DG, Ullrick SR, Kijowski R, et al. MR Arthrography of the Hip: Comparison of IDEAL-SPGR Volume Sequence to Standard MR Sequences in the Detection and Grading of Cartilage Lesions. Radiology 2011;261(3):863–71.

61. Knuesel PR, Pfirrmann CW, Noetzli HP, et al. MR arthrography of the hip: diagnostic performance of a dedicated water-excitation 3D double-echo steady-state sequence to detect cartilage lesions. AJR Am J Roentgenol 2004;183(6):1729–35.

62. Ullrick SR, Blankenbaker DG, Davis KW, et al. MR arthrography of the hip: comparison of an IDEAL-SPGR sequence with standard MR sequences in the detection of cartilage lesions. American Roentgen Ray Society Annual Meeting. Boston (MA), April 21, 2009.

63. Gold SL, Burge AJ, Potter HG. MRI of hip cartilage: joint morphology, structure, and composition. Clin Orthop Relat Res 2012;470(12):3321–31.

64. Chhabra A, Soldatos T, Chalian M, et al. Current concepts review: 3T magnetic resonance imaging of the ankle and foot. Foot Ankle Int 2012;33(2): 164–71.

65. Bauer JS, Barr C, Henning TD, et al. Magnetic resonance imaging of the ankle at 3.0 Tesla and 1.5 Tesla in human cadaver specimens with artificially created lesions of cartilage and ligaments. Invest Radiol 2008;43(9):604–11.

66. Schmid MR, Pfirrmann CW, Hodler J, et al. Cartilage lesions in the ankle joint: comparison of MR arthrography and CT arthrography. Skeletal Radiol 2003; 32(5):259–65.

67. Welsch GH, Mamisch TC, Weber M, et al. High-resolution morphological and biochemical imaging of articular cartilage of the ankle joint at 3.0 T using a new dedicated phased array coil: in vivo reproducibility study. Skeletal Radiol 2008;37(6):519–26.

68. Song IH, Althoff CE, Hermann KG, et al. Knee osteoarthritis. Efficacy of a new method of contrast-enhanced musculoskeletal ultrasonography in detection of synovitis in patients with knee osteoarthritis in comparison with magnetic resonance imaging. Ann Rheum Dis 2008;67(1):19–25.

69. Keen HI, Conaghan PG. Ultrasonography in osteoarthritis. Radiol Clin North Am 2009;47(4):581–94.

70. Guermazi A, Eckstein F, Hellio Le Graverand-Gastineau MP, et al. Osteoarthritis: current role of imaging. Med Clin North Am 2009;93(1):101–26, xi.

71. Walther M, Harms H, Krenn V, et al. Correlation of power Doppler sonography with vascularity of the synovial tissue of the knee joint in patients with osteoarthritis and rheumatoid arthritis. Arthritis Rheum 2001;44(2):331–8.

72. Walther M, Harms H, Krenn V, et al. Synovial tissue of the hip at power Doppler US: correlation between vascularity and power Doppler US signal. Radiology 2002;225(1):225–31.

73. Fernandez-Madrid F, Karvonen RL, Teitge RA, et al. Synovial thickening detected by MR imaging in osteoarthritis of the knee confirmed by biopsy as synovitis. Magn Reson Imaging 1995;13(2):177–83.

74. Hill CL, Gale DG, Chaisson CE, et al. Knee effusions, popliteal cysts, and synovial thickening: association with knee pain in osteoarthritis. J Rheumatol 2001; 28(6):1330–7.

75. Hill CL, Hunter DJ, Niu J, et al. Synovitis detected on magnetic resonance imaging and its relation to pain and cartilage loss in knee osteoarthritis. Ann Rheum Dis 2007;66(12):1599–603.

76. Roemer FW, Guermazi A, Zhang Y, et al. Hoffa's Fat Pad: evaluation on unenhanced MR images as a measure of patellofemoral synovitis in osteoarthritis. AJR Am J Roentgenol 2009;192(6):1696–700.

77. Loeuille D, Rat AC, Goebel JC, et al. Magnetic resonance imaging in osteoarthritis: which method best reflects synovial membrane inflammation? Correlations with clinical, macroscopic and microscopic features. Osteoarthritis Cartilage 2009;17(9):1186–92.

78. Loeuille D, Chary-Valckenaere I, Champigneulle J, et al. Macroscopic and microscopic features of synovial membrane inflammation in the osteoarthritic knee: correlating magnetic resonance imaging findings with disease severity. Arthritis Rheum 2005; 52(11):3492–501.

79. Regatte RR, Schweitzer ME. Ultra-high-field MRI of the musculoskeletal system at 7.0T. J Magn Reson Imaging 2007;25(2):262–9.

80. Jordan CD, Saranathan M, Bangerter NK, et al. Musculoskeletal MRI at 3.0T and 7.0T: a comparison of relaxation times and image contrast. Eur J Radiol 2011. http://dx.doi.org/10.1016/j.ejrad.2011.09.021.

81. Greaves LL, Gilbart MK, Yung A, et al. Deformation and recovery of cartilage in the intact hip under physiological loads using 7T MRI. J Biomech 2009; 42(3):349–54.

82. Greaves LL, Gilbart MK, Yung AC, et al. Effect of acetabular labral tears, repair and resection on hip cartilage strain: a 7T MR study. J Biomech 2010; 43(5):858–63.

83. Chang G, Wiggins GC, Xia D, et al. Comparison of a 28-channel receive array coil and quadrature volume coil for morphologic imaging and T2 mapping of knee cartilage at 7T. J Magn Reson Imaging 2012;35(2):441–8.

84. Madelin G, Jerschow A, Regatte RR. Sodium relaxation times in the knee joint in vivo at 7T. NMR Biomed 2012;25(4):530–7.

85. Juras V, Welsch G, Bar P, et al. Comparison of 3T and 7T MRI clinical sequences for ankle imaging. Eur J Radiol 2012;81(8):1846–50.

86. Du J, Takahashi AM, Chung CB. Ultrashort TE spectroscopic imaging (UTESI): application to the imaging of short T2 relaxation tissues in the musculoskeletal system. J Magn Reson Imaging 2009; 29(2):412–21.

87. Kurtz S, Mowat F, Ong K, et al. Prevalence of primary and revision total hip and knee arthroplasty in the United States from 1990 through 2002. J Bone Joint Surg Am 2005;87(7):1487–97.

88. Chen CA, Chen W, Goodman SB, et al. New MR imaging methods for metallic implants in the knee: artifact correction and clinical impact. J Magn Reson Imaging 2011;33(5):1121–7.

89. Wendt RE 3rd, Wilcott MR 3rd, Nitz W, et al. MR imaging of susceptibility-induced magnetic field inhomogeneities. Radiology 1988;168(3):837–41.

90. Butts K, Pauly JM, Gold GE. Reduction of blurring in view angle tilting MRI. Magn Reson Med 2005;53(2): 418–24.

91. Cho ZH, Kim DJ, Kim YK. Total inhomogeneity correction including chemical shifts and susceptibility by view angle tilting. Med Phys 1988;15(1): 7–11.

92. Lu W, Pauly KB, Gold GE, et al. SEMAC: slice encoding for metal artifact correction in MRI. Magn Reson Med 2009;62(1):66–76.

93. Koch KM, Lorbiecki JE, Hinks RS, et al. A multispectral three-dimensional acquisition technique for imaging near metal implants. Magn Reson Med 2009;61(2):381–90.

94. Koch KM, Brau AC, Chen W, et al. Imaging near metal with a MAVRIC-SEMAC hybrid. Magn Reson Med 2011;65(1):71–82.

Index

Note: Page numbers of article titles are in **boldface** type.

Radiol Clin N Am 51 (2013) 547–554
http://dx.doi.org/10.1016/S0033-8389(13)00033-X

radiologic.theclinics.com

Moving?

Make sure your subscription moves with you!

To notify us of your new address, find your **Clinics Account Number** (located on your mailing label above your name), and contact customer service at:

Email: journalscustomerservice-usa@elsevier.com

800-654-2452 (subscribers in the U.S. & Canada)
314-447-8871 (subscribers outside of the U.S. & Canada)

Fax number: 314-447-8029

Elsevier Health Sciences Division
Subscription Customer Service
3251 Riverport Lane
Maryland Heights, MO 63043

*To ensure uninterrupted delivery of your subscription, please notify us at least 4 weeks in advance of move.

ELSEVIER